Polymers in Drug Delivery

Polymers in Drug Delivery

EDITED BY

Ijeoma F. Uchegbu

Andreas G. Schätzlein

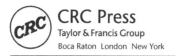

CRC Press
Taylor & Francis Group
Boca Raton London New York

CRC Press is an imprint of the
Taylor & Francis Group, an **informa** business

Cover illustration by Meilan Fang, Simon Fraser University, Vancouver, Canada.

CRC Press
Taylor & Francis Group
6000 Broken Sound Parkway NW, Suite 300
Boca Raton, FL 33487-2742

ISBN 13: 978-0-367-45359-6 (pbk)
ISBN 13: 978-0-8493-2533-5 (hbk)

Library of Congress Card Number 2005046684

Library of Congress Cataloging-in-Publication Data

Polymers in drug delivery / edited by Ijeoma Uchegbu, Andreas Schatzlein.
    p. cm.
   Includes bibliographical references and index.
   ISBN 0-8493-2533-1 (alk. paper)
   1. Polymeric drug delivery systems. 2. Polymeric drugs. 3. Polymers. 4. Drug delivery systems. I. Uchegbu, Ijeoma F. II. Schatzlein, Andreas.

RS201.P65P6444 2006
615'.3--dc22   2005046684

Visit the Taylor & Francis Web site at
http://www.taylorandfrancis.com

and the CRC Press Web site at
http://www.crcpress.com

Preface

H. Ringsdorf and R. Duncan

Drug Delivery — Yesterday and Today

Not only from a science–historical standpoint but even starting with the question of how science evolves and grows, it is very interesting to note that the field of drug delivery parallels or is even part of a paradigmatic development of polymer chemistry during the last 50 years. The evolution moved from synthetic macromolecules as plastic materials to the molecular engineering of pharmacologically active polymer systems. This paradigm shift is helping to bridge the gap between materials science and life science.

When in 1953 Hermann Staudinger was honored with the Nobel Prize "for his discoveries in the field of macromolecular chemistry" [1], the classical materials science-oriented polymer community at that time hardly recognized that, at the very same Nobel Prize celebration [2], H.A. Krebs and F.A. Lipmann reported on enzymes and coenzymes as important biological macromolecules. It was probably even more like news from another star for them that in the same year J.D. Watson and F.H. Crick rang in molecular biology with their *Nature* articles on the DNA-model [3]. Systematically developed in the 1920s, the field of synthetic macromolecules gained worldwide rapid acceptance in the chemical industry and included fibers, plastics, and rubber as valuable materials in industry as well as for our daily use. The "Plastics Age" was born. The Second World War accelerated the development of useful new materials. These already included the first applications in the medical field, e.g., as bone replacement, synthetic fibers as degradable and nondegradable surgical materials, and even their use intravenously (i.v.) injectable macromolecules like PVP (polyvinylpyrrolidone) as plasma expanders used widely on both sides of the front during the Second World War.

The possibilities for synthetic polymers in the biomedical field changed drastically after the 1950s with the rapid development of modern biochemistry and biomedicine. Molecular and cell biology, proteomics, and genetics led to paradigm shifts in several fields [4]. Information about molecular recognition and molecular self-organization, the development of molecular engineering, and the evolution of supramolecular chemistry [5] based on guest–host interaction opened doors in many directions. It is thus not amazing that already in 1981 Hermann Mark — one of the eminent fathers of polymer science — on the occasion of the 100th anniversary of the birth of Hermann Staudinger, reflected upon the future of polymer science [6]. In his essay "Macromolecular Chemistry Today — Aging Roots, Sprouting Branches" he, among other topics, spoke on stabilized and synthetic cells as long-term objectives. Discussing future perspectives, e.g., a possible cooperation of polymer chemistry and cell biology, Hermann Mark wrote: "… there is a multilingual borderland beyond which only a well established interdisciplinary team can expect to progress. This cooperation may give rise to an entirely new discipline which survives the old ones. Materials science thus originated from metallurgy, ceramics, and plastic technology. What about 'life science'? Can polymer chemistry and medicine overlap and strive together for new goals?" Even much earlier, already in 1959, in another context J. Lederberg wrote a contribution that paralleled the dreams of Hermann Staudinger whose focus was always synthetic polymer chemistry but never gave up dreaming about "his" macromolecules in biology and medicine [1]: "If the ingenuity and craftsmanship so successfully directed at the fabrication of organic polymers for the practical needs of mankind were to be concentrated on the problem of constructing a self-replicating assembly along these lines, we predict that the construction of an artificial molecule having the essential functions of primitive life would fall within the grasp of our current knowledge of organic chemistry." [7] What a compliment for and what a trust in chemists! Did our generation of scientists already reach this or similar far-sighted goals? [8] Not yet. But we are certainly on the way, and in this respect the cooperative development of polymer therapeutics [9] and polymers in drug delivery is definitely one of the avenues in modern science to be pursued. Thus, the present book is a very timely one.

Drug delivery yesterday was mainly the application of polymer matrices to regulate the release of drugs (formulation, chronomers, etc.). This is still a very important field. Nevertheless, drug delivery today, in an era of nanotechnology, and molecular biology have already based its new directions on the biological rationale. The rise of polymer therapeutics [9,10] is a perfect example of science at the crossroads of different disciplines, bridging gaps and growing on the intensive cooperation at the interfaces between physics, chemistry, biology, pharmacy, and medicine. The time when pharmacy could just be based on the linear development of research of known pharmaca and their body uptake is long over. The time is not far off when most — or all? — therapeutics will have to be not only tissue- and cell- but even cell-organelle-specific. Fantasy? Impossible? Not at all. Mother Nature, having had more time than we, has developed all her systems up to the point of fulfilling these requirements simultaneously. This is demonstrated perfectly by her biological pharmaceuticals and her biological drug delivery systems. Whenever different functions and properties, such as specific recognition, controlled cell-uptake, local release, and cell-organelle selective activity need to be combined, Mother Nature uses macromolecules. She still develops new selective biopolymers, e.g., by building new antibodies against foreign invaders and even against completely unknown "modern" compounds.

We are certainly still far away from the ingenuity and skill of Mother Nature and from the self-regulating properties of cells and cell organelles, constantly adjusting their functions to new duties on a molecular level. On the other hand, the possibility of synthesizing new drugs and new polymers has reached dazzling heights. Nowadays, basically every compound that is needed, and basically every surface property that is desired, can be synthesized. New polymer types and new polymer structures — even more than Mother Nature ever used — are on the market. New colloidal polymer amphiphiles, new functional multiblock copolymers, highly branched macromolecules, dendrimers with a wide variation of surface characteristics, peptides hybrids, and easily degradable and non-degradable systems have opened new possibilities for the biopharmaceutical and biomedical field. In addition, modern colloid science, as well as the characterization possibilities for polymers in bulk, in solution, and as single molecules, has reached a level scientists could not even dream of 50 years ago. In the meantime, supramolecular chemistry also developed into supramolecular science [11,12], powerfully and creatively opening new fields in science. It also should be mentioned — and it is very visible — that presently the most beloved scientific "nanogames" (nanoscience, nanotechnology, nanochemistry, nanobiology, nanopharmacy, nanomedicine, etc.) are gaining ground: The "new field" of nanoscience seems to pull many of the abovementioned disciplines into its vortex. Even if one remains a little sceptical, it has to be mentioned that coining the term *nanomedicine* has had a very positive effect, helping to overcome barriers between disciplines and scientists who, independent of many attempts to interact, still remained in their "boxes" [13]. In this context and accepting nanomedicine as a "figurehead" for the modern field of biomedicine, one should nevertheless not forget that polymers, micelles, liposomes, cells, cell-organelles, and cell membranes have been "nano-sized systems" long before the word *nanoscience* was coined, and the field was claimed to be a new one.

If we now summarize and concentrate the remarkably broad scale of possible developments for polymers in drug delivery under the framework of *nanomedicine*, will this lead us to the next paradigm shift, to the next generation of polymer therapeutics, of polymers for drug delivery and to new developments in the whole field of biomedicine? Not directly. And certainly not if we only develop results from yesterday linearly. The next paradigm shift is necessary, and it will be possible, but it will only be possible if we will base all new concepts and plans on strictly biological rationales.

Is this a new point? Not at all [9]. To cite André Gide, the famous French writer: "All this has been said before — but because nobody has listened, it all has to be said again." Only on the basis of a biological rationale will we be able to use the modern information volcanos of cell and membrane biology, of polymer and colloid science, of organic and supramolecular chemistry, and of modern characterization methods to reach one of our goals, namely, a wide variety of tissue, cell- and cell-organelle-specific polymer therapeutics and drug delivery systems within our lifespan. In this respect this book may play an important role to interest and to stimulate scientists with very different backgrounds and expertise. As Ijeoma F. Uchegbu wrote in the introduction: "This volume is primarily pitched at the nonspecialist reader, but the wide spectrum of opinion contained herein should also offer food for thought for the specialist." Thus, the book not only wants to present new results, but it combines new concepts with classical expertise and essential old methods. Is it a textbook already?

History always has a prehistory. The history of polymer science started officially with H. Staudinger and his contemporaries in the 1920s [1,14]. There was a prehistory, too: Synthetic and various natural polymers were known before, and by the 1880s were in public use as plastics [14]. And as far as synthetic "biopolymers" are concerned, it was Emil Fischer who in 1902 had described the first systematic synthesis of oligopeptides. He talked about tri- and tetrapeptides [15]. In a similar way, the history of textbooks on polymers in drug delivery may be said to have started with the present text: a "pre-textbook" to stimulate young scientists from different disciplines to enter the field of polymers in drug delivery. What about the prehistory of such a book? Many reviews have been written and will be cited in the different chapters. Honoring the importance of the field and its rapid development cannot be better demonstrated than by the fact that during the last 40 years at least one book appeared per decade that concentrated on biomedical polymers [16–20]. They are not all textbooks. They are either based on scientific meetings or put together as a "Festschrift" to celebrate elderly scientists, or are just summarizing actual and important results in the biomedical field. They are essential and interesting books: all the modern buzzwords for biomedicine can already be found in them. However, they are not written for students. They are all written to excite the specialists. Thus, most of them are stored away in the specialist sections of science libraries.

The present book — slanted to the level of the final year undergraduates — is written to excite young scientists about polymers in drug delivery and to pull them into the game. What we hope for this pre-textbook is that it may reach the textbook section of libraries. It should not only to be found in schools of pharmacy but also as a first introductory book for organic and polymer chemists, for biophysicists, and even for the basic science education of medical students.

REFERENCES AND NOTES

1. H. Ringsdorf, Hermann Staudinger and the future of polymer research: jubilees — beloved occasions for cultural piety, *Angew. Chem. Int. Ed.*, 43, 1064–1076, 2004.
2. The cover: Nobel ceremony honors chemists, *Chem. Eng. News*, 32, 162–163, 1954.
3 J.D. Watson and F.H. Crick, *Nature,* 171, 737, 964, 1953.
4. How does science develop? The essential progress in science does not happen through the continuous collection of facts but by revolutionary processes that induce the replacement of existing models (paradigms) by a new concept: a paradigm shift. Paradigm shifts do not always have to be revolutionary. They only describe a stepwise development of science, where linear thinking and "only logical continuation" of known facts and experiences do not lead necessarily to the next plateau of science; intuition and creativity are part of the game.

    The first two figures following this section illustrate paradigm shifts in science. The first one shows the beginning of a next step: a scientist on the way to new objectives.

    Figure A. And the question, in connection with this book, is: materials science or life science? The following pictures from G. Mordillo show how well this Argentinian caricaturist knows the "classical" polymer chemists: materials science or life science?

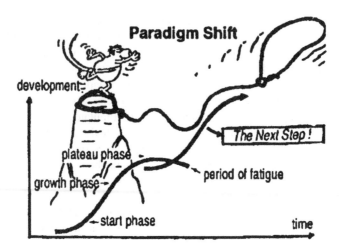

FIGURE A

Figure B. Just to give the interested reader a chance to look at the original — a little bit more complicated — information about paradigm shifts, the first book of Thomas S. Kuhn has to be cited: *The Structure of Scientific Revolutions*, University of Chicago Press, 1962; 2nd ed., 1970; German translation: *Die Struktur wissenschaftlicher Revolutionen*, Suhrkamp Verlag, Frankfurt/Main, 3. Auflage, 1978.

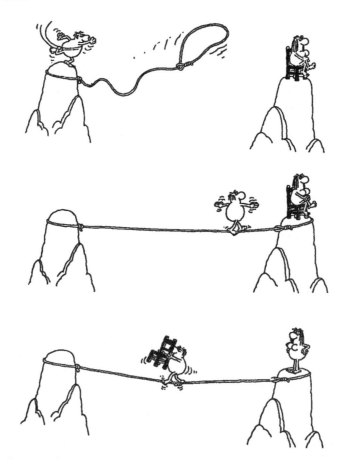

FIGURE B

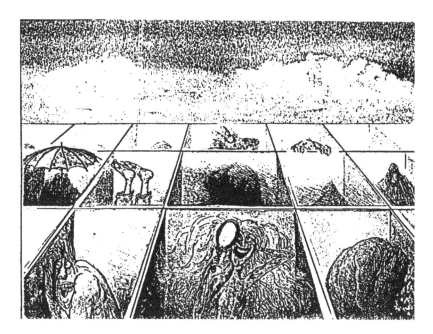

FIGURE C

5. J.M. Lehn, *Supramolecular Chemistry: Concepts and Perspectives*, VCH, New York, 1995.
6. H.F. Mark, Macromolecular chemistry today — aging routes, sprouting branches, *Angew. Chem. Int. Ed.*, 20, 303–304, 1981.
7. J. Lederberg, A view of genetics, *Science*, 131, 275, 1960. (This publication is based on Lederberg's lecture on the occasion of his receiving the Nobel Prize in Medicine in 1958.)
8. Not based on J. Lederberg's prediction but already in 1987, an interdisciplinary workshop on synthesis and simulation of living systems took place in Los Alamos, New Mexico: C.G. Langton, Ed., *Artificial Life*, Addison-Wesley, CA, 1989.
9. R. Duncan, The dawning era of polymer therapeutics, *Nat. Rev. Drug Discovery*, 2, 347–360, 2003.
10. R. Duncan, R. Satchi-Fainavo, Eds., Polymer therapeutics I and II, *Advances in Polymer Science*, Vol. 192 and Vol. 193, Springer Verlag, Berlin, 2005.
11. Jean-Paul Behr, Ed., *The Lock and Key Principle: The State of the Art — 100 Years On*, John Wiley & Sons, New York, 1994.
12. David N. Reinhoudt, Ed., *Supramolecular Materials and Technologies*, John Wiley & Sons, New York, 1999.
13. Figure C. Ronald Searle, The British cartoonist, called the following caricature "Human Beings." As an analogy, we scientists usually very much enjoy sitting in the "boxes" of our speciality areas. Naturally, we are interested to hear what is going on next door! But beyond that?
14. H. Morawetz, *Polymers: The Origins and the Growth of a Science*, Wiley Interscience, New York, 1985.
15. F. Hofmeister, 74. Versammlung der Gesellschaft Deutscher Naturforscher und Ärzte: Über den Bau der Eiweissmoleküle, *Chem. Z.*, 26, Heft 79, 920, 1902, E. Fischer, Über die Hydrolyse der Proteinstoffe, *Chem. Z.* 26, Heft 80, 939 1902, In this paper Emil Fischer talks about synthetic tri- and tetrapeptides.
16. L.G. Donaruma and O. Vogl, Ed., *Polymer Drugs*, Academic Press, New York, 1978.
17. C.G. Gebelein and C.E. Carraher, Eds., *Bioactive Polymer Systems. An Overview*, Plenum Press, New York, 1985.
18. S.L. Cooper, C.H. Bamford, and T. Tsuruta, Eds., *Polymer Biomaterials in Solution, as Interfaces and as Solids*, VSP, Utrecht, 1995.
19. S. Dumitriu, Ed., *Polymeric Biomaterials*, Marcel Dekker, New York, 2002.
20. H. Maeda, A. Kabanov, K. Kataoka, and T. Okano, Eds., *Polymer Drugs in the Clinical Stage. Advantages and Prospects*, Kluwer Academic/Plenum Press New York, 2003.

About the Editors

Ijeoma Uchegbu, Ph.D., is professor of drug delivery in the Department of Pharmaceutical Sciences, University of Strathclyde in Glasgow, and a director of the Nanomedicines Research Centre at the University of Strathclyde. Ijeoma obtained her pharmacy degree from the University of Benin in Nigeria and her Ph.D. from the School of Pharmacy, University of London. Her research has provided insights into the polymer architecture parameters which control the formation, size, and drug delivery capability of various self-assembled nanostructures. Ijeoma Uchegbu, in collaboration with Andreas Schätzlein of the Department of Medical Oncology, University of Glasgow, was also the first to demonstrate that gene transfer activity resided within the lower generation polypropylenimine dendrimers.

Andreas Schätzlein, Ph.D., is head of the Experimental Therapeutics and Gene Medicines Group at the Cancer Research U.K. Centre for Oncology and Applied Oncology, University of Glasgow. He is also a director of the Nanomedicines Research Centre and the Analytical Services Unit. He obtained his first degree as BVMS (Tierarzt) from the University of Munich. During his Ph.D. project in the Department of Medical Biophysics of the Technical University of Munich he joined the biotech start-up IDEA (Innovative Dermal Applications) where he was involved in the preclinical development of the company's transdermal products. His research focuses on the pharmacology of anticancer nanomedicines, specifically on the challenges of gene and drug delivery to solid tumors.

Contributors

Shona Anderson
Department of Pharmaceutical Sciences
University of Strathclyde
Glasgow, United Kingdom

Abdul W. Basit
Department of Pharmaceutics
School of Pharmacy
University of London
London, United Kingdom

Camille Bouissou
Department of Pharmaceutical Sciences
University of Strathclyde
Glasgow, United Kingdom

Anthony Brownlie
Department of Pharmaceutical Sciences
University of Strathclyde
Glasgow, United Kingdom

Patrick Couvreur
Faculté de Pharmacie
Université Paris-Sud
Chatenay-Malabry, France

Vaikunth Cuchelkar
Department of Bioengineering
University of Utah
Salt Lake City, Utah

Christine Dufes
Nanomedicines Research Centre
Centre for Oncology and Applied Pharmacology
University of Glasgow
Glasgow, United Kingdom

Ruth Duncan
Centre for Polymer Therapeutics
Welsh School of Pharmacy
Cardiff University
Cardiff, United Kingdom

Patrick J. Ginty
School of Pharmacy
University of Nottingham
Nottingham, United Kingdom

Hervé Hillaireau
Faculté de Pharmacie
Université Paris-Sud
Chatenay-Malabry, France

Allan S. Hoffman
Bioengineering Department
University of Washington
Seattle, Washington

Steven M. Howdle
School of Chemistry
University of Nottingham
Nottingham, United Kingdom

Kang Moo Huh
Department of Industrial and Physical
  Pharmacy
Purdue University
West Lafayette, Indiana

Seong Hoon Jeong
Department of Industrial and Physical
  Pharmacy
Purdue University
West Lafayette, Indiana

Richard A. Kendall
Department of Pharmaceutics
School of Pharmacy
University of London
London, United Kingdom

Jindřich Kopeček
Department of Pharmaceutics
  and Pharmaceutical Chemistry
University of Utah
Salt Lake City, Utah

Pei Lee Kan
Department of Pharmaceutics
School of Pharmacy
University of London
London, United Kingdom

Kinam Park
Department of Industrial
  and Physical Pharmacy
Purdue University
West Lafayette, Indiana

Helmut Ringsdorf
Universitat Mainz
Mainz, Germany

Felicity R.A.J. Rose
School of Pharmacy
University of Nottingham
Nottingham, United Kingdom

Andreas Schätzlein
Nanomedicines Research Centre
Centre for Oncology and Applied
  Pharmacology
University of Glasgow
Glasgow, United Kingdom

Kevin Shakesheff
School of Pharmacy
University of Nottingham
Nottingham, United Kingdom

Vladmir Torchilin
Department of Pharmaceutical Sciences
Northeastern University
Boston, Massachusetts

Ijeoma F. Uchegbu
Nanomedicines Research Centre
Department of Pharmaceutical Sciences
University of Strathclyde
Glasgow, United Kingdom

Chris van der Walle
Department of Pharmaceutical Sciences
University of Strathclyde
Glasgow, United Kingdom

Wei Wang
MI Production Chemicals
Altens Industrial Estate
Aberdeen, United Kingdom

Table of Contents

1 Introduction

Ijeoma F. Uchegbu

CONTENTS

1.1 DRUG DELIVERY

The science of drug delivery may be described as the application of chemical and biological principles to control the *in vivo* temporal and spatial location of drug molecules for clinical benefit. When drugs are administered, only a very small fraction of the dose actually hits the relevant receptors or sites of action, and most of the dose is actually wasted either by being taken up into the "wrong" tissue, removed from the "right" tissue too quickly, or destroyed en route before arrival. Scientists researching drug delivery seek to address these issues in order to (1) maximize drug activity and (2) minimize side effects [1].

Drug delivery is becoming an extremely demanding science. The reasons are essentially threefold: (1) the emergence of the more challenging low-molecular-weight molecules and biomacromolecules with either poor aqueous solubility, poor tissue permeation, or both, (2) the increased use of biological materials with poorly understood physical properties or questionable shelf life issues, and (3) the realization that if the portion of the dose responsible for adverse events could be directed away from sites where they originate, toxic side effects would become less frequent, thus benefiting the therapeutic index. Today's world requires that drug delivery systems be precise in their control of drug distribution and, preferably, respond directly to the local environment of the pathology in order to achieve a dynamic and beneficial interaction with the host pathology or physiology.

1.2 POLYMERS IN DRUG DELIVERY

Whether the control of oral absorption is desired [2] or the delivery of genes to the interior of specific cells is sought [3,4], the drug delivery macromolecule has emerged the most ubiquitous entity. In the current volume, macromolecules and their "younger (and sometimes smaller) cousins," dendrimers, are presented as components extraordinaire of a variety of drug delivery systems. Scientific reports are peppered with polymer- or dendrimer-containing systems that:

- Prolong drug action by entrapping the drug within matrices [5]
- Shift drug distribution in the direction of tumors [6]
- Shunt therapeutic genes [4] or oligonucleotides [7] into cells

- Enable drug absorption at optimum gastrointestinal tract absorptive sites, [8]
- Make the drug available only when there is a defined change in temperature [9,10] or pH [10] or when activated by an enzyme (as described in Chapter 10 of this volume)

In fact, recent reports show that polymers and dendrimers themselves demonstrate intrinsic bioactivity [3,11]. The drug delivery macromolecule is alive and well, and now has both drug and drug carrier properties [3].

The beauty of this discipline, polymers in drug delivery, is its longevity and self-transforming quality. Polymers have, for decades, performed a valuable function as excipients in tablet and capsule formulations [12–14], moved steadily into the parenteral arena as blood circulation time enhancers [1,15], and are now capable of offering advanced and sophisticated functions (such as drug targeting) [16] to medicines. Polymers have unique cooperative properties that are not found with low-molecular-weight compounds, and therein lies the root of their success. The chemical influence of one molecule may extend not to a few angstroms but to tens of angstroms, enabling it to control events over a comparatively wide three-dimensional (or four-dimensional, including time) continuum. With the intermolecular cooperativity enjoyed by some polymers, the spatial influence of polymers extends even further. A simple example of this capability is the ability of polymers to restrict the diffusion of low-molecular-weight compounds in matrix or nanomedicine arrangements.

Simple manipulation of the water solubility of polymers, by increasing their chain length through cross-linking or by hydrophobising or hydrophilizing them with copolymers and other groups, yields a wealth of materials with a wide spectrum of possible applications. The resulting materials are capable of a variety of drug-enhancing functions. Polymers are able to:

- Prolong drug availability if medicines are formulated as hydrogels [17,18] or micro-particles [19]
- Favorably alter biodistribution if formulated into dense nanoparticles [20]
- Enable hydrophobic drug administration if formulated as micelles [21]
- Transport a drug to its usually inaccessible site of action if formulated as gene medicines [3]
- Make drugs available in response to stimuli [9]

With these wonderful systems comes the inevitable task of polymer characterization. Efficient and thorough characterization will advance our understanding of these materials. In each vial of a "homogenous" polymer there may reside a number of different molecules each of which have roughly the same monomer type, but not necessarily in the same order (if a random copolymer) or connected in the same chain length. To overcome what would otherwise be a major limitation, statistical definitions are used to characterize the mixtures: the mean molecular weight, average level of copolymer A in relation to that of copolymer B, the average number of drug substituents, and so on. This strategy has allowed the advancement of drug delivery polymers because it has been acknowledged that the precise control of atomic composition and molecular weight, applied to low-molecular-weight drug delivery agents or low-molecular-weight drugs, need not be applied to polymeric excipients. However, as scientists endeavor to imitate nature, it must be appreciated that the future will most likely belong to the macromolecules that closely resemble nature's tools, i.e., the proteins and glycoproteins, with a definite polymer sequence and defined and precisely controlled polymer lengths.

What about tolerability? Are these molecules safe? Safety is a concept that is easy to understand but a little difficult to define. A variety of polymers such as the cellulose derivatives and poly(ethylene oxide) derivatives are already routinely used in medicine and appear to pose no identifiable hazard. However, with the new tailored molecules having targeting ability and cell-based activity, there is much to understand with respect to safety, and if we are to exploit the huge potential of the many polymeric materials that science has to offer, the issue of safety will have to be addressed for these new molecules and presumably on a case-by-case basis. Well-designed tests that are relevant to their final purpose will be needed for these new polymer-containing systems.

1.3 THIS VOLUME

This volume is primarily aimed at the nonspecialist reader, but the wide spectrum of opinion contained herein should also offer food for thought to the specialist. An eminent group of international experts have contributed to the volume, and it is hoped that the reader will judge this effort to be a richly sourced, informative, and ultimately rewarding read.

The aim of Chapter 1 is to introduce the subject matter in as jargon-free a manner as possible. Chapters 2 outlines the issues that must be considered when selecting a polymer for biomedical applications: i.e., for fabricating a drug delivery agent, surgical suture, prosthetic implant, or medical device. A number of exemplar polymers and their critical properties are discussed. It is important to understand that these biomaterials may be fabricated into biomedical entities that serve a dual purpose. The use of biomaterials to produce a combined prosthetic device and drug delivery system has been recently demonstrated by the emergence of a new therapeutic entity — the drug-eluting stent [22]. Chapter 3 focuses on polymer characterization and outlines the methods by which polymers may be characterized prior to use. It is impossible to detail all possible characterization techniques, and so only the more commonly used techniques are presented, e.g., methods to measure molecular weight and thermally controlled transitions.

Chapters 4 to 6 profile polymer matrices that have been used in the formulation of solid oral dosage forms, tissue-engineering drug delivery scaffolds, and hydrogels. These matrix systems effectively retard the diffusion of drug molecules, trapping them within a three-dimensional network of polymer chains. Polymers form the basis of technologies, such as tablet matrices and tablet coatings, aimed at modifying drug release in the gastrointestinal tract. A deeper understanding of the effect of diseases of nongastrointestinal origin on gastrointestinal physiology and pathology is required for the advancement of polymers and other oral drug delivery agents. The emerging areas of tissue engineering and tissue reconstruction (Chapter 6) have harnessed the polymer matrix and made it do more than just regulate the release of drug. The mechanical properties of the polymers are an important consideration when fabricating these systems, with a good match between tissue and polymer properties being an essential requirement.

Chapter 7 moves the matrix into the micrometer domain — small spheres with an amorphous and porous matrix into which drugs may be deposited. These matrices benefit from their small size and are thus injectable, implantable, and useful in the oral route. The main staple of this technology is the polymer poly(L-lactide-co-glycolide), a copolymer of glycolic acid and lactic acid monomers. Because the pharmaceutical industry is predicted to rely to a greater extent on drugs of biological origin-biologics, in the future, this chapter focuses on the issues surrounding the encapsulation of biologics within microspheres.

More particulates appear in Chapter 8 to Chapter 13, where nanoparticulates are presented. These structures are important constituents of the new nanomedicines, and they essentially exert control on drug biodistribution by utilizing both active (when bearing homing devices, termed *targeting ligands*) and passive (when controlled by the host pathology or physiology) targeting mechanisms. Chapter 8 profiles solid nanoparticles and nanocapsules prepared from largely-water-insoluble cyanoacrylate polymers and Chapter 9 discusses polymeric micelles; the latter made from essentially water-soluble polymers with both hydrophobic and hydrophilic regions. The nanospheres detailed in Chapter 8 may once again be used to target drugs to tumours for example and they are also able to target vaccines to the gut-associated lymphoid tissue for vaccination purposes. The micellar self-assemblies, which arise from the polymers with both hydrophobic and hydrophilic moieties, may be used for the delivery of hydrophobic drugs for example, and in essence both micellar and nanoparticle systems are able to beneficially alter drug bioavailability. Polymeric vesicles are detailed in Chapter 9 and arise when polymers, which are essentially insoluble in water but have hydrophilic and hydrophobic regions, self-assemble into closed membranes (vesicles). Some of these vesicles such as phospholipid vesicles containing poly(ethylene oxide)-based polymers have been used in licensed medicines for the treatment of cancer (Doxil® or Caelyx®). Stimuli responsive and toughened systems are possible with these technologies, and they could find applications in the future.

In Chapter 11 we move away from any obvious kind of self-assembly and really see the potential of soluble polymer prodrugs — tiny polymer nanomedicines. These polymeric systems allow the targeting of medicines by either keeping them in the blood for prolonged periods or exercising control on their biodistribution to various organs. Recently, bioactive polymers and dendrimers, which are devoid of the conjugated low-molecular-weight drug, emerged. The use of such drug macromolecules should provide the field of medicine with a rich and diverse array of tools in the future [3,11].

The final two chapters of this volume, Chapter 12 and Chapter 13, detail the contribution made by polymers and dendrimers to the gene delivery effort. Including such topics is always a risk as this particular area is fast developing, fuelled by the need to harness the potential offered by therapeutic genes. Therapeutic genes could theoretically cure largely incurable diseases if only genes could be efficiently and safely delivered. It seems almost surreal that such an elegant science as gene therapy should be stalled by a lack of suitable delivery options, but at the time of writing this is precisely the situation. Chapter 13 also provides evidence that dendrimers may one day be used for the controlled delivery of low-molecular-weight drug molecules.

1.4 THE FUTURE

What does the future hold for drug delivery? The future is extremely bright. Although drug delivery technologies, if appropriately applied, should be able to improve therapeutic outcomes, these technologies are required in some instances to simply enable therapy, as is the case with gene therapy and drug targeting. Drug delivery is also intuitively the logical and sensible thing to do. Depositing billions of drug molecules in the blood or gut and allowing the hapless molecules to locate their target, by uncontrolled diffusion, is surely a therapeutic strategy of yesterday and not of tomorrow. Guiding sufficient numbers of molecules in sufficient time directly to their targets, is the future. Polymers have helped this endeavor and will continue to enable this effort in the foreseeable future.

REFERENCES

1. Allen, T. and Cullis, P., Drug delivery systems: entering the mainstream, *Science, 303, 1818–1822, 2004.*
2. Vansavage, G. and Rhodes, C.T., The sustained-release coating of solid dosage forms — a historical review, *Drug Dev. Ind. Pharm.,* 21, 93–118, 1995.
3. Dufes, C., Keith, N., Bisland, A., Proutski, I., Uchegbu, I.F., and Schatzlein, A.G., Synthetic anti-cancer gene medicine exploiting intrinsic anti-tumor activity of cationic vector to cure established tumors, *Cancer Res.,* 65, 8079–8084, 2005.
4. Kircheis, R., Wightman, L., Kursa, M., Ostermann, E., and Wagner, E., Tumor-targeted gene delivery: an attractive strategy to use highly active effector molecules in cancer treatment, *Gene Ther.,* 9, 731–735, 2002.
5. Perry, C.M. and Brogden, R.N., Goserelin — a review of its pharmacodynamic and pharmacokinetic properties, and therapeutic use in benign gynecological disorders, *Drugs,* 51, 319–346, 1996.
6. Brigger, I., Morizet, J., Aubert, G., Chacun, H., Terrier-Lacombe, M.J., Couvreur, P., and Vassal, G., Poly(ethylene glycol)-coated hexadecanoylcyanoacrylate nanospheres display a combined effect for brain tumor targeting, *J. Pharmacol. Exp. Ther.,* 303, 928–936, 2002.
7. Hollins, A.J., Benboutera, M., Omidi, Y., Zinselmeyer, B., Schatzlein, A.G., Uchegbu, I.F., and Akhtar, S., Evaluation of generation 2 and 3 poly(propylenimine) dendrimers for the potential cellular delivery of antisense oligonucleotides targeting epidermal growth factor receptor, *Pharm. Res.,* 21, 458–466, 2004.

8. van den Mooter, G., Maris, B., Samyn, C., Augustijns, P., and Kinget, R., Use of azo polymers for colon-specific drug delivery, *J. Pharm. Sci.,* 86, 1321–1327, 1997.

9. Bromberg, L.E. and Ron, E.S., Temperature-responsive gels and thermogelling polymer matrices for protein and peptide delivery, *Adv. Drug Delivery Rev.,* 31, 197–221, 1998.

10. Yuk, S.H., Cho, S.H., and Lee, S.H., pH/temperature-responsive polymer composed of poly((N,N-dimethylamino)ethyl methacrylate-co-ethylacrylamide), *Macromolecules,* 30, 6856–6859, 1997.

11. Shaunak, S., Thomas, S., Gianasi, E., Godwin, A., Jones, E., Teo, I., Mireskandari, K., Luthert, P., Duncan, R., Patterson, S., Khaw, P., and Brocchini, S., Polyvalent dendrimer glucosamine conjugates prevent scar tissue formation, *Nat. Biotechnol.,* 22, 977–984, 2004.

12. Kumar, M. and Kumar, N., Polymeric controlled drug-delivery systems: perspective issues and opportunities, *Drug Dev. Ind. Pharm.,* 27, 1–30, 2001.

13. Kumar, V. and Banker, G.S., Chemically-modified cellulosic polymers, *Drug Dev. Ind. Pharm.,* 19, 1–31, 1993.

14. Luo, Y. and Prestwich, G.D., Novel biomaterials for drug delivery, *Expert Opin. Ther. Patents,* 11, 1395–1410, 2001.

15. Blume, G. and Cevc, G., Liposomes for the sustained drug release in vivo, *Biochim. Biophys. Acta,* 1029, 91–97, 1990.

16. Duncan, R., The dawning era of polymer therapeutics, *Nat. Rev. Drug Discovery,* 2, 347–360, 2003.

17. Park, K., Shalaby, W.S.W., and Park, H., *Biodegradable Hydrogels for Drug Delivery.* Lancaster, PA: Technomic Publishing, 1993.

18. Hoffman, A.S., Hydrogels for biomedical applications, *Adv. Drug Delivery Rev.,* 54, 3–12, 2002.

19. Park, J.H., Ye, M.L., and Park, K., Biodegradable polymers for microencapsulation of drugs, *Molecules,* 10, 146–161, 2005.

20. Mathiowitz, E., Jacob, J.S., Jong, Y.S., Carino, G.P., Chickering, D.E., Chaturvedi, P., Santos, C.A., Vijayaraghavan, K., Montgomery, S., Bassett, M., and Morrell, C., Biologically erodable microsphere as potential oral drug delivery system, *Nature,* 386, 410–414, 1997.

21. Torchilin, V.P., Lukyanov, A.N., Gao, Z.G., and Papahadjopoulos-Sternberg, B., Immunomicelles: targeted pharmaceutical carriers for poorly soluble drugs, *Proc. Natl. Acad. Sci. USA,* 100, 6039–6044, 2003.

22. Doggrell, S.A., Sirolinnus- or paclitaxel-eluting stents to prevent coronary artery restenosis, *Expert Opin. Pharmacother.,* 5, 2209–2220, 2004.

2 Selecting the Right Polymer for Biomaterial Applications

Allan S. Hoffman

CONTENTS

2.1 INTRODUCTION

Where does one start when trying to select the right polymer for use in a medical implant or therapeutic device? Clearly, for any particular application, one needs to screen a group of polymers on the basis of the most important properties needed in that end use. For example:

1. An intraocular lens (IOL) must be transparent and dimensionally stable. Protein and lipid absorptions are issues that also should be probed, but only after selecting a group of materials for an IOL that are transparent and dimensionally stable.
2. The ball in a ball-in-cage heart valve (such as the Star-Edwards® valve) must be both dimensionally and mechanically stable during the cyclic movements up against the top of the metal stents and back down to the bottom of the cage where it must make a good seal. A related, key factor is that the ball should absorb minimal amounts of water or lipids, which would change both its dimensions and mechanical properties. Blood compatibility is a secondary concern for this application, because the patient will probably have to take an anticoagulant drug on a chronic basis.
3. A blood oxygenator membrane must have good permeability to oxygen and CO_2. Blood interactions are secondary here especially as the patient's blood is probably going to be anticoagulated with heparin during bypass oxygenation.
4. A dental cement must have good adhesive properties, both to the surfaces of the tooth and to the filling material, and must be water resistant once cured. If the cement is going to be subjected to chewing stresses, then both the adhesive bond strength and cohesive

strength under cyclic compressive stresses will be critical to the success of a dental cement. Protein adsorption or bacterial adhesion are not critical.

5. A drug delivery device or system must release the drug at the desired rate, and in order for clinical success, the polymer components of the delivery vehicle must swell (or not), or degrade (or not), or dissolve (or not), or be retrieved (if necessary) after the drug is depleted. The demands on these key properties of the polymer components of a drug delivery system are critical to its success.

One can imagine many such different and widely varying applications of biomaterials in therapeutic implants and devices, where each material in each application must have those one or two critical properties that are key to its success in that particular end use. Therefore, when selecting materials for an implant or therapeutic device, it is important to establish a "priority" list of desirable properties and then to identify the one or two of its most critical properties. This chapter discusses the composition and structure–property relationships of synthetic polymers that are critical to their applications as biomaterials in implants and therapeutic devices, and describes many of the common polymeric biomaterials to exemplify these principles [1,2].

2.2 COMPOSITION AND STRUCTURE–PHYSICAL PROPERTY RELATIONSHIPS FOR SYNTHETIC POLYMERS

Polymers used in implants and therapeutic devices are shown in Figure 2.1 to 2.5. The molecular weights of the different polymers span a very wide range, e.g., from 3 to 5 kDa for poly(ethylene oxide), which is also known as poly(ethylene glycol) (PEG; Figure 2.4) and is used in a variety of drug

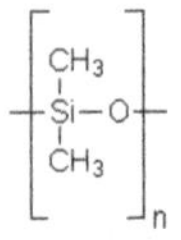

Poly(dimethyl siloxane) (PDMS)
(When lightly crosslinked = Silicone Rubber)

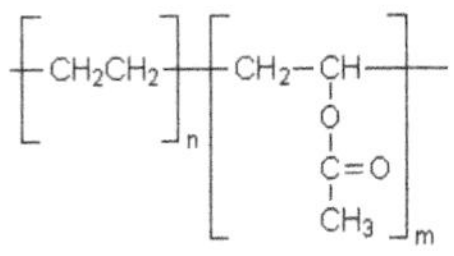

Ethylene-Vinyl Acetate (EVA) copolymers

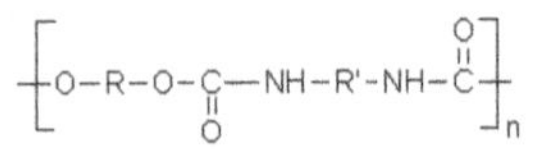

Polyurethanes (where R = polyether [soft segment] and R' = aromatic or cyclic groups [hard segment])

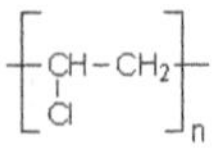

Poly(vinyl chloride) (PVC) (soft when plasticised)

FIGURE 2.1 Soft plastics and rubbers.

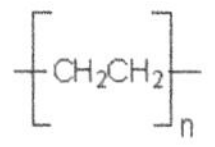

Poly(ethylene) (PE)

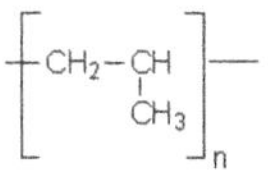

Poly(propylene) (PP)

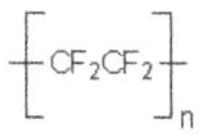

Poly(tetrafluoroethylene) (PTFE)

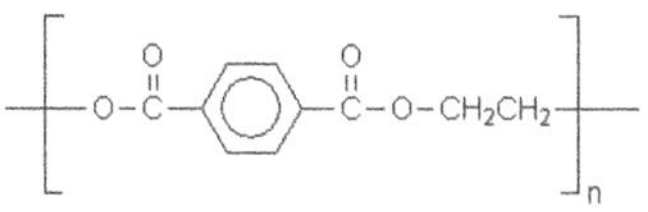

Poly(ethylene terephthalate) (PET)

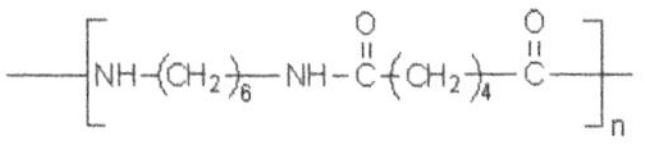

Poly(hexamethylene adipamide) (Nylon 6-6®)

FIGURE 2.2 Crystalline plastics and fiber-forming polymers.

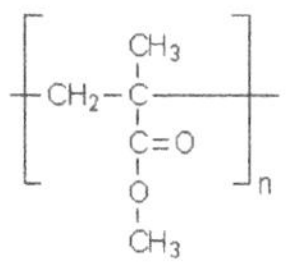

Poly(methylmethacrylate) (PMMA)

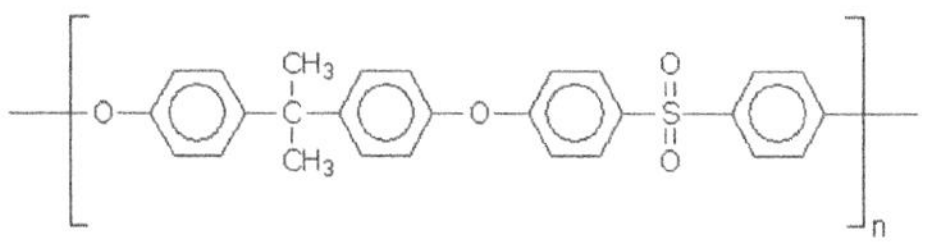

Polysulphone

FIGURE 2.3 Glassy plastics.

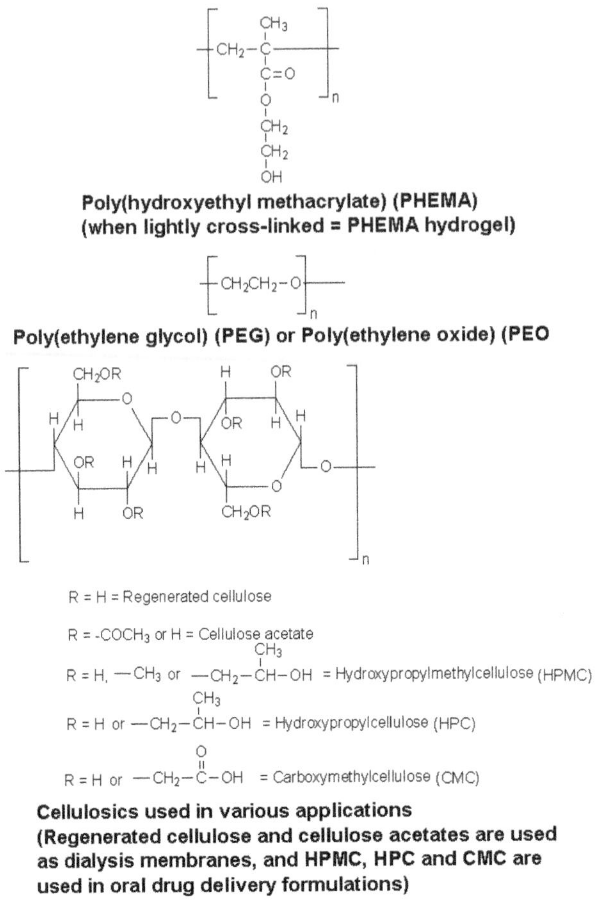

Poly(hydroxyethyl methacrylate) (PHEMA)
(when lightly cross-linked = PHEMA hydrogel)

Poly(ethylene glycol) (PEG) or Poly(ethylene oxide) (PEO

R = H = Regenerated cellulose

R = -COCH$_3$ or H = Cellulose acetate

R = H, —CH$_3$ or —CH$_2$—CH—OH = Hydroxypropylmethylcellulose (HPMC)
                                    CH$_3$

R = H or —CH$_2$—CH—OH = Hydroxypropylcellulose (HPC)
                          CH$_3$

R = H or —CH$_2$—C—OH = Carboxymethylcellulose (CMC)
                        O

Cellulosics used in various applications
(Regenerated cellulose and cellulose acetates are used
as dialysis membranes, and HPMC, HPC and CMC are
used in oral drug delivery formulations)

FIGURE 2.4 Water soluble and water swelling polymers and hydrogels.

delivery formulations, to perhaps as much as a million kDa for the ultra-high molecular weight polyethylene (UHMWPE) (Figure 2.2) used in hip and knee prostheses (UHMWPE differs from low-density PE in that it has less branching, allowing molecules to pack tightly and form a material with high crystallinity and wear resistance). Besides the molecular weight, there are three molecular parameters that control the two major transitions of polymers, the glass transition temperature (Tg) and the melting point temperature (Tm). All polymers have a Tg, but not all have a Tm as only those that are semicrystalline exhibit a melting transition. Tg is a kinetic transition, and it is always lower than Tm, which is a thermodynamic first-order transition. Tg has been estimated to occur at the onset of rotation around main-chain atoms that are about 30 to 40 atoms apart. Tg along with Tm (when present) essentially define the physical and mechanical properties of a polymeric material in the solid state, and those properties at ambient or body temperature will direct the end use of the polymer as a biomaterial. For example, a tough, rubbery material is needed as a pumping bladder in a left ventricular assist device, whereas a strong, highly crystalline material is needed as a fiber for use in a woven vascular graft or as a suture. The biological environment can have a major influence on Tg for polymers that absorb significant amounts of water. Lipid absorption from blood can also influence the physical and mechanical properties of nonpolar polymers. Extraction of soluble components from a polymer are also potentially important, such as in the case of extraction of plasticizer from PVC into blood, e.g., when PVC is used as a blood storage bag.

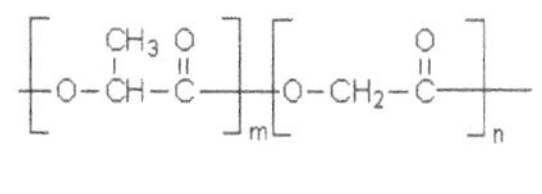

Poly(lactide-co-glycolide) (PLGA)

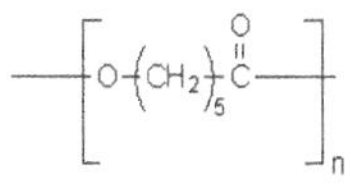

Poly(caprolactone) (PCL)

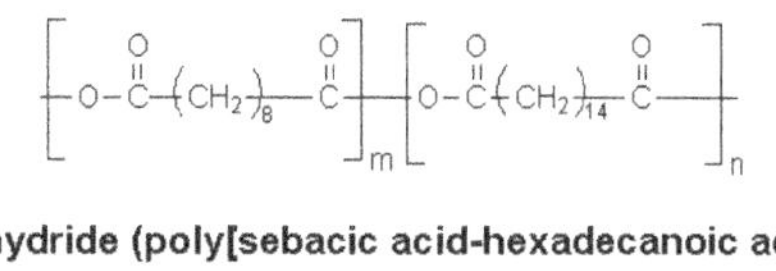

Polyanhydride (poly[sebacic acid-hexadecanoic acid] anhydride)

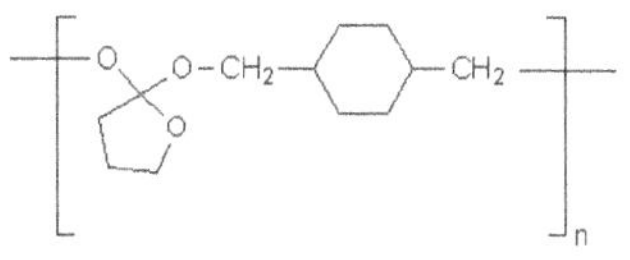

Poly(orthoester) (POE)

FIGURE 2.5 Hydrolytically-degradable polymers.

The three key molecular properties of a polymer that control its Tg (and Tm), and thus its physical and mechanical properties between ambient and body temperatures, are chain stiffness, chain polarity, and chain architecture. *Chain stiffness* is measured by the magnitude of the energy barrier for rotation around main-chain bonds. *Chain polarity* is related to the presence of polar groups (especially H-bonding groups) along the backbone or in pendant groups. *Chain architecture* relates to the presence or absence of bulky side groups, because small side groups lead to a "smooth" or "streamlined" shape for the backbone, which facilitates packing of the chains in crystallites. Most polymeric biomaterials have random bond configurations along the backbone chain and are not stereo-regular. Exceptions are (a) polypropylene (PP, Figure 2.2), which is a useful fiber only when it has the isotactic bond configuration (where the pendant methyl groups are all oriented in the same configuration along the main chain) that forms a helical chain conformation, and (b) L- or D,L-lactic acid polymers (PLA, Figure 2.5), which are biodegradable polyesters with stereo-specific bond configurations of the pendant methyl groups along the main chain.

The three molecular parameters of chain stiffness, polarity, and architecture act together to control Tg (and Tm). Because Tm is due to a thermodynamic transition, at the melting point there is equilibrium between the crystalline state and the amorphous molten state, and therefore the free energy of melting, $\Delta Gm = 0$. This results in the definition of the melting temperature as:

$$Tm = \Delta Hm/\Delta Sm \qquad (2.1)$$

The enthalpy of melting, ΔHm, is mainly related to the ability of the chains to pack closely in crystallites, and the entropy of melting, ΔSm, is related to the gain in randomness upon melting. If the chains are very symmetrical and polar, they will pack well in the crystallites and ΔHm will be large. On the other hand, if the chains are not very symmetrical or polar, they will not pack so well in the crystallite and ΔHm will be lower. However, the major factor controlling

Tm for many polymers is ΔSm, which is the gain in conformational "freedom" of the chain as it goes from the crystalline to the melt phase. If the chain is stiff, there is relatively small gain in conformational freedom because it is already in an extended conformation in the crystallite and ΔSm will be small, leading to a high Tm; if the chain is very flexible, ΔSm should be large as it goes from the extended conformation in the crystallite to a random, flexible coil in the melt, leading to a low Tm [3,4].

The interactions of polar groups on different chains will tend to increase the rotational energy barrier, leading to a higher Tg, and, assuming a symmetrical chain backbone, the polymer will also form crystallites with a high ΔHm and low ΔSm of melting. Polyamides have a streamlined architecture and H-bonding groups along their backbones, leading to a high-melting semicrystalline material that also has a relatively high Tg (e.g., Tm = ~267°C and Tg = 45°C for Nylon® 6-6; Figure 2.2). If the chain is both streamlined and has stiff groups along the backbone, such as seen in the poly(ethylene terephthalate) chain (PET; Figure 2.2), then this polymer will also be a high-melting (Tm = 270°C) useful fiber. PET also has a high Tg of 69°C. It is often seen that the molecular factors that increase one of the transitions will also increase the other. Thus, a plot of Tg vs. Tm that includes data for many polymers rises in an approximately linear fashion with some broadening ("fanning out") at the higher temperatures.

The presence of bulky side groups, whether polar or not, will increase the stiffness of the chain, raising its Tg. This is especially true for bulky polar groups. The bulky side groups will also inhibit packing of the chains in crystallites, and such a polymer will be glassy and amorphous at body temperature. An example of such a polymer is poly(methyl methacrylate) (PMMA; Figure 2.1b), which is used in hard contact lenses and IOLs. If the polymer lacks significant polar interactions and has a low energy barrier for the rotation of main-chain bonds, Tg will be well below the ambient temperature and the polymer will exhibit rubbery behavior at conditions the biomaterials are used. For such rubbers, the flexibility of the main chain is much more important than chain architecture, so even streamlined chains will be amorphous, rubbery materials at body temperature. An example of this is the chain architecture of silicone rubber poly(dimethylsiloxane) (PDMS; Figure 2.1), which is so streamlined that the chains can readily pack together in crystallites. However, chain flexibility is very high, ΔSm is very large, the Tm of PDMS is –43°C, and PDMS is a noncrystalline, amorphous rubber at ambient conditions [3–5].

Table 2.1 shows Tg and Tm for common polymeric biomaterials. PEG and poly(vinyl chloride) (PVC) are shown without the effect of water or plasticizer, respectively, on their two key transition temperatures.

As mentioned earlier and as indicated in Table 2.1, water absorption can have a significant influence on Tg. Polarity in the polymers will lead to absorption of water, and that can convert a rigid, glassy polymer to a soft hydrogel. For example, soft contact lenses are made from a lightly

TABLE 2.1
Tg and Tm of Common Polymeric Biomaterials

Polymer	Chemical Structure	T_g (°C)	T_m (°C)
Poly(dimethyl siloxane) (PDMS)	Figure 2.1	−127	− 43
Polyethylene (PE)	Figure 2.2	−100	130
Poly(ethylene oxide) (PEO or PEG) (dry)	Figure 2.4	−41	66
Poly(hexamethylene adipamide) (Nylon 6-6)	Figure 2.2	45	267
Poly(ethylene terephthalate) (PET)	Figure 2.2	69	270
Poly(vinyl chloride) (PVC) (no plasticizer)	Figure 2.1	81	273
Poly(methyl methacrylate) (PMMA)	Figure 2.3	105	—
Poly(tetrafluoroethylene) (PTFE)	Figure 2.2	127	327

crosslinked poly(hydroxyethyl methacrylate) (PHEMA; Figure 2.4), which swells significantly in water. The polymer has a large and bulky polar side group (a hydroxyethyl ester group), which makes it amorphous and glassy at body temperature when dry (as soft contact lens wearers can attest if they accidentally leave the lenses out to dry) and becomes a soft hydrogel when swollen in water (absorbing about 35 to 40% water).

Water absorption is also important if there are hydrolyzable bonds in the backbone of the polymer, such as ester groups. When these bonds hydrolyze, the polymer backbone degrades, and eventually the polymer itself will break up into pieces and disappear. Degradable poly(lactide-*co*-glycolide) (PLGA; Figure 2.5) sutures are the best example of this type of polymer. Although most degradable polymers break down *in vivo* by hydrolysis of main-chain bonds, water absorption may also permit enzymes to penetrate and attack polymers that are enzymatically susceptible. The composition of degradable polymers will determine their Tg and Tm before implantation, and that will control their key physical and mechanical properties, such as the crystalline state needed for a strong degradable suture. The composition of degradable polymers will also control their degradation rate, usually by controlling their absorption of water. The more hydrophobic, degradable polyesters, such as poly(caprolactone) (PCL; Figure 2.5) and poly(lactic acid) (PLA; Figure 2.5), degrade much more slowly than PLGA with a 1: 1 ratio of lactic acid and glycolic acid [1,2].

2.3 THE INFLUENCE OF COMPOSITION AND STRUCTURE OF CERTAIN POLYMERS ON THEIR APPLICATIONS AS BIOMATERIALS: SOME EXAMPLES

2.3.1 SILICONE RUBBER

Lightly crosslinked PDMS (Figure 2.1; Figure 2.6 shows a schematic of a crosslinked network) is one of the most commonly used polymeric biomaterials, particularly when a rubbery material is called for [5–8]. Other elastomers such as natural latex rubber, polyisoprene, and thermoplastic rubbers such as styrene-butadiene block polymers all have unsaturation in their backbones, so they are unsuitable for long-term implantation. Natural latex may also have protein impurities that can cause allergic or even immunogenic responses. The backbone composition and structure of PDMS is the most flexible backbone known among all the synthetic polymers. The —Si—O—Si— bond angle is 143°, which is much greater than the —C—C—C— bond angle in most other polymers, and the oxygen atom is so small and unhindered relative to the adjacent silicon atoms that the chain is essentially freely rotating. Thus, PDMS has the lowest Tg (~ –120°C) of any polymer. However, its physical strength

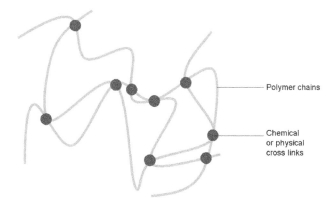

Polymer chains

Chemical or physical cross links

FIGURE 2.6 Sketch of a crosslinked network.

is poor, even when cross-linked, so it is usually used only when it is both cross-linked and reinforced with silica [5,6].

The hardness and toughness of lightly crosslinked PDMS (Silicone Rubber) may be enhanced by increasing the cross-link density (increasing the number of cross-links per unit volume). Silicone chains are crosslinked by replacing some of the $-Si-CH_3$ groups with $-Si-H$ and $-Si-CH=CH_2$ groups, and adding platinum, which catalyses the addition of the two, forming $-Si-CH_2-CH_2-Si-$ crosslinks between different chains. (5) Other ways to stiffen and toughen Silicone Rubber besides increasing the crosslink density, include increasing the silica filler content and/or substituting $-Si-CH_3$ groups with Si-phenyl groups. The ability to "molecularly engineer" its mechanical properties, plus its inertness in biologic media, make PDMS eminently suitable as a substitute for stiffer tissues such as the ear, nose, and chin. Its use as a breast implant has been controversial [9,10]. The most attractive and successful breast implant was composed of a silicone rubber bag or capsule filled with a gel-like silicone polymer. It had the right "feel" of the tissue it was replacing, and was widely successful. Only a small percent of implants had to be removed, for a variety of reasons. It should be noted that finite failure rates are to be expected with all man-made devices, even implants. However, on the basis of a relatively few failures of the silicone gel-encapsulated silicone breast implants, lawyers filed class action liability suits claiming that patients were not properly informed about many potential undesirable effects before implantation. One claim made was that the outer surface of the PDMS capsule was supposed to have caused immune responses, leading to formation of antibodies to PDMS, but this claim was never demonstrated scientifically. In those rare cases when the silicone gel leaked out of the capsule, the plaintiffs claimed that it caused a variety of problems, including diseases ranging from lupus to lymphatic tumors [10]. Most of these claims have not been found to be statistically significant by scientific studies, but nevertheless some are still possible in a large patient population. However, the large awards handed down to plaintiffs by some judges have caused changes in the currently available implants, which now use a saline solution inside the PDMS capsule instead of a silicone gel. Silicone remains the material of choice for the outer capsule used for breast implants. A variety of outer capsule modifications have also been developed, such as incorporation of perfluorinated components in the PDMS composition, to reduce the permeability of the capsule wall to lower MW components in the silicone gel, and surface roughening to promote formation of a thin fibrous collagen capsule around the implant.

In the early days of PDMS usage as a ball in the Star-Edwards ball-in-cage heart valve, the silicone ball absorbed lipids from the blood, swelled, and became brittle [11–13]. This caused it to break up, and the fragments escaped the cage and flowed downstream in the arterial blood, causing vessel blockages that killed the patient. The cross-linking chemistry was changed and the silica content may also have been changed; today, the result continues to be a successful heart valve.

The remarkably high oxygen and CO_2 permeability of PDMS has made it the material of choice for a blood oxygenator membrane [6]. Oxygen and CO_2 are apolar gases, and as such they dissolve and permeate best in hydrophobic media. Other hydrophobic rubbers do not match the high permeability of PDMS; because of its highly flexible backbone chain, it is amorphous (i.e., noncrystalline) and has a low density that allows very high permeation to those two gases. Its low density is reflected in its unusually low melt viscosity. Fluorocarbons also have high permeability to these gases, and perfluoro groups have been incorporated into PDMS networks to achieve enhanced oxygen permeation. Microporous polymers prepared from polysulfones (Figure 2.3) and other polymers have replaced PDMS membranes in blood oxygenators. The coagulation of blood at the entry to the gas-filled pores forms a thin protein film that acts as the barrier membrane, and it is so thin that it has an even higher permeability to oxygen and CO_2 than PDMS with perfluoro segments. Silicone Rubber is used in the more recent, long-wear contact-lens compositions to provide enhanced oxygen permeability to the underlying corneal tissues; poly(vinyl pyrrolidone) is entrapped within the Silicone Rubber to provide good wettability and lubricity for the lens on the eye surface [6].

The hydrophobic and amorphous low-density properties of PDMS have also made it the material of choice in the drug delivery implant called Norplant®. In this implant, a silicone rubber tube is loaded with a PDMS rod filled with particles of the hydrophobic contraceptive steroid, Norgestrel, a synthetic progestin, and this drug permeates the tube wall and delivers a constant, steady state rate over a period as long as five years [6].

One application in which PDMS has *not* been useful is as the pumping bladder in the left ventricular assist device or the total artificial heart. It simply does not have the necessary flex life, even when cross-linked and reinforced with silica. Polyurethanes have much greater flex lives and are currently the pump bladder of choice [8] (see the following text for more details about polyurethanes).

2.3.2 POLY(ETHYLENE TEREPHTHALATE)

Poly(ethylene terephthalate) (PET) (Figure 2.2) has a backbone that is stiff because of the —(C = O)—phenyl—(C = O)— groups, which rotate as a single unit. Its chain architecture is also very streamlined, and therefore PET packs well into crystallites, resulting in a high Tm. It is also hydrophobic, so water absorption is minimal, and therefore the terephthalate ester groups are stable against degradation. These properties result in an inert, high-melting crystalline polymeric biomaterial that has become the material of choice for implant fabrics such as those used in vascular grafts and tissue fixation fabrics for anchoring implants by sutures to the surrounding tissues [14–20]. PET is also used in film form as the backing film for some transdermal drug delivery patches.

2.3.3 POLYETHYLENE AND POLY(TETRAFLUOROETHYLENE)

In the early to mid-1950s John Charnley, orthopedic surgeon, in the U.K. conceived of the prosthetic hip implant that combined a metal stem and ball as the femoral component and a plastic cup as the acetabular, i.e., the hip socket component [21,22]. His first choice for the cup was the polymer with the lowest known surface friction, PTFE (Figure 2.1). However, he did not realize that a more important property than low surface friction for the cup material was its surface wear resistance. PTFE rapidly wore, and produced many small particles that created a significant and undesirable inflammatory response, resulting in the need to retrieve all the implanted hip prostheses [23]. PE (Figure 2.2) is a simple polymer chain, streamlined in shape (when it is polymerized with catalysts that avoid branching reactions), with high flexibility, and has no polar groups, so it has a low Tg and a Tm of about 135°C when it is in the ultra-high molecular weight, high-density, and high-crystallinity form Charnley heard about UHMWPE, and he tried the product of Ruhr-Chemie in Germany, and that particular UHMWPE became the standard polymeric articulating surface for hip and knee implants. The key property of UHMWPE that PTFE lacked is a high wear resistance [24]. Today materials scientists are still trying to improve that property by radiation-cross-linking UHMWPE.

PE is also a major component of ethylene vinyl acetate (EVA; Figure 2.1) copolymers, in which ethylene is copolymerized with vinyl acetate (VA) in varying ratios. These copolymers are used as rate-controlling membranes in skin patches and in earlier reservoir drug delivery devices. The addition of VA as a comonomer interferes with PE crystallization within the EVA polymer matrix; therefore, the higher the VA content in EVA, the less the crystalline content. The lower the crystallinity of EVA, the higher the permeability of a drug through the EVA matrix. EVA polymers of 20 to 50% VA are currently used as rate-controlling membranes in transdermal skin patches.

PTFE has been fabricated as an expanded, microporous material known as expanded PTFE (e-PTFE), which has proven to be very successful in tubular form as a synthetic vascular graft. Surgeons like the "feel" of it as a vascular graft, and it is an alternate choice instead of PET for that application [25]. Early attempts to make a woven graft of PTFE were unsuccessful because of the low burst strength of the woven fabric, as noted earlier. However, its use in the form of a tube of e-PTFE proved to be successful as a vascular graft, particularly when the graft was reinforced with fibrils of PTFE wound around its outer circumference. Thus, PTFE's failure owing to its poor wear resistance as a solid acetabular hip cup or its poor burst strength as a woven fabric tube stand out in contrast to its success as an expanded, microporous PTFE tube for use as a vascular graft.

This is one more example of how the key properties required for a particular application will determine success or failure of a particular biomaterial (and sometimes the physical form of the material) in that particular use [26].

2.3.4 ACRYLIC POLYMERS AND COPOLYMERS

PMMA (Figure 2.3) was the first successful acrylic polymer used as a biomaterial. It is a glassy, transparent material at body temperature because of the large pendant, bulky ester group combined with the methyl group that are both linked to the alpha-carbon. PMMA is transparent, dimensionally stable, and non-water-absorbing, and it has proven useful as an IOL. (It has been known commercially as Perspex®, Lucite®, or Plexiglas®.) Furthermore, because it is hydrophobic, it does not absorb significant amounts of water, and therefore the pendant ester group is stable over a long term. The application of PMMA as an IOL was developed just after World War II when ophthalmologist, Dr. Harold Ridley, was examining British RAF airmen who had in their eyes fragments of Perspex® PMMA from blown-out airplane cockpit canopies and windows. Ridley noticed that the material was inert within the eye tissues [27]. The dimensional stability and transparency of PMMA also made it useful as a hard contact lens. A wide variety of contact lenses are now available, with oxygen gas permeability as an additional key property for the long-wear lenses. This property was first achieved by copolymerizing perfluoro- or siloxane-modified acrylic monomers with the MMA monomer and more recently the long wear lenses have evolved to soft, transparent PDMS blends and interpenetrating networks (IPNs) with hydrophilic polymers, as noted above [28,29].

PMMA also contributed to the success of the hip implant (see earlier discussion). Acrylic polymers were already in use as dental cements when Dennis Smith, polymer chemist, suggested to John Charnley that he try to use them as a cement in the hip implant in order to hold the femoral stem in place within the femur [30–32]. In this system, liquid MMA monomer containing one part (e.g., dimethyl toluidine) of a two-part polymerization catalyst that is active at ambient temperature, is mixed with a solid powder of PMMA containing the second part of the catalyst (e.g., benzoyl peroxide), and the viscous mixture polymerizes to a hard solid in a few minutes. This addition to the protocol, plus the substitution of the low-wear-resistant PTFE by the high-wear-resistant UHMWPE, led to the ultimate success of the hip implant. One could say that this novel collaboration of a polymer chemist and an orthopedic surgeon was one of the earliest examples of a successful interdisciplinary bioengineering team [21,22].

The soft contact lens was developed in Czechoslovakia in the late 1960s by Wichterle and Lim [33]. They replaced the pendant methyl ester group of PMMA with a hydroxyethyl ester group, forming the novel polymer PHEMA (Figure 2.1d). Because the hydroxy group absorbed water, they had to cross-link the chains with ethylene glycol dimethacrylate (EGDMA) in order to retain the dimensional stability needed for the contact lens. This was one of the first, if not the first, hydrogels to be used in a biomedical application.

Another important acrylic polymeric hydrogel is a copolymer of a methacrylate ester such as MMA with an acrylic acid monomer such as methacrylic acid (MAA). This copolymer is hydrophobic and water insoluble at acidic pHs such as those found in the stomach, but, depending on the MAA content, it will swell and slowly dissolve at pHs of 7 to 8, such as those found in the intestines. These types of copolymers are used as enteric coatings for oral drug formulations in which the drug (e.g., aspirin) may irritate the stomach lining and, therefore, will only be released in the enteric or intestinal region.

There has also been widespread interest in acrylic polymers and hydrogels that are responsive to other stimuli besides pH, such as temperature. These so-called "smart" polymers have a balance of hydrophobic and hydrophilic groups that lead to their stimuli-responsive behaviors. They have been conjugated or complexed with proteins, nucleic acid drugs, and other biomolecules, in a wide variety of applications. These types of polymers may have significant future uses in the area of drug delivery, cell culture, microfluidic assays, affinity separations, and enzyme bioprocesses [34–46].

Photopolymerizable acrylic hydrogels that also have degradable poly(lactic acid) (PLA) sequences in their structures have been developed as sealants and antiadhesion gels for surgical applications [47].

2.3.5 CELLULOSICS

Regenerated cellulose and cellulose acetate (Figure 2.4) membranes are the materials of choice for blood dialyzers [48–53]. Regenerated cellulose may be obtained by treating cellulose with sodium hydroxide, followed by carbon disulfide to form soluble cellulose xanthate. Cellulose is then regenerated from cellulose xanthate by dissolving in sodium hydroxide and treating with sulfuric acid, sodium sulfate, and zinc ions. Cuprammonium cellulose may also be used to produce regenerated cellulose and in this procedure cellulose is solubilized in water by treating with copper, ammonia, and sodium hydroxide. Cellulose is then regenerated by the removal of copper and ammonia and neutralization of the sodium hydroxide. The purpose of the blood dialysis separation process is to remove small- and middle-molecular-weight toxins in the blood that the kidneys have failed to remove, but not to remove proteins or salt ions. The osmolarity of the dialyser extraction fluid is balanced with that of the blood in order not to remove the salt ions in the blood along with the toxins. Dialysis membranes must have the right-sized pores and fluxes and must be suitable for dialyzing patients several times a week. The original membrane used by the inventor of the artificial kidney, Willem Kolff, MD, was a sausage casing, which was all he could get at the time he developed the first dialyzer during World War II in The Netherlands.

Today, dialysis membranes are categorized in three groups: low-, medium-, and high-flux membranes. Low-flux membranes are the traditional regenerated cellulose (e.g., using cuprammonium or xanthate processes) or "thin-skin" cellulose acetate hollow fibers. These low-flux membranes do not efficiently remove the so-called "middle molecules" such as beta-2-microglobulins, which cause amyloidosis complications among long-term dialysis patients. The medium-flux membranes have greater pore volumes and diameters, which provide higher flux along with some removal of the "middle" molecules. The high-flux membranes are prepared from porous polysulfone coated to make the pores more hydrophilic; they shorten the dialysis times, but they remove more than the microglobulins, which tends to distress older patients. The key to the choice of membrane is finding, for each patient, the right balance between reducing the complications from amyloidosis and minimizing the load on the patient. Dialysis membranes are another example of how it is so important to apply the right polymer for the right end use, and in this case, that end use is the "right patient" [52,53].

Cellulose acetates have also been used as the rate-controlling membrane in oral osmotic pump delivery devices. Other cellulose derivatives are used in pills and tablets as binders that act as swelling agents that control enteric and colonic release of drugs in oral drug delivery formulations. These polymers include hydroxypropyl methylcellulose (HPMC), hydroxypropyl cellulose (HPC), and carboxymethyl cellulose (CMC) (Figure 2.4). Each of these polymers has a balance of hydrophilic and hydrophobic groups on the cellulosic backbones that determines the ultimate swelling and gelling or dissolution rates that control the rate of drug release in the upper intestines. These cellulosic compositions also have to be tailored to the ultimate desired rate of release.

2.3.6 POLYURETHANES

Polyurethanes (PUs; Figure 2.1) are tough polymers that are used as pumping bladders in heart-assist devices, including the total artificial heart, and also in pacemaker leads [19,26]. They are most often constructed from polyether diols such as poly(tetramethylene oxide) (PTMO) that have been reacted with an excess of diisocyanates and with chains extended either with diamines to form poly(ether-urea-urethanes) (PEUUs) or with diols to form poly(ether-urethanes) (PEUs). Secondary reactions can also lead to branching of the main chains. Thus, PUs are modular polymers with physical properties that can be controlled by varying the molecular weights, compositions, and relative amounts of the original diol, the diisocyanate, and the chain extenders in order to best match the demands of the end-use application. One example of this principle is the use of PUs as the rate-controlling membrane for water permeation into the osmotic LHRH delivery system, called the Duros® implant of Alza Corp. Potential *in vivo* oxidative degradation of the ether groups in the soft, R segment in polyurethanes have been a major issue with their use as pacemaker leads. Silicones have been incorporated into polyurethanes to impart better surface resistance to degradation [8,54–59].

2.3.7 DEGRADABLE POLYESTERS

There is a family of degradable polyesters that are synthesized by ring-opening polymerization of cyclic lactones. The polyesters in this family that have achieved success in the clinic as degradable sutures and drug delivery matrices are copolymers of lactide and glycolide, also known as lactic-acid–glycolic-acid copolymers (Figure 2.5) or PLGA. Each of the homopolymers is crystalline and degrades relatively slowly, but the copolymers tend to have less crystallinity, and thus they degrade more rapidly. One composition used in drug delivery microparticles is prepared from a 50:50 mixture of lactide and glycolide, but other ratios have been used, especially in sutures, where the strength of the suture and its retention during the early time period of wound healing is a more important factor than degradation rate. The half-life of such a degradable polyester can be length-ened by adding a more hydrophobic comonomer, such as poly(caprolactone) PCL (Figure 2.5), which slows down the degradation rate by its lower water uptake. This component is not yet approved for clinical use by the U.S. Food and Drug Administration (FDA). The PLGA family of copolymers is another good example of how the composition of the polymeric biomaterial can be tailored to the end use. Degradable polymers have uses that range from sutures to drug delivery, surgical sealants and antiadhesive coatings, and tissue-engineering scaffolds [63–79].

REFERENCES

1. Ratner, B.D., Hoffman, A.S., Schoen, F.J., and Lemons, J.E., Eds., *Biomaterials Science*, 2nd ed., Elsevier/Academic Press, New York, 2004.
2. Cooper, S.L., Visser, S.A., Hergenrother, R.W., and Lamba, N.M.K., Polymer, in *Biomaterials Science*, 2nd ed., Ratner, B.D., Hoffman, A.S., Schoen, F.J., and Lemons, J.E., Eds., Elsevier/Academic Press, New York, 2004, p. 67, chap. 2.2.
3. Billmeyer, F.W., Jr., *Textbook of Polymer Science*, 3rd ed., Wiley-Interscience, New York, 1984.
4. Rodriquez, F., *Principles of Polymer Systems*, 4th ed., Hemisphere, New York, 1996.
5. Colas, A. and Curtis, J., Silicone biomaterials: history and chemistry, in *Biomaterials Science*, 2nd ed., Ratner, B.D., Hoffman, A.S., Schoen, F.J., and Lemons, J.E., Eds., Elsevier/Academic Press, New York, 2004, p. 80, chap. 2.3.
6 Curtis, J. and Colas, A., Medical applications of silicones, in *Biomaterials Science*, 2nd ed., Ratner, B.D., Hoffman, A.S., Schoen, F.J., and Lemons, J.E., Eds., Elsevier/Academic Press, New York, 2004, p. 698, chap. 7.19.
7. Smith, A.L., Introduction to silicones, *The Analytical Chemistry of Silicones*, John Wiley & Sons, New York, 1991.
8. Ward, R.S., Thermoplastic silicone-urethane copolymers: a new class of biomedical elastomers, *Medical Device and Diagnostic Industry Magazine*, April 2000.
9. Swanson, J.W. and LeBeau, J.E., The effect of implantation on the physical properties of silicone rubber, *J. Biomed. Mater. Res.*, 8, 357, 1974.
10. Herdman, R.C. and Fahey, T.J., Silicone breast implants and cancer, *Cancer Invest.*, 19(8), 821, 2001.
11. McHenry, M.M., Smeloff, E.A., Fong, W.Y., Miller, G.E., and Ryan, P.M. Critical obstruction of prosthetic heart valves due to lipid absorption by Silastic, *J. Thorac. Cardiovasc. Surg.*, 59(3), 413, 1970.

12. Carmen, R. and Mutha S.C., Lipid absorption by silicone rubber heart valve poppets — *in vivo* and *in vitro* results, *J. Biomed. Mater. Res.*, 6, 327, 1972.

13. Swanson, A.B., Silicone rubber implants for replacement of arthritic or destroyed joints in the hand, *Surg. Clin. N. Am.*, 48, 1113, 1968.

14. Hall, C.W., Liotta, D., Ghidoni, J.J., DeBakey, M.E., and Dressler, D.P., Velour fabrics applied to medicine, *J. Biomed. Mater. Res.*, 1, 179–196, 1967.

15. Hoffman, A.S., Medical application of polymeric fibers, *J. Appl. Polym. Sci., Appl. Polym. Symp.*, 31, 313, 1977.

16. Shalaby, S.W., Fibrous materials for biomedical applications, in *High Technology Fibers*, Part A, Lewin, M. and Preson, J., Eds., Marcel Dekker, New York, 1985.

17. King, M.W., Designing fabrics for blood vessel replacement, *Can. Text. J.*, 108(4), 24–30, 1991.

18. Shalaby, S.W., Fabrics, in *Biomaterials Science*, 1st ed., Ratner, B.D., Hoffman, A.S., Schoen, F.J., and Lemons, J.E., Eds., Academic Press, Boston, MA, 1996, pp. 118–124, chap. 2.10.

19. Padera, R.F. Jr. and Schoen, F.J., Cardiovasuclar medical devices, in *Biomaterials Science*, 2nd ed., Ratner, B.D., Hoffman, A.S., Schoen, F.J., and Lemons, J.E., Eds., Elsevier/Academic Press, New York, 2004, p. 470, chap. 7.3.

20. Weinberg, S. and King, M.W., Medical fibers and biotextiles, in *Biomaterials Science*, 2nd ed., Ratner, B.D., Hoffman, A.S., Schoen, F.J., and Lemons, J.E., Eds., Elsevier/Academic Press, New York, 2004, p. 86, chap. 2.4.

21. Charnley, J., *Low Friction Arthroplasty of the Hip, Theory and Practice*, Springer-Verlag, Berlin, 1979.

22. Hallab, N.J., Jacobs, J.J., and Katz, J.L., Orthopedic applications, in *Biomaterials Science*, 2nd ed., Ratner, B.D., Hoffman, A.S., Schoen, F.J., and Lemons, J.E., Eds., Elsevier/Academic Press, New York, 2004, p. 527, chap 7.7.

23. Jacobs, J.J., Shanbhag, A., Glant, T.T., Black, J., and Galante, J.O., Wear debris in total joints, *J. Am. Acad. Orthopaed. Surg.*, 2, 212–220, 1994.

24. McKellop, H., Shen, F.W., Lu, B., Campbell, P., and Salovey, R., Effect of sterilization method and other modifications on the wear resistance of acetabular cups made of ultra-high molecular weight polyethylene. A hip-simulator study, *J. Bone Joint Surg. Am.*, 82-A, 1708–1725, 2000.

25. Jansen, J.A., Von Recum, A.F., Textured and porous materials, in *Biomaterials Science*, 2nd ed., Ratner, B.D., Hoffman, A.S., Schoen, F.J., and Lemons, J.E., Eds., Elsevier/Academic Press, New York, 2004, p. 218, chap. 2.15.

26. Wagner, W.R., Borovetz, H.S., and Griffith, B.P., Implantable cardiac assist devices, in *Biomaterials Science*, 2nd ed., Ratner, B.D., Hoffman, A.S., Schoen, F.J., and Lemons, J.E., Eds., Elsevier/Academic Press, New York, 2004, p. 494, chap. 7.4.

27. Ridley, H., Intra-ocular acrylic lenses, *Trans. Ophthalmol. Soc. U.K.*, 71, 617–621, 1951.

28. Patel, A.S., Intraocular lens implants: a scientific perspective, in *Biomaterials Science*, 2nd ed., Ratner, B.D., Hoffman, A.S., Schoen, F.J., and Lemons, J.E., Eds., Elsevier/Academic Press, New York, 2004, p. 592, chap. 7.11

29. Refojo, M.F., Ophthalmalogical applications, in *Biomaterials Science*, 2nd ed., Ratner, B.D., Hoffman, A.S., Schoen, F.J., and Lemons, J.E., Eds., Elsevier/Academic Press, New York, 2004, p. 584, chap. 7.10.

30. Charnley, J., The bonding of prosthesis to bone by cement, *J. Bone Joint Surg. Br.*, 46, 518, 1964.

31. Charnley, J., *Acrylic Cement in Orthopedic Surgery*, E.S. Livingstone, Edinburgh, 1970.

32. Smith, D.C., Adhesives and sealants, in *Biomaterials Science*, 2nd ed., Ratner, B.D., Hoffman, A.S., Schoen, F.J., and Lemons, J.E., Eds., Elsevier/Academic Press, New York, 2004, p. 573, chap. 7.9.

33. Wichterle, O. and Lim, D., Hydrophilic gels for biological use, *Nature*, 185, 117–118, 1960.

34. Hoffman, A.S., Intelligent polymers, in *Controlled Drug Delivery*, Park, K., Ed., ACS Publications, ACS, Washington, D.C., 1997.

35. Hoffman, A.S., Applications of smart polymers as biomaterials, in *Biomaterials Science*, 2nd ed., Ratner, B.D., Hoffman, A.S., Schoen, F.J., and Lemons, J.E., Eds., Elsevier/Academic Press, New York, 2004, p. 107, chap. 2.6.

36. Ratner, B.D. and Hoffman, A.S., Synthetic hydrogels for biomedical applications, in *Hydrogels for Medical and Related Applications*, Andrade, J.D., Ed., Vol. 31, ACS Symposium Series, American Chemical Society, Washington, D.C., 1976, pp. 1–36.

37. Korsmeyer, R.W. and Peppas, N.A., Effects of the morphology of hydrophilic polymeric matrices on the diffusion and release of water soluble drugs, *J. Membrane Sci.*, 9, 211–227, 1981.

38. Hoffman, A.S., Applications of thermally reversible polymers and hydrogels in therapeutics and diagnostics, *J. Controlled Release*, 6, 297–305, 1987.

39. Okano, T., Bae, Y.H., Jacobs, H., and Kim, S.W., Thermally on-off switching polymers for drug permeation and release, *J. Controlled Release*, 11, 255–265, 1990.

40. Dong, L.C. and Hoffman, A.S., A novel approach for preparation of pH-sensitive hydrogels for enteric drug delivery, *J. Controlled Release*, 15, 141–152, 1991.

41. Kim, S.W., Temperature-sensitive polymers for delivery of macromolecular drugs, in *Advanced Biomaterials in Biomedical Engineering and Drug Delivery Systems*, Ogata, N., Kim, S.W., Feijen, J., and Okano, T., Eds., Springer-Verlag, Tokyo, 1996, pp. 125–133.

42. Peppas, N.A., Hydrogels and drug delivery, *Crit. Opin. Colloid Interface Sci.*, 2, 531–537, 1997.

43. Peppas, N.A., Gels for drug delivery, in *Encyclopedia of Materials: Science and Technology*, Elsevier, New York, 2001, pp. 3492–3495.

44. Peppas, N.A., Huang, Y., Torres-Lugo, M., Ward, J.H., and Zhang, J., Physicochemical foundations and structural design of hydrogels in medicine and biology, *Annu. Rev. Biomed. Eng.*, 2, 9–29, 2000.

45. Hoffman, A.S. et al., Really smart bioconjugates of smart polymers and receptor proteins, *J. Biomed. Mater. Res.*, 52, 577–586, 2000.

46. Okano, T., Kikuchi, A., and Yamato, M., Intelligent hydrogels and new biomedical applications, in *Biomaterials and Drug Delivery toward the New Millennium*, Han Rim Won Publishing, Seoul, Korea, 2000, pp. 77–86.

47. Alleyne, C.H. Jr., Cawley, C.M., Barrow, D.L., Poff, B.C., Powell, M.D., Sawhncy, A.S., and Dellehay, D.L., Efficacy and biocompatibility of a photo-polymerized synthetic, absorbable hydrogel as a dural sealant in a canine craniotomy model, *J. Neurosurg.*, 88, 308–313, 1998.

48. Michaels, A.S., Operating parameters and performance criteria for hemodialyzers and other membrane separation devices, *Trans. Am. Soc. Artif. Intern. Organs*, 12, 387, 1966.

49. Henderson, L.W., Historical overview and principles of hemofiltration, *Dialysis Transpl.*, 9, 220, 1980.

50. Malchesky, P.S. and Nosé, Y., Control in plasmapheresis, in *Control Aspects of Biomedical Engineering*, Nalecz, M., Ed., *Int. Fed. Automatic Control*, Pergamon Press, Oxford, 1987, pp. 111–122.

51. Sueoka, A., Applications of membrane technologies for therapeutic apheresis, *Ther. Apheresis*, 2, 252, 1998.

52. Malchesky, P.S., Membrane processes for plasma separation and plasma filtration: guiding principles for clinical use, *Ther. Apheresis*, 5, 270–282, 2001.

53. Malchesky, P.S., Extracorporeal artificial organs, in *Biomaterials Science*, 2nd ed., Ratner, B.D., Hoffman, A.S., Schoen, F.J., and Lemons, J.E., Eds., Elsevier/Academic Press, New York, 2004, p. 514, chap. 7.6.

54. Padera, R.F. Jr., and Schoen, F.J., Cardiovascular medical devices, in *Biomaterials Science*, 2nd ed., Ratner, B.D., Hoffman, A.S., Schoen, F.J., and Lemons, J.E., Eds., Elsevier/Academic Press, New York, 2004, p. 470, chap. 7.3.

55. Wagner, W.R., Borovetz, H.S., and Griffith, B.P., Implantable cardiac assist devices, in *Biomaterials Science*, 2nd ed., Ratner, B.D., Hoffman, A.S., Schoen, F.J., and Lemons, J.E., Eds., Elsevier/Academic Press, New York, 2004, p. 494, chap. 7.4.

56. Stokes, K., Coury, A., and Urbanski, P., Autooxidative degradation of implanted polyether polyurethane devices, *J. Biomater. Appl.*, 1, 412–448, April 1987.

57. Stokes, K., Polyether polyurethanes: biostable or not? *J. Biomater. Appl.*, 3, 228–259, October 1988.

58. Ratner, B.D., Gladhill, K.W., and Horbett, T.A., Analysis of in vitro enzymatic and oxidative degradation of polyurethanes, *J. Biomed. Mater. Res.*, 22, 509–527, 1988.

59. Santerre, J.P., Labow, R.S., Duguay, D.G., Erfle, D., and Adams, G.A., Biodegradation evaluation of polyether- and polyester urethanes with oxidative and hydrolytic enzymes, *J. Biomed. Mater. Res.*, 28, 1187–1199, 1994.

60. Santerre, J.P., Meek, E., Tang, Y.W., and Labow, R.S., Use of fluorinated surface modifying macromolecules to inhibit the degradation of polycarbonate-urethanes by human macrophages, *Trans. 6th World Biomaterials Congress*, 77, 2000.

61. Takahara, A., Coury, A.J., Hergenrother, R.W., and Cooper, S.L., Effect of soft segment chemistry on the biostability of segmented polyurethanes, I. in vitro oxidation, *J. Biomed. Mater. Res.*, 25, 341–356, 1991.

62. Ward, R.S.,Thermoplastic silicone-urethane copolymers: a new class of biomedical elastomers, *Med. Dev. Diagnost. Ind.*, April, 2000.
63. Frazza, E.J. and Schmitt, E.E., A new absorbable suture, *J. Biomed. Mater. Res.*, 1, 43–58, 1971.
64. Williams, D.F., Review: biodegradation of surgical polymers, *J. Mater. Sci.*, 17, 1233–1246, 1982.
65. Kopecek, J. and Ulbrich, K., Biodegradation of biomedical polymers, *Prog. Polym. Sci.*, 9, 1–58, 1983.
66. Barrows, T.H., Degradable implant materials: a review of synthetic absorbable polymers and their applications, *Clin. Mater.*, 1, 233–257, 1986.
67. Ratner, B.D., Introduction: degradation of materials in the biological environment, in *Biomaterials Science*, 2nd ed., Ratner, B.D., Hoffman, A.S., Schoen, F.J., and Lemons, J.E., Eds., Elsevier/Academic Press, New York, 2004, p. 411, chap. 6.1.
68. Chu, C.C., Classification and general characteristics of suture materials, in *Wound Closure Biomaterials and Devices*, Chu, C.C., Von Fraunhofer, J., and Greisler, H.P., Eds., CRC Press, Boca Raton, FL, 1997, pp. 39–63, chap. 4.
69. Roby, M.S. and Kennedy, J., Sutures, in *Biomaterials Science*, 2nd ed., Ratner, B.D., Hoffman, A.S., Schoen, F.J., and Lemons, J.E., Eds., Elsevier/Academic Press, New York, 2004, p. 615, chap. 7.13.
70. Weinberg, S. and King, M.W., Medical fibers and biotextiles, in *Biomaterials Science*, 2nd ed., Ratner, B.D., Hoffman, A.S., Schoen, F.J., and Lemons, J.E., Eds., Elsevier/Academic Press, New York, 2004, p. 86, chap. 2.4.
71. Kohn, J., Abramson, S., and Langer, R., Bioresorbable and bioerodible materials, in *Biomaterials Science*, 2nd ed., Ratner, B.D., Hoffman, A.S., Schoen, F.J., and Lemons, J.E., Eds., Elsevier/Academic Press, New York, 2004, p. 115, chap. 2.7.
72. Coury, A.J., Chemical and biochemical degradation of polymers, in *Biomaterials Science*, 2nd ed., Ratner, B.D., Hoffman, A.S., Schoen, F.J., and Lemons, J.E., Eds., Elsevier/Academic Press, New York, 2004, p. 411, chap. 6.2.
73. Heller, J., Polymers for controlled parenteral delivery of peptides and proteins, *Adv. Drug Delivery Rev.*, 10, 163–204, 1993.
74. Heller, J. and Hoffman, A.S., Drug delivery systems, in *Biomaterials Science*, 2nd ed., Ratner, B.D., Hoffman, A.S., Schoen, F.J., and Lemons, J.E., Eds., Elsevier/Academic Press, New York, 2004, p. 629, chap. 7.14.
75. Jeong, B., Choi, Y.K., Bae, Y.H., Zentner, G., and Kim, S.W., New biodegradable polymers for injectable drug delivery systems, *J. Controlled Release*, 62, 109–114, 1999.
76. Jeong, B., Bae, Y.H., and Kim, S.W., Biodegradable thermosensitive micelles of PEG-PLGA-PEG triblock copolymers, *Colloids Surf. B: Interfaces*, 16, 185–193, 1999.
77. Sawhney, A.S., Pathak, C.P., and Hubbell, J.A., Bioerodible hydrogels based on photopolymerized poly(ethylene glycol)-co-poly(x-hydroxy acid) diacrylate macromers, *Macromolecules*, 26, 581–587, 1993.
78. Langer, R. and Vacanti, J.P., Tissue engineering, *Science*, 260, 920–926, 1993.
79. Mikos, A.G., Lu, L., Temenoff, J.S., Synthetic bioresorbable polymer scaffolds, in *Biomaterials Science*, 2nd ed., Ratner, B.D., Hoffman, A.S., Schoen, F.J., and Lemons, J.E., Eds., Elsevier/Academic Press, New York, 2004, p. 735, chap. 8.4.

3 Polymer Characterization Techniques

Wei Wang

CONTENTS

3.1 INTRODUCTION

For decades polymer materials have been used for the administration of pharmaceuticals, and they are now playing an increasingly important role in the fabrication of various controlled-release and drug-targeting systems. The use of a polymer for drug delivery is guided by its molecular and bulk properties. Molecular variables that control the function include: the nature of the monomers and monomer linkers, monomer sequence distribution along chains, the average molecular weight and molecular weight distribution, molecular conformation, and molecular architecture. For drug delivery systems, the important polymer bulk properties, which indeed derive from the polymer's molecular properties, are solubility, biocompatibility, biodegradability, and stability. In drug delivery, as in any application, it is essential that the materials are fit for the purpose. Nontoxicity and biocompatibility are crucial attributes for polymers chosen for biomedical applications as are the polymer's functional properties. In considering the polymer's functional properties, it is of utmost importance that adequate polymer characterization is available for materials selection.

There are many methods available for the characterization of macromolecules and polymer-based materials. The purpose of this chapter is to present an overview of the more common techniques that are used to characterize polymers and polymer-based materials. Wherever possible, the overview in this chapter is also illustrated with specific examples. It is impossible to cover every analytical technique available to the polymer analyst or even to cover selected techniques in specific detail. However, the reader is directed to the bibliography and references at the end of this chapter for more details of the various techniques highlighted.

3.2 MOLECULAR WEIGHT DETERMINATION

The average molecular weight (MW) is a fundamental characteristic of a polymer sample. Most properties of a polymer material are more or less related to its molecular weight. Molecular weight also essentially controls the function of biomedical polymers.

A pure polymer sample is composed of molecules differing only in the degree of polymerization (DP). There are various ways in which the molecular weight of a polymer may be defined: the number-averaged molecular weight (M_n), the weight-averaged molecular weight (M_w), the z-averaged molecular weight (M_z), and the viscosity-averaged molecular weight (M_v).

M_n is the average molecular weight on the basis of the number of molecules (N_i) in a particular weight class (M_i):

$$M_n = \Sigma N_i M_i / \Sigma N_i \tag{3.1}$$

An average on the basis of the weight fraction (W_i) of molecules in a particular weight class (M_i) is M_w:

$$M_w = \Sigma N_i M_i^2 / \Sigma N_i M_i \tag{3.2}$$

Mathematically, M_z is defined by

$$M_z = \Sigma N_i M_i^3 / \Sigma N_i M_i^2 \tag{3.3}$$

Finally, M_v is defined by the equation:

$$M_v = \{\Sigma N_i M_i^{1+\alpha} / \Sigma N_i M_i\}^{1/\alpha} \tag{3.4}$$

where α is a parameter in Mark–Houwink equation and a constant for a given polymer, solvent, and temperature. This constant is discussed further in Subsection 3.2.3.

The ratios of different average molecular weights are useful indicators of molecular weight distribution, and a parameter known as the *polydispersity index* (n) is expressed as:

$$n = M_w / M_n \tag{3.5}$$

For an idealized monodisperse polymer sample, the molecular weight averages are identical, i.e., $M_n = M_w = M_z = M_v$.

When the polymer is polydisperse, the following relation holds: $M_n < M_v \leq M_w < M_z$.

Various methods of determining polymer molecular weight are summarized in Table 3.1. In more common practice, light scattering (LS), gel permeation chromatography (GPC), gel permeation chromatography plus light scattering (GPC/LS), and viscometry are the techniques used. GPC/LS is especially useful as it may be performed quickly and gives results for M_n, M_z, M_w, and molecular size [1,2].

TABLE 3.1
Methods for the Determination of Polymer Molecular Weight

Methods	Measured Parameter	Molecular Weight Measured	Upper Limit (g mol^{-1})
End-group assay	Number of end groups in a known amount of polymer	M_n	2×10^4
Cryoscopy	Freezing point of dilute polymer solution	M_n	2×10^4
Ebulliometry	Boiling point of dilute polymer solution	M_n	2×10^4
Vapour-pressure osmometry	Temperature difference between drops of polymer solution and solvent in saturated solvent vapour	M_n	4×10^4
Membrane osmometry	Osmotic pressure of polymer solvent	M_n	5×10^4
Ultracentrifugation	Concentration of polymer after controlled centrifugation	M_w, M_z	1×10^7
Light scattering (LS)	Intensity of light scattered by dilute polymer solutions	M_w	1×10^8
Gel permeation chromatography (GPC)	Elution volume of the polymer solution through a GPC column packed with porous microparticles	M_n, M_w, M_z	1×10^8
GPC/LS	Elution volume of the polymer solution through a GPC column packed with porous microparticles and intensity of light scattered by dilute polymer solution	M_n, M_w, M_z	1×10^8
Viscometry	Flow time of polymer solution through a capillary	M_v	1×10^8

3.2.1 LIGHT SCATTERING

When a parallel beam of light passes through a transparent system, a small part of the light is scattered elastically (Rayleigh scattering). The scattering arises because of optical discontinuities in the medium. For solutions of polymer molecules, additional scattering arises from the presence of the solute molecules, and this may be shown to be a function of the concentration of the polymer molecules, as well as their size and shape. When measurements are made of the differences in intensity of the scattered light between the solvent and a series of dilute polymer solutions, then it is possible to determine the averaged size of polymer solutes and hence their molecular weights. The results of the measurement are usually expressed as the weight-average molecular weight. The theoretical basis of light scattering from polymer solutions was first established by Zimm in the 1940s [3]. The equation relating scattering of light to molecular weight is given as:

$$Kc/R_\theta = 1/M_w + 1/M_w(16\pi^2/3\lambda^2)\sin^2(\theta/2) <S^2>z + A_2c \qquad (3.6)$$

where c is the polymer concentration; R_θ, the Rayleigh ratio, i.e., the excess intensity of scattered light at the angle θ; λ, the wavelength of light; θ, π, the scattering angle; $<S>z$, the z-averaged mean radius of gyration, i.e., the molecular size in solution; and A_2, the second virial coefficient, which quantifies the interaction between the macromolecule and the solvent. K is given by the equation:

$$K = 2\pi^2 n^2 (dn/dc)^2/N_0 \lambda^4 \qquad (3.7)$$

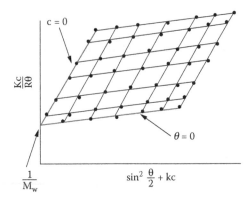

$c = 0$

$\dfrac{Kc}{R\theta}$

$\theta = 0$

$\dfrac{1}{M_w}$ $\sin^2 \dfrac{\theta}{2} + kc$

FIGURE 3.1 Schematic representation of a Zimm plot. M_w is obtained from the intercept on the y axis.

N_0 is Avogadro s number; n, the refractive index of the solvent, and dn/dc, the refractive index increment of the solute, i.e., the change in refractive index per unit change in polymer concentration (a constant for a polymer—solvent combination at a particular temperature).

In order to determine M_w, $<S>_z$, and A_2, the scattering intensities of various dilute polymer solutions of differing concentrations are determined at various scattering angles (typically from 35° to 150°). R_θ is then calculated and Kc/R_θ plotted against $(\sin^2(\theta/2) + kc)$, where k is an arbitrary constant chosen to produce a reasonable spread of data points. This plot is termed a *Zimm plot* (Figure 3.1). Using this method, M_w is obtained as the inverse of the value of the intercept (Kc/R_θ) as shown in Figure 3.1. From the Equation 3.6, $<S^2>_z$ and A_2 are estimated from the slopes of the $c = 0$ and $\theta = 0$ lines, respectively, as shown in Figure 3.1.

3.2.2 GEL PERMEATION CHROMATOGRAPHY

GPC or size exclusion chromatography (SEC) is a very convenient and simple way of measuring polymer molecular weights and the distribution of these values about their mean. The polymer solution is injected into a solvent stream that flows through one or more columns packed with highly porous microparticles, and polymer molecules are separated according to their size. The small molecules enter the deep pores, and their progress is retarded relative to the large molecules. Detection of the polymer mass in the eluent is accomplished using either a refractive index (RI) or ultraviolet absorption (UV) detector. The RI detector detects solutes based on the difference between the refractive index of the solution and the solvent, and the UV detector detects solutes based on their absorption of light of a particular wavelength. Before any molecular weight determination, the GPC system needs to be calibrated with a series of standard samples of known molecular weights and a very narrow molecular weight distribution ($M_w/M_n < 1.1$). Standard samples of polystyrene, poly(ethylene glycol), and dextran are usually used. It is necessary to mention that polymer molecules are separated by GPC according to their hydrodynamic volume, which is not only dependent on molecular weight but also on molecular conformation in solution. Calibration curves thus differ for different polymer types. This may be problematic if one is measuring the molecular weight of a new type of polymer that is structurally unrelated to the standards. Ideally, the test polymer samples should have the same hydrodynamic properties as the calibration standards.

GPC/LS is a particularly useful method of determining polymer molecular weight. In this method, a light-scattering detector is connected to a GPC system just prior to the connection of an RI detector (see Figure 3.2). By combining the outputs from both the detectors, absolute molecular weights can be obtained rapidly and independently of column calibration standards. At the same time, polymer molecular weight distribution and molecular size in solution can be determined.

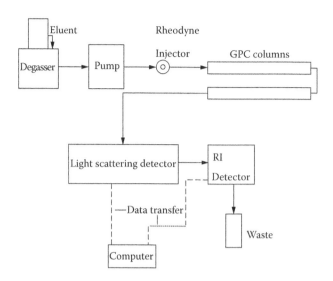

FIGURE 3.2 Schematic diagram of a gel permeation chromatography/light scattering setup for the measurement of polymer molecular weight.

For copolymers, polymer composition information can also be obtained if a UV, RI, and light-scattering detector are combined [4].

3.2.3 VISCOMETRY

Viscometry may also be used to determine polymer molecular weight. This method is based on the Mark–Houwink equation (Equation 3.8),

$$[\eta] = K\,M^{\alpha} \tag{3.8}$$

where K and α are constants for a particular polymer–solvent system and can be found by using a series of samples of known molecular weights and fitting the viscometry data to Equation 3.9.

$$\text{Log }[\eta] = \log K + \alpha \, \text{Log } M \tag{3.9}$$

where $[\eta]$ is known as the *intrinsic viscosity*, which is measured using a fairly simple Ubbelodhe viscometer. Experimentally, one would measure the flow time of the pure solvent (t_0) and the flow time (t) of several concentrations (c) of dilute polymer solutions, and use the resulting data to determine the polymer specific viscosity (η_{sp}) as given in the following text:

$$\eta_{sp} = (t - t_0)/t_0 \tag{3.10}$$

One would then proceed to plot η_{sp}/c *vs.* c to yield a straight line, the intercept of which would give $[\eta]$ according to Equation (3.11)

$$\eta_{sp}/c = [\eta] + k[\eta]^2\,c \tag{3.11}$$

where k is the Huggins constant and is dependent on the interaction between the polymer and solvent molecules. The molecular weight measured by viscometric methods (Equation 3.9) is termed the *viscosity-averaged molecular weight* (M_v) and has a magnitude between M_w and M_n, but is usually much closer to the M_w value [5].

3.3 VIBRATIONAL SPECTROSCOPY — INFRARED AND RAMAN SPECTROSCOPY

A molecule can undergo various modes of vibration, each often consisting of a complex mixture of bond stretches and deformations. At low temperatures, such a molecule will exist in its ground vibrational state and will be excited to a higher vibrational state if radiant energy is absorbed, which coincides with the energy difference (ΔE) between the excited and ground states of the molecule. ΔE is related to the frequency of radiation (μ) absorbed, and the relationship is described by Equation 3.12:

$$\Delta E = h\mu \tag{3.12}$$

where h is Planck's constant (6.626×10^{-27} erg sec). It is the detection of this absorbed energy that forms the basis of infrared (IR) spectroscopy. In practice, the spectral transitions are detected by scanning through the entire IR frequency while continuously monitoring the transmitted light intensity. The energies of molecular vibrations of interest for analytical work mostly correspond to wavelengths in the range 2.5 to 25 μm (or 400–4000 cm^{-1} in terms of wave number). The frequency and intensity of vibrations are sensitive to the chemical and physical structures, and so provide qualitative and quantitative means of characterizing the composition and geometry of the molecules and materials. Characterization using IR spectroscopy often results in the identification of the functional groups and the modes of their attachment to the polymer backbone, and in some cases the absorption spectrum constitutes a molecular fingerprint. Table 3.2 lists the absorption bands of some functional groups.

This method has been extensively applied to characterize the polymer's molecular and material structure. An example of its use is for the determination of the level of amine groups in chitosan. Chitosan is an increasingly interesting polysaccharide in the drug delivery field, and the amine content of chitosan is very important for various applications. The absorption band ratios of amide II at 1655 cm^{-1} to the hydroxyl group at 3450 cm^{-1}, i.e., A_{1655}/A_{3450}, has been used for amine content determination [6].

Raman spectroscopy is another useful vibrational spectroscopy tool that provides structural information by detecting the inelastic scattering of photons by molecules. The energy of the scattered photon is related to the vibrational energy of the molecule in the ground state.

TABLE 3.2
Absorption Wavelengths and Wave Numbers of Some Functional Groups

Group	Wavelength (μm)	Wave Number (cm^{-1})	Group	Wavelength (μm)	Wave Number (cm^{-1})
—OH	2.84–3.22	3520–3100	C=C	6.06–6.25	1650–1600
—NH	2.86–3.23	3500–3100	C≡N	4.17–4.76	2400–2100
≡CH	3.02–3.12	3310–3200	C=O	5.4–6.3	1850–1582
=CH$_2$	3.25	3080	C—O—C	7.9–8.3	1260–1200
=CH—	3.31	3020	C—F	7.4–8.3	1350–1200
Ar—H	3.24–3.33	3090–3000	C—Cl	13.7–15.9	730–630
—CH$_3$	3.36–3.39	3960	Si—O	8.1–9.8	1220–1020
—CH$_2$—	3.41–3.43	3920	Si—C	11.63–13.28	860–700
$\overset{\mid}{\underset{\mid}{-\text{CH}}}$	3.46	2890	Si—CH$_3$	7–9.4	1260
C≡C	4.4–4.7	2250–2150	Si—H	4.46	2240

Vibrational spectroscopy techniques are relatively simple, nondestructive, and versatile, and they may be used to analyze films, powders, and solutions [7,8]. In addition to structural information, IR and Raman spectra may be used to study polymer crystallinity, macromolecular orientation, and average molecular weight. Average molecular weight is measured by quantifying the end groups.

3.4 NUCLEAR MAGNETIC RESONANCE SPECTROSCOPY

NMR is a most powerful tool for the study of the microstructure and chain configuration of polymers, both in solution and in the solid state. The importance of NMR as a technique stems from the fact that the NMR signals can be assigned to specific atoms along the polymer backbone and side chains. The identification of certain atoms or groups in a polymer molecule as well as their positions relative to each other can be obtained by one-, two- and three-dimensional NMR spectra [1,8,9].

The NMR technique utilizes the property of spin possessed by nuclei such as ^{1}H, ^{13}C, ^{15}N, ^{17}O, and ^{19}F. When a strong external magnetic field (the strength H_0 is at least 10,000 G) is applied to material containing such nuclei, they behave like bar magnets and can orientate themselves in two energy states, a low-energy state, in which the alignment is parallel to the field, and a high-energy state, in which the alignment is opposed to the field. The transition of a nucleus from one energy state to another occurs if a discrete amount of energy is absorbed from an electromagnetic radiation whose frequency is v, such that:

$$E = hv = 2\mu H_0 \tag{3.13}$$

where μ is magnetic moment of the nucleus, and h is Planck's constant. For ^{1}H in a magnetic field of 14,000 G, the frequency v of such energy is 60 MHz. NMR is thus a form of absorption spectroscopy. It measures the absorption intensity of a peak on the scale of radiation frequency or magnetic field strength.

If the resonance frequency for all nuclei of the same type in a molecule were identical, only one line or peak would be observed; for example, the protons of a methyl group would resonate at the same frequency as those in an aromatic ring. Thankfully, this is not the case, and subtle differences in NMR frequencies are observed because of the differing molecular environments of the nuclei. Surrounding electrons shield the nuclei to different extents, depending on the chemical nature of such surrounding chemical groups or atoms. These changes or displacements in the resonance are called *chemical shifts*. They are measured in parts per million (ppm) at a particular frequency (or the equivalent field strength) on a scale labeled δ. Chemically inert material, mostly tetramethylsilane (TMS), is used as a chemical-shift standard reference, and its chemical-shift position is assigned a value 0. Typically, for ^{1}H nuclei, a range of 10 ppm can cover most polymer molecules. The corresponding range for ^{13}C nuclei is much greater, i.e., up to about 600 ppm.

^{1}H NMR spectral information for a cetyl poly(ethylenimine) [10] best illustrates the utility of this technique (Figure 3.3).

3.5 MICROSCOPY

Microscopy is a major tool for the characterization of polymer material ultrastructure. In the field of drug delivery, microscopical examinations enable an understanding of a number of variables that govern delivery. Such imaging techniques may be used to examine the detailed shape, size, and distribution of polymeric micro- and nanoparticles, as well as their interactions with biological environments. There are a variety of microscopy techniques available, and these include traditional optical microscopy, scanning electron microscopy (SEM) and transmission electron microscopy (TEM) [8], and scanning probe microscopy (SPM) [11].

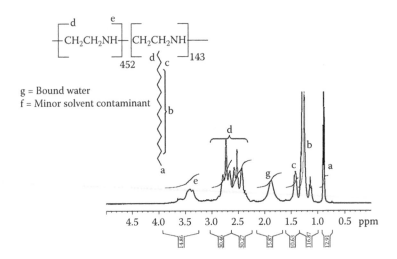

FIGURE 3.3 ¹H NMR of cetyl poly(ethylenimine). (From Wang, W., Qu, X., Gray, A.I., Tetley, L., and Uchegbu, I.F., *Macromolecules*, 37, 9114–9122, 2004.)

3.5.1 OPTICAL MICROSCOPY

Optical microscopy provides microstructural information with a resolution on the order of 1 μm. Imaging is carried out using both reflected and transmitted light. If the absorption coefficient varies regionally within a sample, when a beam of light travels through such a sample, contrasting regions of intensity will be obtained in the final image. For a specimen that can be prepared as a thin film, for instance, by casting on the microscope slide, examination using transmitted light is most useful, but little detail can be observed without some type of contrast enhancement. Two common techniques available to achieve contrast are polarized-light microscopy and phase-contrast microscopy. The former exploits the ability of crystalline materials to rotate the plane of polarized light; thus, structural information may be obtained using crossed polarizers. For example, the melting point of a crystal may be obtained by observing the sample on a heated stage and noting the temperature at which the last trace of crystallinity disappears. The structure of polymer liquid crystals may also be studied using polarizing microscopy. Reflected-light microscopy is useful for examining the topographical features of solid polymer materials.

Other more specialized techniques exist for the optical microscopy examination and study of polymeric biomaterials, such as confocal laser scanning microscopy, infrared microscopy, fluorescence microscopy, and Raman microscopy.

3.5.2 TRANSMISSION ELECTRON MICROSCOPY

Transmission electron microscopy (TEM) involves transmitting a beam of electrons instead of light through a sample in a high-vacuum environment. The images and associated contrasts arise from regional differences in electron densities. TEM has a resolution of about 1 to 100 nm, and it can thus provide very detailed structural information on polymeric materials, even down to the molecular level. The TEM specimen needs to be very thin in order to transmit electron beams through the sample. Normally, the specimens are placed on copper grids or carbon-coated copper grids and viewed through the holes in the grid. Techniques such as replication, heavy-metal staining, and solvent etching are widely used to increase image contrast. An example of polymeric bilayer vesicles stained with methylamine tungstate [12] is shown in Figure 3.4. The unstained white peripheries

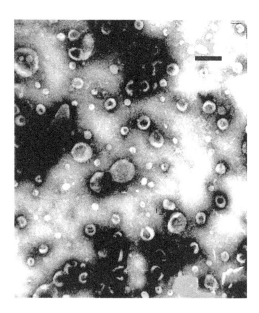

FIGURE 3.4 Transmission electron micrographs of palmitoyl glycol chitosan vesicles. Vesicles were prepared by the probe sonication of palmitoyl glycol chitosan (8 mg) and cholesterol (4 mg) in water (4 ml). (From Wang, W., McConaghy, A.M., Tetley, L., and Uchegbu, I.F., *Langmuir*, 17, 631–636, 2001.)

of the vesicles are clearly seen. In this case, vesicles were prepared by probe sonication of palmitoyl glycol chitosan (8 mg) and cholesterol (4 mg) in water (4 ml).

A further advantage of TEM is that it can be rapidly adjusted to provide an electron diffraction pattern from a selected area, facilitating the investigation of crystal structure and orientation and enabling particular morphological features to be identified.

3.5.3 SCANNING ELECTRON MICROSCOPY

Scanning electron microscopy (SEM) is another very valuable electron microscopy technique with a resolution of about 5 nm. In SEM, a fine beam of electrons is scanned across the surface of an opaque specimen, and an appropriate detector collects the electrons emitted from each point. In this way, an image having a great depth of field and a remarkable three-dimensional appearance is built up line by line. To produce stable images, the specimen is usually coated with a conducting film prior to examination. In most cases, a gold or gold–palladium alloy is used to coat the surface either by evaporation or by sputtering. The typical film thickness is about 20 nm. Another advantage of coating is that coating materials can give a high secondary electron yield and thus increase image contrast.

3.5.4 SCANNING PROBE MICROSCOPY

The term scanning probe is employed because when a probe tip is brought very close to a surface, the physical phenomenon, such as the interaction force between the tip and surface for AFM and the weak electrical current flowing between tip and sample for STM, may be exploited to produce a three-dimensional topographical image of the surface. The resolution is at the nanometer level. The most popular scanning probe microscopy (SPM) techniques include scanning tunneling microscopy (STM) and atomic force microscopy (AFM). AFM is a particularly popular technique and operates by measuring attractive or repulsive forces between a tip and the sample surface, and unlike electron microscopy, AFM can image samples both in air and in liquids [11].

3.6 THERMAL ANALYSIS

This is a group of techniques in which some structure-dependent physical properties of the polymer are measured as a function of temperature or time, while a polymer is subjected to a controlled temperature program. The most common techniques are differential scanning calorimetry (DSC), thermal gravimetry (TG), and dynamic mechanical analysis (DMA) [13]. These techniques can be used to identify and characterize both polymers and drug-loaded polymeric delivery systems.

3.6.1 DIFFERENTIAL SCANNING CALORIMETRY

Whenever a polymer undergoes a phase transition such as melting or a glass transition from the rigid "glass state" to the soft "rubber state," the temperature tends to remain constant while energy is taken into the system. Differential scanning calorimetry (DSC) is essentially a technique that compares the differences between the energy acquired or released by a sample and a suitable reference as a function of temperature or time while the sample and reference are subject to a controlled temperature rise. DSC is useful for recording thermal transitions such as the glass transition temperature T_g, melt temperature T_m, and degradation or decomposition temperature T_D. DSC may also be used to characterize the liquid crystal state of organization and other forms of self-assembly. For example, Figure 3.5 gives DSC data on some polymeric cetyl poly(ethylenimine) self-assemblies. Cetyl poly(ethylenimines) with 3 mol% cetylation (curve 1) and 49 mol% cetylation (curve 6) do not form vesicular self-assemblies and a thermal-gel-to-liquid-crystalline-phase transition is thus not seen at 33 to 40°C. However, polymers with between 18 and 49 mol% cetylation (curve 2 to curve 5) do form unilamellar bilayer vesicle assemblies and a gel-to-liquid phase transition is seen in their DSC curves at 33 to 40°C [14].

3.6.2 THERMAL GRAVIMETRY

This method is used to measure the change in weight of a polymer sample while it is heated, using a sensitive balance. Such a weight change would indicate a physical or chemical change in the material and is used for the characterization of drug-containing polymeric materials.

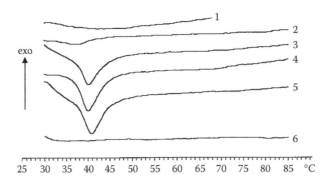

FIGURE 3.5 Differential scanning calorimetry plots from samples of self-assembled cetylated poly(ethylenimines). Curve 1 — 3 mol% cetylation, curve 2 — 18 mol% cetylation, curve 3 — 33 mol% cetylation, curve 4 — 24 mol% cetylation, curve 5 — 37 mol% cetylation, and curve 6 — 49 mol% cetylation.

3.6.3 DYNAMIC MECHANICAL ANALYSIS

In this technique, the properties of a polymer are studied as it goes through a time-dependent mechanical change. This analytical technique is able to give important information on polymer relaxation processes and phase morphologies. It is a useful method for identifying segmental and side-chain motion within a chain and can also be used to study copolymers and polymer blends.

3.7 X-RAY DIFFRACTION METHODS

X-ray diffraction is a useful method for investigating the arrangements of atoms or molecules within a material. If there is an orderly arrangement of substructures within a material with repeat distances of a similar magnitude to the wavelength of light used (0.05–0.25 nm), interference patterns are produced, and such patterns provide information on the geometry of the polymer structures. Two primary diffraction methods are used to study polymers, i.e., wide-angle x-ray scattering (WAXS) and small-angle x-ray scattering (SAXS). WAXS (5° to 120°) is useful for studying the semicrystalline polymers with a range of interatomic distances of 0.1 to 5 nm. From the measurement of relative intensities of diffraction peaks in the crystalline part and the diffusion halo from the amorphous part, the crystalline content of the polymer may be obtained. WAXS can also be used to get information on helical polymers, such as the number of repeat units per turn in helical structures of linear polymers and the length of the repeat unit along the fiber axis. The value of the angles used in SAXS is from 1° to 5°. SAXS is useful in detecting large periodicities from 5 to 70 nm in a structure such as lamellae or the distribution of particles or voids in the materials [15].

3.8 MECHANICAL AND RHEOLOGICAL ANALYSES

The mechanical and rheological properties of polymers are a reflection of the polymers' molecular (molecular weight, molecular weight distribution, conformation, architecture, and crystallinity) properties. An assessment of a polymer's mechanical and rheological properties is often carried out in order to establish if the polymer is fit for the purpose [8].

The tensile properties of solid polymers can be characterized by their deformation behavior, which is obtained by measuring stress–strain responses. Rubbery polymers are soft and reversibly extensible and exhibit a lower modulus or stiffness. Glass and semicrystalline polymers have higher moduli and lower extensibility. If network structures are achieved from the cross-linking of polymers, large-scale movement or flow is prevented, because the freedom of motion of the polymer chain is restricted [13].

Rheological testing is used to obtain information related to the flow behavior of polymer melts and polymer solutions. Capillary and rotational rheometers are available to study the viscosity and viscoelasticity of polymers. Polymer fluids are non-Newtonian in behavior, mostly being shear-thinning or pseudoplastic (a reversible decrease in viscosity with increasing shear rate). Viscoelasticity is a unique property of certain polymers, which display both viscous- and elastic-type behavior at ordinary temperatures and loading rates. The extent of each component mainly depends on the structure and morphology of polymer molecules. Rheological characterization is a very useful way of assessing hydrogels. Hydrogels are either chemically or physically cross-linked water-soluble polymers with a network-type structure, and these materials swell in water without dissolving. Figure 3.6 is a dynamic mechanical characterization of a cross-linked hyaluronan injectable hydrogel showing that elastic modulus G′, viscous modulus G″, and phase angle δ are very weakly dependent on frequency. G′ is much higher than G″, and both are almost parallel to each other because of the strong covalently cross-linked network structure [16].

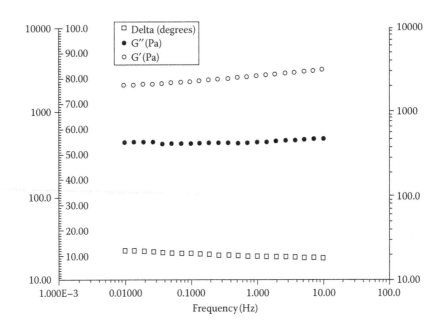

FIGURE 3.6 Dynamic mechanical properties of injectable hyaluronan hydrogel.

REFERENCES

1. Young, R.J. and Lovell, P.A., *Introduction to Polymers,* 2nd ed., London: Chapman and Hall, 1991.
2. Fried, J.R., *Polymer Science and Technology,* Upper Saddle River, NJ: Prentice Hall, 1995.
3. Zimm, B.H., The scattering of light and the radial distribution function of high polymer solutions, *J. Chem. Phys.,* 16(12), 1093–1099, 1948; Apparatus and methods for measurement and interpretation of the angular variation of light scattering: preliminary results on polystyrene solutions, *J. Chem. Phys.,* 16(12), 1099–1116, 1948.
4. Harald, P. and Trathnig, B., *HPLC of Polymers,* Berlin: Springer-Verlag, 1998.
5. Tompa, H., *Polymer Solutions,* London: Butterworths, 1956.
6. Baxter, A., Dilllon, M., Taylor, K.D.A., and Roberts, G.A.F., Improved method for I.R determination of the degree of N-acetylation of chitosan, *Int. J. Biol. Macromol.,* 14, 166–169, 1992.
7. Siesler, H.W. and Holland-Moritz, K., *Infrared and Raman Spectroscopy of Polymers,* New York: Marcel Dekker, 1980.
8. Hunt, B.J. and James, M.I., *Polymer Characterisation,* Glasgow, London: Blackie Academic and Professional, 1993.
9. Kotayama, T. and Hatada, K., *NMR Spectroscopy of Polymer,* Berlin: Springer-Verlag, 2004.
10. Wang, W., Qu, X., Gray, A.I., Tetley, L., and Uchegbu, I.F., Self-assembly of cetyl linear polyethylenimine to give micelles, vesicles and nanoparticles is controlled by the hydrophobicity of the polymer, *Macromolecules,* 37, 9114–9122, 2004.
11. James, D.B., Chris, A.M., and Gilbert, C.W., *Applications of Scanned Probe Microscopy to Polymers,* Oxford: Oxford University Press, 2005.
12. Wang, W., McConaghy, A.M., Tetley, L., and Uchegbu, I.F., Controls on polymer molecular weight may be used to control the size of palmitoyl glycol chitosan polymeric vesicles, *Langmuir,* 17, 631–636, 2001.
13. Mark, J., Ngai, K., Graessley, W., Mandelkern, L., Samulski, E., Koenig, J., and Wignall, G., *Physical Properties of Polymers,* 3rd ed., Cambridge: Cambridge University Press, 2004.
14. Wang, W. and Uchegbu, I.F., Unpublished work.
15. Alexander, L.E., *X-Ray Diffraction Methods in Polymer Science,* New York: John Wiley & Sons, 1970.
16. Osada, Y. and Khokhlov, A.R., *Polymer Gels and Network,* New York: Marcel Dekker, 2002.

4 The Role of Polymers in Solid Oral Dosage Forms

Richard A. Kendall and Abdul W. Basit

CONTENTS

4.1 INTRODUCTION

Despite increasing research into alternative routes and methods of drug delivery, the oral route remains the most popular one, accounting for 70% of all forms of drug therapy. The reasons for this are readily apparent — the oral route, being the most convenient and acceptable one to the patient, improves compliance. Furthermore, owing to the well-established manufacturing methods used to produce solid oral dosage forms (e.g., tablets and capsules), such dosage forms are cheaper to produce, making them the most cost-effective choice, in light of the importance of reducing overall prescribing costs, for prescribers and healthcare providers.

Solid oral dosage forms can be divided into two main categories: immediate-release dosage forms, where disintegration and subsequent drug release and dissolution occurs in the stomach, and the (non-immediate) modified-release technologies, which utilize polymers to alter the site or time of drug release within the gastrointestinal tract.

The need for modified-release technologies arose from an understanding that disintegration of a dosage form in the stomach, resulting in immediate release of drug, is not always desirable. In recent years there has been an increasing tendency to deliver drug entities as modified-release formulations, and although it can be appreciated that the unit cost of a modified-release formulation will be greater than the equivalent immediate-release variety, the former version may confer a reduction in overall healthcare costs. This may be in terms of a reduction in the number of doses to be taken to achieve the desired therapeutic effect, therefore reducing overall medication costs, or the subsequent improvement in compliance, negating the implications of ineffective therapy, or the need for further medication needed to treat drug-induced side effects of the original treatment.

4.2 FATE OF DOSAGE FORMS IN THE GASTROINTESTINAL TRACT

It is necessary to describe the structure and physiology of the gastrointestinal tract (see Figure 4.1 and Table 4.1) in order to understand the *in vivo* fate of dosage forms. The major functions of the gastrointestinal tract are to break down ingested food into nutrients, which are absorbed into the systemic circulation, and to eliminate waste products. An oral dosage form will be subjected to the same physiological processes of secretion, motility, digestion, absorption, and excretion that food-stuffs are. Once swallowed, with an adequate volume of water, conventional immediate-release dosage forms will leave the oral cavity and rapidly pass along the esophagus into the stomach, where disintegration of the dosage form will occur within minutes. The released drug will then dissolve in the liquid contents, and the drug solution will pass directly into the small intestine, the optimal site for the absorption of most drugs into the systemic circulation. Absorption is normally complete from the small intestine, although on some occasions drug enters the large intestine where absorption of certain drugs is possible [1]. In contrast, modified-release dosage forms are generally formulated to move through some portion, or the entirety, of the gastrointestinal tract intact. Transit is then dictated by whether the dosage form is single-unit (tablet or capsule) or multiple-unit (pellets or granules, approximately 1 mm in diameter) in design.

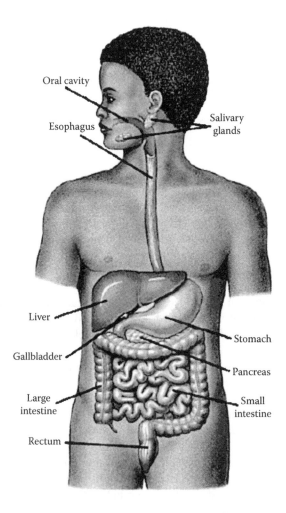

FIGURE 4.1 Anatomy of the human gastrointestinal tract. (Adapted from Martini, F.H., *Fundamentals of Anatomy and Physiology* (5th ed.), Prentice Hall, NJ, 2002, p. 847.)

TABLE 4.1
Physiology of the Human Gastrointestinal Tract

Region	Length (m)	Surface Area (m²)	pH	Bacterial Count (cfu/ml)	Residence Time (h)
Stomach	0.20	0.10	1.0–2.5	10^2	0–2 h (fasted)
					Highly variable (fed)
Small intestine					3–5 h
Duodenum	0.25	1.9	5.5–6.0	10^2	
Jejenum	2.80	184	6.0–7.0	10^5	
Ileum	4.20	276	7.0–7.5	10^7	
Large intestine					Variable, in the range
Cecum	0.20	0.05	6.4–7.0	10^8	20–30 h
Colon	1.50	0.25	7.0–7.5	10^{12}	

The transit of modified-release dosage forms has been largely elucidated thanks to imaging techniques, in particular, gamma scintigraphy. Gamma scintigraphy involves the radiolabeling of a dosage form with a short-lived radionuclide and the subsequent location of its position in the gastrointestinal tract by using a gamma camera at regular time points. Although the technique provides no anatomical detail, the dosage form can be visualized leaving the stomach, arriving at the colon, and the disintegration and dispersal followed [2–4].

Gastric emptying of single-unit and multiple-unit modified-release dosage forms is markedly different and highly influenced by whether the dosage form is administered before or after food. In the fasted state, the contractile activity of the stomach is characterized by the migrating myoelectric complex (MMC), which are cycles of contractions that can be divided into four phases, repeating every 2 h. The gastric emptying of modified-release dosage forms from the fasted stomach is directly related to the timing of administration relative to the MMC. Large single-unit dosage forms can only empty during phase III contractions (intense contractions designed to empty the stomach of indigestible debris). Pellets may empty more rapidly during the less intense contractions of the MMC.

If administered after food, single-unit modified-release dosage forms will not empty until after all the food has been broken down to particles of a size small enough to empty through the pylorus, the stomach has returned to fasted state activity, and phase III MMC contractions have recommenced. Owing to their smaller size, pellets have been shown to empty with the food, and hence they empty more rapidly from the stomach in the fed state, generally after a slight lag time, progressively emptying through the pylorus with digestible material [5].

Post-gastric-emptying, single-unit systems generally move through the small intestine intact, whereas multiple-unit systems spread out as discrete units. The spreading out of the multiple-unit system results in a more reproducible gastrointestinal transit, drug release, and plasma concentration–time profile, with a reduced incidence of dose dumping or incomplete release. A faster onset of action of multiparticulates, which is due to a more rapid gastric emptying and larger surface-area-to-volume ratio is a further advantage, as is the slower colonic transit due to the effects of "streaming" [5]. Multiple-unit systems, despite being more complicated to manufacture, are now the preferred platform for modified-release oral dosage forms.

Gamma scintigraphy is particularly useful when correlated with pharmacokinetic data (pharmacoscintigraphy) obtained from blood or urine sampling and enables the relationship between biodistribution of the dosage form and drug absorption to be examined [6]. The technique is a useful tool in product development and for obtaining regulatory approval for modified-release dosage forms, whereby a pharmaceutical company must demonstrate that a dosage form performs *in vivo* according to its proposed rationale. The need for *in vivo* proof of efficacy is born from an increased understanding that no amount of *in vitro* testing can accurately predict how a new drug entity or delivery system is going to perform in humans. Recently, there has been much research into *in vitro* testing methodologies that will achieve good *in vivo–in vitro* correlations [7]. This is of particular importance for drugs that exhibit poor solubility and/or permeability.

4.3 IMMEDIATE-RELEASE DOSAGE FORMS

4.3.1 Tablets

Polymers have been used for many years as excipients in conventional immediate-release oral dosage forms, either to aid in the manufacturing process or to protect the drug from degradation upon storage. The judicious choice of excipients is also necessary to enhance the *in vivo* behavior of the dosage form. Disintegration and subsequent drug release and dissolution and, therefore, absorption and bioavailability (i.e., pharmacokinetics) can, to a certain extent, be controlled by the choice of excipients. Microcrystalline cellulose is often used as an alternative to carbohydrates as diluents in tablet formulations of highly potent low-dose drugs. Starch and cellulose are used as disintegrants in tablet formulations, which swell on contact with water, resulting in the tablet "bursting," increasing the exposed surface area of the drug, and improving the dissolution characteristics of a formulation. Polymers including polyvinyl-pyrrolidone and hydroxypropyl methylcellulose (HPMC) also find uses as binders that aid the formation of granules that improve the flow and compaction properties of tablet formulations prior to tableting. Occasionally, dosage forms must be coated with a "nonfunctional" polymeric film coating in order to protect a drug from degradation, mask the taste of an unpalatable drug or excipient, or improve the visual elegance of the formulation, without affecting the drug release rate [8,9]. Low-viscosity grades of HPMC or polyvinyl-pyrrolidone are suitable for such applications.

4.3.2 Capsules

Capsules are used as an alternative to tablets, for poorly compressible materials, to mask the bitter taste of certain drugs, or sometimes to increase bioavailability. Many of the polymeric excipients used to "bulk out" capsule fills are the same as those used in immediate-release tablets. Gelatin has been used almost exclusively since the 1830s as a shell material for hard (two-piece) and soft (one-piece) capsules. This is due in part to its ready availability but primarily because of its near-to-ideal physicochemical properties for the encapsulation of solid and semisolid material, that is, its ability to form thin but tough and flexible films that gel at an appropriate temperature, and remain stable over long-term storage but dissolve readily in biological fluids at 37°C. As a further advantage, gelatin being odorless and tasteless is acceptable to most palates.

However, as gelatin is derived from the skin, tendons, and ligaments of animals, it is not an acceptable pharmaceutical excipient for all patient groups, and is precluded from use by patients with religious or dietary restrictions. Furthermore, gelatin is not universally compatible with all active ingredients as it has a high residual water content (13 to 15%), which renders it unsuitable for the encapsulation of hydrolyzable or hygroscopic drugs or excipients. The amino groups of gelatin are also prone to reaction with some drugs, resulting in discoloration and retardation of capsule dissolution. Additionally, gelatin is a rather brittle material, prone to cracking on long-term storage in dispensing jars containing a desiccant when the moisture content falls below 10%. It has been attempted to overcome these limitations by the use of gelatin alternatives for capsule shell manufacture.

HPMC is a versatile pharmaceutical excipient available as different grades and used in oral and topical formulations. At low concentrations (2 to 6%), HPMC has been used as a binder in wet granulation and dry, direct compression tableting processes, as well as for film-coating, as mentioned earlier. At concentrations of 15 to 35%, HPMC can also be used to produce extended-release formulations (see Subsection 4.4.1).

HPMC has recently been developed and accepted as an alternative material for the manufacture of hard (two-piece) capsules. It holds many of the advantages of gelatin (comparable, rapid *in vivo*

TABLE 4.2
Comparative *In Vivo* Disintegration Times of Coadministered HPMC and Gelatin Capsules in Eight Fasted Human Volunteers, Evaluated Using Gamma Scintigraphy

Volunteers	Disintegration Time of HPMC Capsules (min)	Disintegration Time of Gelatin Capsules (min)
1	9	11
2	6	4
3	7	7
4	11	13
5	10	4
6	8	5
7	11	7
8	8	3
Mean (±S.D.)	9 (±2)	7 (±4)

disintegration time (see Table 4.2) [10], tasteless, and odorless) while overcoming its limitations. Holding a much lower residual water content (4 to 6%) [11], while remaining flexible and resistant to cracking, even when the water content falls below 1%, HPMC is also chemically unreactive, and so it is compatible with all active ingredients. Finally, being of plant origin, HPMC capsules are suitable for all patient groups, and although they have only been available for a relatively short period of time, HPMC capsules have already caught on in the nutraceuticals market in the U.S. because of their shorter time to market. Pharmaceutical HPMC capsule products are also in the pipeline and should reach the market soon. The limiting factor at present to the use of HPMC capsules as an alternative to gelatin is primarily cost, which is due to the higher cost of raw materials, slower gelling of HPMC relative to gelatin thus increasing production time, and the fact that HPMC capsule production is a more recent and less well-established process.

4.4 MODIFIED-RELEASE DOSAGE FORMS

It is now generally accepted that, for many therapeutic agents, drug delivery using immediate-release dosage forms results in suboptimal therapy and/or systemic side effects. Pharmaceutical scientists have attempted to overcome the limitations of conventional oral dosage forms by developing modified-release dosage forms. With regard to oral drug delivery, modified release can be described as an alteration in the site or timing of drug release within the gastrointestinal tract, and can be further divided into extended release and delayed release.

4.4.1 EXTENDED-RELEASE DOSAGE FORMS

The therapeutic effect of drugs that have a short biological half-life may be enhanced by formulating them as extended- or sustained-release dosage forms. Extended- and sustained-release dosage forms prolong the time that systemic drug levels are within the therapeutic range and, thus, reduce the number of doses the patient must take to maintain a therapeutic effect, thereby increasing compliance. Drugs with a narrow therapeutic index are also suitable for incorporation into an extended-release dosage form, where the peaks associated with C_{max} can often be dampened, reducing the possibility of systemic side effects occurring when drug levels in blood exceed the minimum toxic concentration. Unlike an immediate-release dosage form, where disintegration and drug release occurs rapidly in the stomach, extended-release formulations release the drug gradually as the dosage moves along the gastrointestinal tract. Extended-release dosage forms are commonly proposed as a formulation tool for achieving zero-order drug release; however, zero-order release *in vitro* rarely translates to constant drug absorbance and drug blood levels *in vivo* because of the heterogeneous composition of, and transit rate through, the gastrointestinal tract (see Table 4.1).

The most commonly used water-insoluble polymers for extended-release applications are the ammoniomethacrylate copolymers (Eudragit RS and RL), cellulose derivatives ethylcellulose and cellulose acetate, and polyvinyl derivative, polyvinyl acetate. Eudragit RS and RL differ in the proportion of quaternary ammonium groups, rendering Eudragit RS less permeable to water, whereas ethylcellulose is available in a number of different grades of different viscosity, with higher-viscosity grades forming stronger and more durable films.

A common approach to producing extended-release dosage forms is to coat the "core" dosage form (single- or multiple-unit) with one of the aforementioned water-insoluble polymers that is semipermeable to water, producing a reservoir system whereby drug release will occur gradually by diffusion as water leaches into the dosage form and the drug solution diffuses out. Release rate can be modified by incorporation of low-molecular-weight pore-forming agents into the water-insoluble film coat.

Because extended-release polymers are water insoluble, they have traditionally been applied as film coatings from organic solutions. However, in recent years, stricter environmental legislation has driven the development of aqueous-based latex or pseudolatex dispersions as an alternative to organic solutions for film coating. Although organic coating solutions are generally thought to produce a better quality film coat (with the polymer being in solution rather than suspension, facilitating molecular diffusion and film formation upon drying), the disadvantage of using aqueous-based systems has been partly overcome by the judicious addition of plasticizers that increase the film flexibility of aqueous-based coatings, improving particle diffusion to form a uniform film upon drying. In some cases, the aqueous dispersion offers advantages over its organic counterpart by possessing a high solid content, therefore reducing coating and drying times. Details of the most popular water-insoluble polymers, along with their aqueous dispersions, are shown in Table 4.3.

An alternative approach for achieving extended release is to incorporate the water-insoluble polymer into the tablet matrix (generally, this approach is not suitable for the production of multiple-unit systems because of their small size). Diffusion of drug solution through pores in the matrix controls drug release and the release rate is determined by the ratio of drug to polymer, drug solubility, the dimensions of the dosage form, and the tortuosity of the fluid-filled pores.

Single-unit hydrophilic matrix tablets composed of high-viscosity HPMC have also been proposed as extended-release formulations; these tablets are capable of swelling upon contact with the gastrointestinal fluid and releasing the drug over a prolonged period of time. This concept has been extended and applied to the versatile Geomatrix tablet (see Figure 4.2), a double- or triple-layered tablet, with the

TABLE 4.3
Water-Insoluble Polymers Commonly Used in the Production of Extended-Release Oral Dosage Forms

Polymer	Classification	Aqueous Dispersion
Ammoniomethacrylate copolymers	Acrylic derivative	Eudragit RS/RL 30D
Ethylcellulose	Cellulose derivative	Aquacoat ECD, Surelease
Cellulose acetate	Cellulose derivative	—
Polyvinyl acetate	Polyvinyl derivative	Kollicoat SR 30D

Note: All polymers are available in powder/granule form for use in organic solutions and in some cases ready-to-use aqueous dispersions.

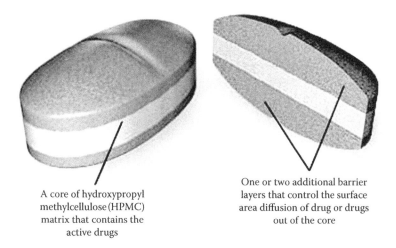

A core of hydroxypropyl
methylcellulose (HPMC)
matrix that contains the
active drugs

One or two additional barrier
layers that control the surface
area diffusion of drug or drugs
out of the core

FIGURE 4.2 A controlled-release Geomatrix trilayered tablet (Image courtesy of SkyePharma www.skyepharma.com).

different layers comprising polymers that swell, gel, or erode at rates that enable a variety of release profiles. Eight types of modified-release are claimed: zero order, binary (two drugs in one formulation), quick–slow, slow–quick, positioned, accelerated, delayed, and multiple-pulse. Pharmacoscintigraphic studies have been carried out on various incarnations of the Geomatrix tablet [12].

A combination of polymers are used in the OROS™ osmotic-pump-type delivery system to produce extended-release profiles [13]. A cellulose acetate polymer membrane allows ingress of fluid into a tablet core, which contains a second, swellable polymer that hydrates, pumping drug solution or suspension through a precision-drilled delivery orifice in the tablet coat. The rate at which the drug leaves the delivery orifice is dictated by the amount of drug within the tablet core, surface area of the tablet, thickness of the coating, and diameter of the delivery orifice. The *in vivo* performance of the OROS delivery system is described in two different volunteers [14], which graphically demonstrates how gastrointestinal physiology can drastically influence the *in vivo* performance of even the most elegantly designed delivery system. Figure 4.3 illustrates how gastrointestinal transit time impacts systemic drug levels, on this occasion for an extended-release dosage form, but the data can be extrapolated for all modified-release formulations, particularly those that are single unit in nature.

4.4.1.1 Gastroretentive Dosage Forms

Gastroretentive dosage forms offer an alternative strategy for achieving extended-release profiles, in which the formulation will remain in the stomach for prolonged periods, releasing the drug *in situ*, which will then dissolve in the liquid contents and slowly pass into the small intestine. Unlike a conventional extended-release dosage form, which gradually releases the drug during transit along the gastrointestinal tract, such a delivery system would overcome the problems of drugs that are absorbed preferentially from specific sites within the gastrointestinal tract (for example, many drugs are absorbed poorly from the distal gut, where an extended-release dosage form may spend the majority of its time), producing nonuniform plasma time profiles.

A variety of strategies have been proposed to extend gastric residence; however, sinking delivery systems of density >2.6 g/cm^3 designed to resist antral mixing and peritalsis [15], and magnetic delivery systems do not rely on polymers, *per se*, to achieve gastroretention. Mucoadhesive [16–20] and low-density [21,22] polymers have been evaluated, with little success so far, for their ability to extend gastric residence time by bonding to the mucus lining of the stomach and floating on top of the gastric contents, respectively.

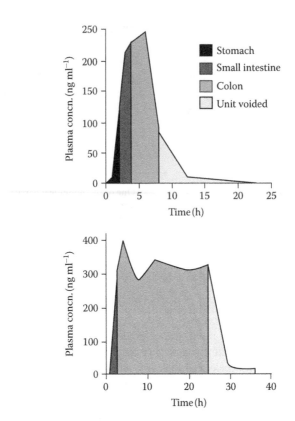

FIGURE 4.3 Plasma concentration–time profiles for oxprenolol delivered from an OROS device in an individual with a short (top diagram) and long (bottom diagram) colon transit time. (From Washington, N., Washington., C., and Wilson, C.G., *Physiological Pharmaceutics: Barriers to Drug Absorption*, 2nd ed., Taylor and Francis, London, 2001, p. 158.)

4.4.2 Delayed-Release Dosage Forms

In contrast to extended-release dosage forms, which release drug over a prolonged period of time, delayed-release formulations release a bolus of drug after a predetermined time or in a predetermined location. In practice, there are two types of delayed-release formulations designed either to target release to the proximal small intestine (enteric coating) or the colon.

4.4.2.1 Enteric Coating

Enteric coating is possibly the most established of all modified-release technologies, first reported in 1884 by Unna [23], and is commonly used to prevent release of a gastric-irritant or acid-labile drug molecule in the stomach. This can be relatively easily achieved by coating the dosage form with a weakly acidic polymer, containing ionizable carboxylic acid groups, that remains intact in the stomach while breaking down at the more neutral pHs encountered in the small intestine as a result of ionization, disruption, and dissolution of the polymer coat.

Early attempts at enteric coating used natural materials such as shellac, gelatin, and keratin. Such materials, being of natural origin, suffered problems with batch-to-batch variability, and for the purposes of enteric coating, they are of historical significance only.

Over the years, polymer chemists have synthesized a variety of pH-sensitive polymers, soluble above a range of threshold pHs (see Table 4.4). The proportion of ionizable monomers in the polymer chain is possibly the major determinant of threshold dissolution pH, but other factors play a role in defining this pH [23].

TABLE 4.4
pH-Sensitive Polymers Commonly Used in the Production of Delayed-Release Oral Dosage Forms

Polymer	Dissolution Threshold pH	Aqueous Dispersion
Cellulose Derivatives		
Cellulose acetate trimellitate	5.0	—
Hydroxypropyl methylcellulose 55	5.5	—
Hydroxypropyl methylcellulose acetate succinate L	5.5	Aqoat AS-L
Hydroxypropyl methylcellulose acetate succinate M	6.0	Aqoat AS-M
Cellulose acetate phthalate	6.0	Aquacoat CPD
Hydroxypropyl methylcellulose acetate succinate H	6.8	Aqoat AS-H
Acrylic Derivatives		
Poly(methacrylic acid, ethyl acrylate) 1:1	5.5	Eudragit L30-D55 Eastacryl 30D Kollicoat MAE30 DP Acryl-eze
Poly(methacrylic acid, methyl methacrylate) 1:1	6.0	—
Poly(methacrylic acid, methyl methacrylate, methyl acrylate) 2.5:6.5:1	6.8	Eudragit FS
Poly(methacrylic acid, methyl methacrylate) 1:2	7.0	—
Polyvinyl Derivatives		
Polyvinyl acetate phthalate	5.0	Sureteric

Note: All polymers are available in powder/granule form for use in organic solutions and in some cases ready-to-use aqueous dispersions.

A polymer with a dissolution threshold pH in the range 5 to 6 is considered ideal for use as an enteric coat; this is based on the premise that the pH of the stomach, even in the fed state, will rarely reach this level but will exceed this level in the duodenum, where secretion of bicarbonate neutralizes the acidic chyme leaving the stomach.

There is no single enteric polymer that is applicable for the enteric coating of all drug molecules. The nature of the core material (acidity or basicity, or permeability through different enteric polymer films) may limit the choice of polymer. The pK_a of the coating polymer must also be carefully considered, and the potential for premature release in the stomach (for polymers with low pK_a values) weighed against the requirement for a rapid release in the small intestine. Because the physicochemical properties of the drug will have a bearing on this, it is important to consider the consequences of premature release in the stomach (drug degradation or risk of mucosal damage) alongside the requirement for a rapid release of a poorly soluble drug in the small intestine in order to optimise bioavailability and achieve the desired therapeutic effect.

Enteric coating is not without its problems. A lag time of 1.5 to 2 h postgastric emptying for complete disintegration of an enteric-coated capsule and tablet has been demonstrated [6,24]. This is slower than reported for *in vitro* disintegration times, and implies that modified-release dosage forms should be designed as multiple-unit systems, in which the increased surface-area-to-volume ratio would reduce the time for intestinal disintegration while minimizing the possibility of total failure of the dosage form and premature release in the stomach. Furthermore, the *in vivo* evidence highlights the need for new enteric polymers to be developed, which will improve the rapidity of intestinal release while remaining intact in the stomach. It is likely that enteric polymers of the future will be available primarily as ready-to-use aqueous-based formulations, with the pharmaceutical industry moving away from traditional organic polymer solutions for film coating.

4.4.2.2 Colonic Drug Delivery

It is only recently that the colon has been accepted as an important site for drug delivery, partly because of the need to better treat localized pathologies (inflammatory bowel diseases and carcinomas) and also in order to achieve systemic absorption of a variety of drugs from this site [1], especially considering a colonic residence time of up to 5 days [25]. As with any form of targeted delivery, a "trigger factor" specific to the organ being targeted must be exploited. These include pH, transit time, pressure, and bacteria [26].

4.4.2.2.1 pH-Responsive Drug Delivery

The pH of the small intestine increases aborally (see Table 4.1), and pH-sensitive polymers with a dissolution threshold pH in the range 6.8 to 7.5 may be considered as candidates for colonic targeting. Although the pH of the terminal ileum is typically around 1 to 2 pH units higher than that in the cecum [27], because of the cecal fermentation of dietary fiber to fatty acid, it is hoped that the pH-sensitive coating would begin to destabilize in the region of the terminal ileum or cecum, minimizing absorption from the small intestine and facilitating delivery of therapeutic agent to the colon.

The limitations of using the pH approach to target the colonic region have also been demonstrated [28]. Using gamma scintigraphy to follow the transit of rapidly disintegrating tablets coated with Eudragit S (pH threshold of 7.0) in seven volunteers, it was demonstrated that there was variability in both time (5 to 15 h) and site (ileocaecal junction to splenic flexure) of drug release. Such variability can be attributed to the inter- and intraindividual variation in gastrointestinal transit times and pH.

The rational design of pH-sensitive polymers in the future may improve the site-specific delivery of drugs to different regions of the gastrointestinal tract by virtue of pH. With the advent of more accurate and sensitive radiotelemetry capsules capable of measuring gastrointestinal pH, it may be possible to define the pH threshold that facilitates colon targeting with a greater degree of certainty. Alternatively, the rate of polymer dissolution may be important. Rohm Pharma have recently developed Eudragit P4135/FS, a polymer that dissolves at approximately the same pH as S100 but at a slower rate, which may reduce the potential for premature drug release before the colon is reached. The possibility of premature drug release and systemic absorption must be weighed against the possibility of the dosage form being voided intact, which would also clearly result in therapeutic failure.

In summary, the use of currently available pH-sensitive polymers to deliver drugs to the colon can be described, at best, as selective. It is for this reason that alternative methods for colonic delivery have been proposed.

4.4.2.2.2 Time-Responsive Delivery

Time has been utilized on the assumption that the small-intestinal transit time is relatively constant, in comparison to gastric emptying and colonic residence time, at 3 to 5 h [29]. Wilding et al. investigated the Pulsincap® device, which consists of a nondisintegrating half capsule shell, sealed at the open end with a hydrogel plug, which hydrates and swells on contact with gastrointestinal fluids and is thus ejected from the capsule shell, effecting drug release [30]. The lag time preceding drug release can be controlled by altering the composition of the hydrogel plug, but a lag time of 5 h is considered appropriate for colon arrival. Variable release positions (which can be partially alleviated by enteric-coating the capsule, thus negating the influence of gastric emptying) and poor spreading of capsule contents have been reported, limiting the effectiveness of Pulsincap® as a colon-specific delivery system.

4.4.2.2.3 Pressure-Responsive Delivery

A pressure-controlled colon delivery capsule (PCDC) has been described [31,32], which utilizes the increase in pressure of the luminal contents to effect drug release. The device comprises the drug, dispersed in a suppository base, coated with the hydrophobic polymer ethylcellulose. The suppository base melts after the PCDC has been swallowed, resulting in the capsule resembling a liquid-filled ethylcellulose balloon, that is capable of remaining intact in the small bowel but which will rupture when exposed to the more intense haustral contractions and luminal contents of higher viscosity encountered in the colon. So far, this delivery system has not been evaluated using gamma scintigraphy, so its *in vivo* targeting potential cannot be fully evaluated. Furthermore, little is known about the luminal pressures along the gastrointestinal tract and whether these are subject to the same inter- and intrasubject variation as pH and transit times.

4.4.2.2.4 Bacteria-Responsive Delivery

The bacterial count in the colon is approximately 10 million times higher than that in the proximal gastrointestinal tract (see Table 4.1). Azo-polymers being selectively degraded by bacterial enzymes present in the large bowel [33], were originally proposed as coatings to achieve colon-specific drug delivery. As azo-polymers are known to be potential carcinogens [34], a variety of naturally occurring polysaccharides have been exploited as alternative bacterial responsive polymers [35] as they are generally regarded as safe (GRAS), and many of them are already used as excipients in solid oral dosage forms or are constituents of the human diet.

Amylose is one polysaccharide that has been rigorously investigated [36–39]. In the glassy state, amylose has good film-forming properties and is resistant to degradation by pancreatic enzymes in the small intestine, although it is fermented by a wide variety of bacterial enzymes in the colon. In combination with the water-insoluble polymer ethylcellulose, which reduces swelling and drug release from the hydrophilic amylose, a film coating can easily be applied to tablets, capsules, or pellets to achieve site-specific delivery to the colon (COLAL technology). The COLAL technology is the only polysaccharide-based system to have successfully undergone phase II clinical trials, in which it was used to deliver prednisolone metasulphobenzoate to the colon of patients with active ulcerative colitis [40]. Figure 4.4 shows a series of scintigraphic images following the transit of a COLAL pellet system in the human gastrointestinal tract.

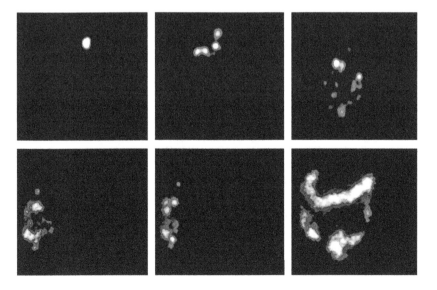

FIGURE 4.4 Scintigraphic images of COLAL pellet system administered to a human volunteer. From the top left to the bottom right: t = 0 h, pellets in stomach; t = 0.25 h, gastric emptying; t = 3 h, pellets dispersed throughout small intestine; t = 7 h and t = 9 h, pellet arrival at caecum and in ascending colon; t = 24 h, complete distribution of pellets in colon. (Images courtesy of author).

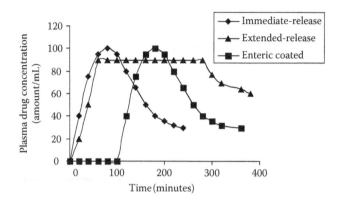

FIGURE 4.5 Theoretical pharmacokinetic profiles for immediate-release, extended-release and enteric-coated tablet formulations (note that a colon-targeted formulation would be similar to the enteric-coated formulation but would be delayed for a further 3 to 4 h).

4.5 CONCLUSION

A variety of immediate-release and modified-release applications, which make use of polymers to influence and optimize the drug-release characteristics from oral formulations, have been discussed. The "ideal" pharmacokinetic profiles for modified-release dosage forms in comparison to immediate-release are summarized in Figure 4.5. Although *in vitro* dissolution profiles are often promising, such results are rarely seen *in vivo*. This is because, irrespective of how well designed a delivery system has been to date its *in vivo* performance can occasionally be defeated by the complexity and variability of gastrointestinal physiology. The challenge for pharmaceutical scientists is, therefore, to improve the knowledge and understanding of gastrointestinal tract physiology or pathology and the behavior of dosage forms within the gastrointestinal tract by using imaging techniques such as gamma scintigraphy. Pharmaceutical scientists also need to develop and evaluate new polymers and delivery systems that offer better *in vivo* performance in terms of a more rapid drug release or that are capable of overcoming the variability in gastrointestinal transit.

REFERENCES

1. Fara, J.W., Colonic drug absorption and metabolism, in *Novel Drug Delivery and Its Therapeutic Application,* Prescott, L.F. and Nimmo, W.S., Eds., John Wiley & Sons, Chichester, U.K., 1989.
2. Digenis, G.A., Sandefer, E.P., Page, R.C., and Doll, W.J., Gamma scintigraphy: an evolving technology in pharmaceutical formulation development — Part 1, *PSTT,* 1(3), 100, 1998.
3. Digenis, G.A., Sandefer, E.P., Page, R.C., and Doll, W.J., Gamma scintigraphy: an evolving technology in pharmaceutical formulation development — Part 2, *PSTT,* 1(4), 160, 1998.
4. Wilding, I.R., Coupe, A.J., and Davis, S.S., The role of gamma scintigraphy in oral drug delivery, *Adv. Drug Delivery Rev.*, 46, 103, 2001.
5. Davis, S.S., Hardy, J.G., Taylor, M.J., Whalley, D.R., and Wilson, C.G., A comparative study of the gastrointestinal transit of a pellet and tablet formulation, *Int. J. Pharm*, 21, 167, 1984.
6. Wilding, I.R. et al., The evaluation of an enteric-coated naproxen tablet formulation using gamma scintigraphy, *Eur. J. Pharm. Biopharm.,* 39(4), 144, 1993.
7. Dressman, J.B. and Reppas, C., In vitro-in vivo correlations for lipophilic, poorly water-soluble drugs, *Eur. J. Pharm. Sci.*, S73, 2000.
8. Hogan, J.E., Film-coating materials and their properties, in *Pharmaceutical Coating Technology*, Cole, G., Hogan, J., and Aulton, M.E., Eds., Taylor and Francis, London, 1995.

9. Van Savage, G. and Rhodes, C.T., The sustained release coating of solid dosage forms: a historical review, *Drug Dev. Industrial Pharm.*, 21(1), 93, 1995.
10. Tuleu, C. et al., A comparative scintigraphic assessment of the disintegration of HPMC and gelatin capsules in fasting subjects, *AAPS J.*, 6(4) Abstract, W5137, 2004.
11. Ogura, T., Furuya, Y., and Matsuura, S., HPMC capsules — an alternative to gelatin, *Pharm. Technol. Eur.*, 10(11), 32, 1998.
12. Wilding, I.R. et al., Pharmacoscintigraphic evaluation of a modified release (Geomatrix®) diltiazem formulation, *J. Controlled Release*, 33, 89, 1995.
13. Palangio, M. et al., Dose conversion and titration in a novel, once-daily, OROS® osmotic technology, extended-release hydromorphone formulation in the treatment of chronic malignant or nonmalignant pain, *J. Pain Symptom Manage.*, 23(5), 355, 2002.
14. Washington, N., Washington, C., and Wilson, C.G., *Physiological Pharmaceutics: Barriers to Drug Absorption*, 2nd ed., Taylor and Francis, London, 2001, p. 158.
15. Clarke, G.M., Newton, J.M., and Short, M.D., Gastrointestinal transit of pellets of differing size and density, *Int. J. Pharm.*, 114, 81, 1993.
16. Longer, M.A., Ch'ng, H.S., and Robinson, J.R., Bioadhesive polymers as platforms for oral controlled drug delivery III: oral delivery of chlorothiazide using a bioadhesive polymer, *J. Pharm. Sci.*, 74(4), 406, 1985.
17. Park, K. and Robinson, J.R., Bioadhesive polymers as platforms for oral-controlled drug delivery: method to study bioadhesion, *Int. J. Pharm.*, 19, 107, 1984.
18. Ch'ng, H.S. et al., Bioadhesive polymers as platforms for oral controlled drug delivery II: synthesis and evaluation of some swelling, water-insoluble bioadhesive polymers, *J. Pharm. Sci.*, 74(4), 399, 1985.
19. Harris, D., Fell, J.T., Sharma, H.L., and Taylor, D.C., Gastrointestinal transit of potential bioadhesive formulations in man: a scintigraphic study, *J. Controlled Release*, 12, 45, 1990.
20. Leung, S.-H.S. and Robinson, J.R., Polymer structure features contributing to Mucoadhesion II., *J. Controlled Release,* 12, 187, 1990.
21. Timmermans, J. and Moes, A.J., How well do floating dosage forms float? *Int. J. Pharm.*, 62, 207, 1990.
22. Whitehead, L. et al., Floating dosage forms: an in-vivo study demonstrating prolonged gastric retention, *J. Controlled Release*, 55, 3, 1998.
23. Agyilirah, G.A. and Banker, G.S., Polymers for enteric coating applications, in *Polymers for Controlled Drug Delivery,* Tarcha, P.J., Ed., CRC Press, Boca Raton, FL, 1991, pp. 39–66.
24. Cole, E.T. et al., Enteric coated HPMC capsules deigned to achieve intestinal targeting. *Int. J. Pharm.*, 231, 83, 2002.
25. Cummings, J.H. et al., Fecal weight, colon cancer risk and dietary intake of non-starch polysaccharides (dietary fibre), *Gastroenterology,* 103, 1783, 1992.
26. Basit, A.W., Advances in colonic drug delivery, *Drugs*, 65, 1991, 2005.
27. Evans, D.F. et al., Measurement of gastrointestinal pH profiles in normal ambulant human subjects, *Gut*, 29, 1035, 1988.
28. Ashford, M. et al., An in vivo investigation into the suitability of pH-dependent polymers for colonic targeting, *Int. J. Pharm.*, 95, 193, 1993.
29. Davis, S.S., Hardy, J.G., and Fara, J.W., Transit of pharmaceutical dosage forms through the small intestine, *Gut*, 27, 886, 1986.
30. Wilding, I.R. et al., Gastrointestinal transit and systemic absorption of captopril from a pulsed-release formulation, *Pharm. Res.*, 9, 654, 1992.
31. Hu, Z. et al., New preparation method of intestinal pressure-controlled colon delivery capsules by coating machine and evaluation in beagle dogs, *J. Controlled Release*, 56, 293, 1998.
32. Takaya, T. et al., Development of a colon delivery capsule and pharmacological activity of recombinant human granulocyte colony-stimulating factor in beagle dogs, *J. Pharm. Pharmacol.*, 47, 474, 1995.
33. Saffran, M. et al., A new approach to the oral administration of insulin and other peptide drugs, *Science*, 233, 1081, 1986.
34. Van den Mooter, G. et al., Use of azo polymers for colon-specific drug delivery, *J. Pharm. Sci.*, 86(12), 1321, 1997.
35. Fish, N.W. and Bloor, J.R., Drug delivery to the colon, *Expert Opin. Ther. Patents*, 9, 1515, 1999.

36. Cummings, J.H. et al., In vivo studies of amylose- and ethylcellulose-coated ^{13}C glucose microspheres as a model for drug delivery to the colon, *J. Controlled Release*, 40, 123, 1996.

37. Basit, A.W., Oral colon-specific drug delivery using amylose-based film coatings, *Pharm. Technol. Eur.*, 12(2), 30, 2000.

38. Tuleu, C. et al., Colonic delivery of 4-aminosalicylic acid using amylose-ethylcellulose-coated hydroxy-propylmethylcellulose capsules, *Aliment. Pharmacol. Ther.*, 16, 1771, 2002.

39. Basit, A.W. et al., The use of formulation technology to assess regional gastrointestinal drug absorption in humans, *Eur. J. Pharm. Sci.*, 21, 179, 2004.

40. Thompson, R.P.H. et al., Preserved endogenous cortisol levels during treatment of ulcerative colitis with COLAL-PRED, a novel oral system consistently delivering prednisolone metasulphobenzoate to the colon, *Gastroenterology*, 122(Suppl. 1): T1207, 2002.

5 Hydrogel Drug Delivery Systems

Seong Hoon Jeong, Kang Moo Huh, and Kinam Park

CONTENTS

5.1 INTRODUCTION

5.1.1 HYDROGELS IN DRUG DELIVERY

Over the past several decades, research on hydrogels has expanded significantly because of the participation of many scientists from a wide range of research fields. The widespread application of hydrogels is linked to their unique property of exhibi ting an intermediate behavior between solid and liquid materials. Hydrogels are three-dimensional networks of hydrophilic polymer chains that do not dissolve but can swell in water [1]. Because of the hydrophilic properties of polymer chains, they are able to retain a large amount of water within their structures. The high biocompatibility of hydrogels results from their high water content and soft-surface properties [2]. In addition, hydrogels are versatile materials because they can be tailor-made to possess various properties by manipulating the synthetic or processing methods. The physicochemical, mechanical, and biological properties, as well as new functional properties, can be easily modulated. For example, hydrogels can be made to respond to environmental stimuli, such as temperature, pH, light, and specific molecules. These interesting properties have made hydrogels useful for various applications ranging from pharmaceutical and biomedical to other industrial applications.

Of the many applications of hydrogels, controlled drug delivery is one of the areas in which hydrogels have played a vital role. The hydrated matrix results in good compatibility with proteins as well as living cells and body fluids. Since the first report on the biomedical use of poly(2-hydroxyethyl methacrylate) hydrogels by Wichterle and Lim in 1960 [3], various other hydrogels have been developed for biomedical and pharmaceutical applications, particularly for the delivery of drugs and bioactive substances.

5.1.2 DEFINITIONS AND CLASSIFICATIONS

More than four decades of research on hydrogels has resulted in a large number of new synthetic hydrogels and modified natural hydrogels. The presence of various hydrogels makes it difficult to classify them using a single criterion. Hydrogels can be classified using various criteria depending on their preparation methods and physicochemical properties, and some of them are listed in Table 5.1.

Hydrogels can be prepared from both natural and synthetic materials. Natural polymers, such as proteins, polysaccharides, and deoxyribonucleic acids (DNAs), can be cross-linked to form hydrogels. As cross-linking polymerization of amino acids, carbohydrates, and nucleic acids is not easy, natural polymers are cross-linked by either physical or chemical bonds. Unlike hydrogels made of natural polymers, synthetic hydrogels can be easily prepared by cross-linking polymerization of synthetic monomers. Because of the availability of various monomer structures, hydrogels can be synthesized to possess virtually any property of choice. Natural polymers can be combined with synthetic polymers to obtain combined properties in one hydrogel. For example, the biodegradable property of natural polymers has been combined with several functionalities of synthetic polymers to give new functional hydrogels with biodegradability [4,5].

One of the criteria for classifying hydrogels is the nature of cross-linking by which individual polymer chains are connected to form a network: chemical and physical cross-linking. When the polymer chains of a hydrogel are connected by covalent cross-linking, they are known as *chemical gels*. Because the polymer chains are covalently linked to each other, hydrogels cannot be reshaped once set. For this reason, chemically cross-linked hydrogels are also called *thermoset hydrogels*. *Physical gels* are defined as continuous, disordered, three-dimensional networks formed by associative forces capable of forming noncovalent cross-links [6]. Such noncovalent cross-links include hydrogen bonding, hydrophobic interaction, stereocomplex formation, ionic complexation, and crystallinity. The resultant associations act as physical junction domains, which are not cross-linking points found in chemical hydrogels but are the chain segments consisting of many monomer units. As noncovalent associations are reversible, physical hydrogels can be processed by solvent casting or heating, therefore they are also referred to as *thermoplastic hydrogels*.

Hydrogels with interconnected pores provide unique properties of fast-swelling kinetics and high swelling ratios. Porous hydrogels can be prepared by a variety of methods, such as the

---

TABLE 5.1
Various Criteria for the Classifications of Hydrogels

Origin	Natural
	Synthetic
Water content or degree	Low swelling
of swelling	Medium swelling
	High swelling
	Superabsorbent
Porosity	Nonporous
	Microporous
	Macroporous
	Superporous
Cross-linking	Chemical (or covalent)
	Physical (or noncovalent)
Biodegradability	Biodegradable
	Nondegradable

---

porosigen technique, phase separation technique, cross-linking of individual hydrogel particles, and gas-blowing (or foaming) technique. Depending on the pore size, porous hydrogels are divided into microporous (10 to 100 nm range), macroporous (100 nm to 10 μm range), and superporous hydrogels (10 to 1000 μm range) [7,8].

5.2 PROPERTIES AND STRUCTURES OF HYDROGELS

Swelling of hydrogels in aqueous media is the most important property for their applications. The swelling property is usually characterized by measuring their capacity to absorb water or aqueous solutions. Measuring the weight of a swollen hydrogel is the simplest way of characterizing the swelling kinetics and swelling equilibrium. The swelling ratio (R_s), which is the most commonly used parameter to express the swelling capacity of hydrogels, is defined as follows:

$$R_s = (W_s - W_d)/W_d \tag{5.1}$$

where W_s and W_d are the weights of swollen and dried hydrogels, respectively.

The swelling properties are determined by many factors, including the type and composition of monomers, cross-linking density, and other environmental factors such as temperature, pH, and ionic strength. The swelling force is counterbalanced by the retractive force induced by the cross-links of the network. When these two counteracting forces become equivalent, swelling of the hydrogel reaches its equilibrium state. The cross-linking density and the swelling property are inversely related. The degree of cross-linking has been often determined by measuring either equilibrium swelling or elastic modulus [6,9].

The cross-linking density of a hydrogel is also closely related to other important properties such as mechanical strength and permeability. The mechanical properties of hydrogels basically depend on their composition and structure. Because of the high water content of fully swollen hydrogels, they are, in general, mechanically very weak. The low mechanical strength can be improved by increasing the cross-linking density, making an interpenetrating network (IPN) structure or copolymerization with hydrophobic comonomers. These approaches are usually accompanied by the decreased swelling property.

Biodegradable hydrogels that can slowly degrade and disappear from the body have attracted significant attention for drug delivery applications. The degradation mechanism is also used to control the kinetics of drug release from the hydrogel formulations. Biodegradation occurs by either simple hydrolysis or enzyme-catalyzed hydrolysis. A large number of biodegradable polymers, such as poly(lactic acid) (PLA), poly(glycolic acid) (PGA), poly(lactic-co-glycolic acid) (PLGA), poly(ε-caprolactone), poly(ortho esters), polyanhydrides, and polyphosphoesters, have been developed for their applications in tissue-engineering temporary scaffolds [10], sutures [11], and matrices for drug delivery systems [12]. Many of the biodegradable polymers are hydrophobic and water insoluble, thus they cannot be directly used to make hydrogels. Recent advances in hydrogel synthesis, however, have made it possible to fabricate various kinds of biodegradable hydrogels, using hydrophobic biodegradable polymers appropriately combined with hydrophilic polymers, to give significant swelling behavior in aqueous environments [13–16].

5.3 HYDROGEL FABRICATIONS

Various methods have been used to synthesize hydrogels. There are generally two different methods to prepare chemical hydrogels as shown in Figure 5.1. Polymerization of water-soluble monomers in the presence of bi- or multifunctional cross-linking agents results in chemical hydrogels. Typical examples of water-soluble monomers include acrylic acid, acrylamide, hydroxyethyl methacrylate, hydroxypropyl acrylate, and vinylpyrrolidone. Chemical hydrogels can also be prepared by cross-linking

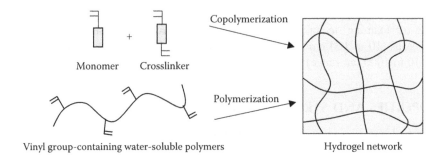

FIGURE 5.1 Synthetic methods for formation of hydrogel networks.

water-soluble polymers using chemical reactions that involve functional groups of the polymers. Functional groups for cross-linking reactions include vinyl, hydroxyl, amine, and carboxyl groups. Many examples and details of cross-linking reactions with different functional groups are described in the literature [6,17,18]. Physical hydrogels are prepared by cross-linking without chemical reactions. Noncovalent bonds can be formed through electrostatic interactions, hydrogen bonding, antigen-antibody interactions, and supramolecular associations [19–22].

5.4 APPLICATIONS OF HYDROGELS IN DRUG DELIVERY

5.4.1 BASIC CONCEPTS OF HYDROGEL DRUG DELIVERY

Drug delivery technologies have advanced to a point where drug release can be achieved for years at relatively constant rates. The benefits of controlled drug delivery are: (1) more effective therapies with reduced side effects, (2) the maintenance of effective drug concentration levels in the blood, (3) patient's convenience as medicines are taken less frequently, and (4) increased patient compliance. Most of the controlled drug delivery technologies are based on utilization of polymers and hydrogels.

Release of drug molecules from a delivery device is controlled by various methods, and the most widely used mechanisms are diffusion, dissolution, osmosis, and ion exchange. For diffusion-controlled drug delivery, drugs are loaded in the water-insoluble polymer matrices (monolithic devices; Figure 5.2a) or in reservoirs that are subsequently covered with a water-insoluble polymer

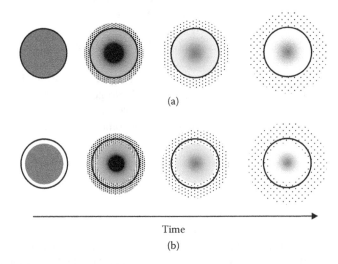

FIGURE 5.2 Schematic representation of drug delivery from: (a) a polymer matrix, (b) a reservoir system.

membrane (reservoir devices; Figure 5.2b). The same monolithic and reservoir devices can be prepared by using water-soluble or biodegradable polymers and hydrogels, in which the drug release is controlled by dissolution of the polymers and hydrogels. As in Figure 5.2a, highly cross-linked hydrogels can be used as monolithic devices, or the hydrogel core can be covered with a water-insoluble polymer membrane to form reservoir devices (Figure 5.2b). In osmosis-controlled drug delivery systems, the core of the devices is often made of hydrogels as a source of osmotic pressure. In ion-exchange-based drug delivery systems, water-soluble polyelectrolytes are highly cross-linked, and these are basically hydrogels with very high cross-linking densities, which prevents the system from swelling.

Controlled drug delivery by diffusion, dissolution, osmosis, and ion exchange allows continuous delivery of drugs at predetermined rates. In many instances, however, drug delivery has to be noncontinuous, or *pulsatile*. For example, delivery of insulin should not be continuous; rather, a bolus of insulin has to be delivered only when the blood glucose level is increased. Such delivery, known as *modulated* or *self-regulated* delivery, requires hydrogels with properties recognizing the changes in environmental conditions, i.e., "environment-sensitive hydrogels."

5.4.2 Environment-Sensitive Hydrogels

Hydrogels can be prepared to possess the properties that can respond to environmental changes, such as temperature, pH, light, and specific molecules such as glucose. Such hydrogels can undergo reversible volume phase transition or sol-gel phase transition upon small changes in the environmental condition. For this additional property, they are called environment-sensitive hydrogels, or more commonly "intelligent" or "smart" hydrogels.

As shown in Figure 5.3, a smart hydrogel can undergo swelling due to a change in the pH of the environment, resulting in easier diffusion of drug molecules through the expanded polymer network. Alternatively, the temperature of the environment can be increased to shrink the temperature-sensitive hydrogels for faster release of the drugs through a squeezing action. Typical examples of the environment-sensitive hydrogels are listed in Table 5.2, and the structures of selected polymers are shown Figure 5.4.

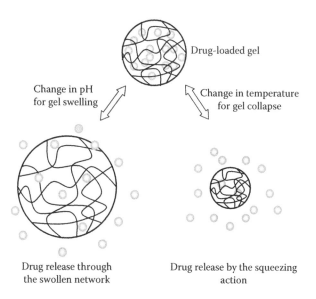

Drug-loaded gel

Change in pH
for gel swelling

Change in temperature
for gel collapse

Drug release through
the swollen network

Drug release by the squeezing
action

FIGURE 5.3 Schematic representation of drug release from hydrogels that are sensitive to environmental factors such as pH and temperature.

TABLE 5.2
Environment-Sensitive Hydrogels Used for Drug Delivery

Environmental Factor	Typical Polymers	Main Mechanism	Applications	References
Temperature	PNIPAAm, PDEAAm, PEO-PPO block copolymers	Competition between hydrophobic interaction and hydrogen bonding	On/off drug release, squeezing device	23–27
pH	Polyelectrolytes, PAA, PDEAEM	Ionization of polymer chains upon pH change	pH-dependent oral drug delivery	31
Glucose	pH-sensitive hydrogels; Concanavalin A-grafted polymers; polymers containing phenylborate groups	pH change caused by glucose oxidase; reversible interaction between glucose-containing polymers and Concanavalin A; reversible solgel transformation	Self-regulated insulin delivery	33–38
Electric signal	Polyelectrolytes (pH-sensitive)	Reversible swelling or deswelling in the presence of electric field	Actuator, artificial muscle, on off drug release	63–65
Light	Copolymer of PNIPAAm and light sensitive chromophore, such as triphenylmethane and leuco derivatives	Temperature change via the incorporated photosensitive molecules; dissociation into ion pairs by UV irradiation	Optical switches, ophthalmic drug delivery	66–68
Antigen	Semi-IPN with grafted antibodies or antigens	Competition between polymer-grafted antigen and free antigen	Modulated drug release in the presence of a specific antigen; sensor for immunoassay and antigen	69

Note: PNIPAAm = poly(*N*-isopropylacrylamide); PDEAAm = poly(*N,N*-diethylacrylamide); PEO-PPO = polyethylene oxide-polypropylene oxide; PAA = poly(acrylic acid); PDEAEM = poly(*N,N*-diethylaminoethyl methacrylate); IPN = interpenetrating network.

Temperature-sensitive hydrogels with the volume phase transition property have been studied extensively for drug delivery [23]. Among the many temperature-sensitive hydrogels, poly(*N*-isopropylacrylamide) (PNIPAAm) is widely used (Figure 5.4A). The water solubility of PNIPAAm and its copolymers is dramatically changed around their lower critical solution temperatures (LCSTs), which can be modulated to be close to the body temperature [23]. It is soluble in water when the temperature is lower than the LCST, but becomes insoluble above the LCST. This inverse (or negative) thermosensitivity in the hydrogel is because of the competition between hydrogen bonding and hydrophobic interactions. Hydrogen bonding between hydrophilic groups of the polymer chains and water molecules is dominant at lower temperatures, resulting in higher water solubility or higher swelling. As the temperature increases, however, hydrophobic interactions among hydrophobic groups become stronger, resulting in shrinking of the hydrogels because of interpolymer chain association through hydrophobic interactions. This property has been used for "on/off" drug delivery systems [24,25]. Cross-linked P(NIPAAm-*co*-butyl methacrylate (BMA))

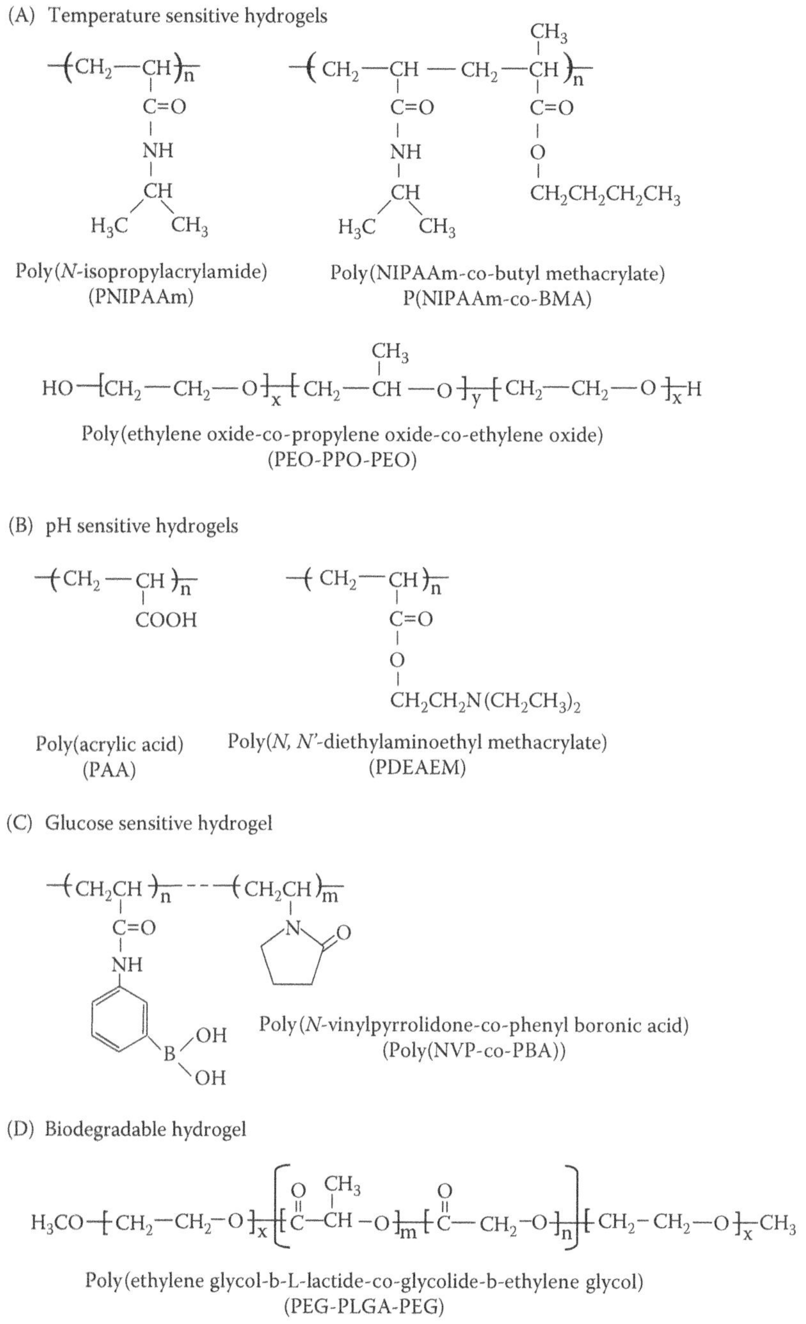

(A) Temperature sensitive hydrogels

Poly(N-isopropylacrylamide)
(PNIPAAm)

Poly(NIPAAm-co-butyl methacrylate)
P(NIPAAm-co-BMA)

Poly(ethylene oxide-co-propylene oxide-co-ethylene oxide)
(PEO-PPO-PEO)

(B) pH sensitive hydrogels

Poly(acrylic acid)
(PAA)

Poly(N, N'-diethylaminoethyl methacrylate)
(PDEAEM)

(C) Glucose sensitive hydrogel

Poly(N-vinylpyrrolidone-co-phenyl boronic acid)
(Poly(NVP-co-PBA))

(D) Biodegradable hydrogel

Poly(ethylene glycol-b-L-lactide-co-glycolide-b-ethylene glycol)
(PEG-PLGA-PEG)

FIGURE 5.4 Molecular structures of selected environment-sensitive hydrogels.

hydrogels and IPNs of PNIPAAm and poly(tetramethylene ether glycol) were also studied extensively for the same applications [26,27].

Positive thermosensitive hydrogels can be formed by IPNs having positive thermosensitivity: swelling at high temperature and shrinking at low temperature. Typical examples are IPNs of poly(acrylic acid) (PAA), polyacrylamide (PAAm), and P(NIPAAm-*co*-BMA) [28]. The reversible swelling in response to a temperature change was dependent on the BMA content in the polymer

[29]. Some thermosensitive hydrogels were investigated for parenteral applications, and biodegradable hydrogels were preferred. In case of triblock copolymers, the propylene oxide (PPO) segment of PEO-PPO-PEO block copolymers was replaced by a biodegradable PLGA segment to give the biodegradable property (Figure 5.4A and Figure 5.4D) [30].

Another important stimulus that greatly influences the states of hydrogels is pH. Polyelectrolytes are pH-sensitive hydrogels containing acidic or basic pendant groups, which can accept or donate protons upon environmental pH changes. For example, as shown in Figure 5.4B, cationic polyelectrolytes such as poly(N,N-diethylaminoethyl methacrylate) dissolve or swell at low pH because of ionization. A relatively-high-swelling behavior of polyelectrolyte hydrogels is because of the electrostatic repulsive interaction among charges present on the polymer chains. Thus, the extent of swelling is dependent on pH, ionic strength, and type of counterions [31]. The pH difference between the stomach and the intestine is large enough to be of use in the case of pH-sensitive hydrogels. As many of the potentially useful pH-sensitive hydrogels swell at high pH and shrink at low pH, drug release can be accelerated when the device reaches the intestine, where pH is near neutral. This type of hydrogel is useful for protecting acid-labile drugs in the stomach.

Hydrogels can be prepared to be responsive to both temperature and pH by incorporating ionizable and hydrophobic functional groups in the same hydrogels. When an anionic monomer, such as acrylic acid, is incorporated into a thermoreversible polymer, the LCST of the resulting hydrogel is dependent on both the temperature and the pH of the environment at the same time. As the pH of the medium increases above the pK_a of the carboxyl groups of polyanions, the LCST increases because of the increased hydrophilicity and charge repulsion.

Various glucose-sensitive hydrogels have been developed as self-regulated insulin delivery systems. The most common method involves adding glucose oxidase to pH-sensitive hydrogels. As shown in Figure 5.5, glucose is converted to gluconic acid by glucose oxidase in the hydrogels, and the resulting pH decrease can induce the swelling of the pH-sensitive hydrogels to release more insulin [32–35]. Concanavalin A (ConA) is also frequently used for modulated insulin delivery.

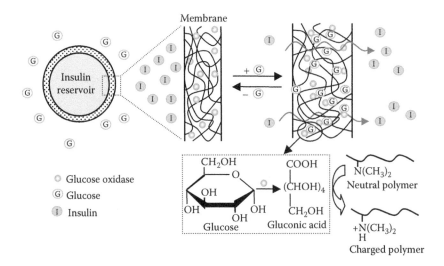

FIGURE 5.5 An example of the self-regulated insulin-release hydrogel membrane system. As glucose molecules go into the membrane, they are converted into gluconic acid by glucose oxidase, resulting in decrease of pH in the hydrogel. This results in ionization of the polymer, poly(N,N-dimethylaminoethyl methacrylate-co-ethylacrylamide), which in turn increases the LCST. This causes swelling of the membrane, and insulin can be released to the surroundings through the swollen membrane. (From Yuk, S.H., Cho, S.H., and Lee, S.H., pH/temperature-responsive polymer composed of poly((N,N-dimethylamino)ethyl methacrylate-co-ethylacrylamide), *Macromolecules,* 30, 6856, 1997.)

ConA is a glucose-binding protein obtained from a plant. In ConA-based systems, insulin can be modified with glucose for interaction with ConA for modulated release in the presence of free glucose [36]. Alternatively, ConA is used as a physical cross-linker of glucose-attached polymer chains. In the absence of free glucose, the system forms a gel to retard the release of insulin. In the presence of free glucose, however, the gel becomes sol for faster release of insulin [37,38]. Phenylboronic acid and its derivatives (Figure 5.4C) have also been used to form complexes with glucose for controlling the insulin release [39].

Although the concept of these environment-sensitive hydrogels is quite promising, significant improvements of the hydrogel properties are still required for practical applications. Response of the hydrogels to environmental changes should be fast for the timely release of insulin. One of the ways to accomplish this is to make thinner or smaller hydrogels, such as films and microparticles. This often results in dimensional limitations and mechanical failures in their practical uses [40].

5.4.3 BIODEGRADABLE HYDROGELS

Biodegradable hydrogels can be broken down into biologically acceptable low-molecular-weight molecules in the body by simple hydrolysis or enzymatic catalysis. Use of biodegradable hydrogels eliminates the need of removing a drug delivery device after release of the drug has been completed [41]. Biodegradable hydrogels can have many advantages in drug delivery, such as improved biocompatibility and flexibility in controlling the release of drugs. Colon-specific hydrogels were developed by using polymers that can be degraded by microbial enzymes in the colon [42,43]. Biodegradable hydrogels can be fabricated into microparticles for injection [44,45]. PLGA has been used most widely for making biodegradable drug delivery systems. The PLGA systems, however, have some intrinsic limitations for protein release. In many cases, toxic organic solvents are used to prepare the dosage form, and a low-pH environment resulting from degradation of PLGA can adversely affect the effectiveness and stability of the protein [46]. To overcome these limitations, a biodegradable dextran hydrogel was investigated [47]. The dextran hydrogels were prepared by mixing aqueous solutions of dextran modified with either L-lactate or D-lactate without using any organic solvents. Also, chemical cross-linking agents were not used to prepare the hydrogels owing to the physical cross-linking by stereocomplex formation between enantiomeric oligomeric lactic acid chains. Biodegradable hydrogels can be designed to demonstrate thermosensitivity, and this makes hydrogels highly suitable for the delivery of proteins or genes. Biodegradable triblock copolymers, such as PEG-PLGA-PEG, have been investigated extensively as a carrier for plasmid DNA and genes [30,48,49].

5.4.4 SPECIFIC APPLICATIONS OF HYDROGELS IN ORAL DRUG DELIVERY

Of the many routes of drug administration, oral administration has been considered to be most convenient, and hence the majority of dosage forms are designed for oral delivery. Different types of hydrogels can be used for delivery of drugs to certain regions in the gastrointestinal tract ranging from the oral cavity to the colon, as shown in Figure 5.6.

In the oral cavity, fast-disintegrating tablets and mucoadhesive hydrogels can be used. One of the ways to make fast-disintegrating tablets is to incorporate appropriate disintegrating agents in the formulation. Microparticles of superporous hydrogels with fast-swelling and superabsorbent properties were applied to develop fast-disintegrating tablet formulations [50]. Superporous hydrogels were ground into microparticles for this particular application. Superporous hydrogel microparticles maintained numerous pores smaller than 1 μm, which were connected to each other to form an open pore structure. This unique porous structure allowed water to move through with capillary forces, resulting in a fast wicking effect into the tablet core. Tablets prepared by direct compression in the presence of superporous hydrogel microparticles disintegrated in about 10 to 20 sec. In case of mucoadhesive hydrogels, buccal drug delivery is known to have a faster onset of drug action and to bypass the hepatic first-pass metabolism and degradation in the gastrointestinal

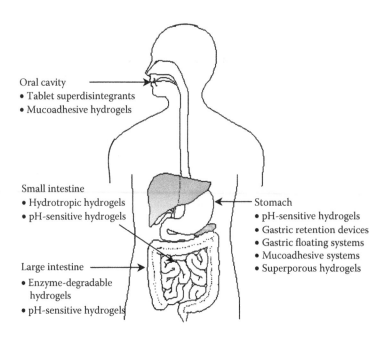

Oral cavity
• Tablet superdisintegrants
• Mucoadhesive hydrogels

Small intestine
• Hydrotropic hydrogels
• pH-sensitive hydrogels

Stomach
• pH-sensitive hydrogels
• Gastric retention devices
• Gastric floating systems
• Mucoadhesive systems
• Superporous hydrogels

Large intestine
• Enzyme-degradable
  hydrogels
• pH-sensitive hydrogels

FIGURE 5.6 Various hydrogels and hydrogel formulations that can be used in different segments of the gastrointestinal tract for drug delivery.

tract [51]. For maximum benefit from buccal drug delivery, bioadhesive dosage forms were developed. Buccal bioadhesive hydrogels can be prepared using (1) hydroxyethylcellulose (HEC), hydroxypropylcellulose (HPC), polyvinylpyrrolidone (PVP), and poly(vinyl alcohol) [52], (2) mixtures of different polymers, such as HPC, hydroxypropylmethylcellulose (HPMC), karaya gum, and PEG 400 [53], or HPC and Carbopol 934 [54].

Despite the advances in drug delivery technologies, development of "once-a-day" oral dosage forms is still a big challenge. This is mainly due to the limited transit time of the formulation through the gastrointestinal tract. As most drugs are absorbed from the upper small intestine, the time period available for effective drug absorption is usually limited to several hours. To overcome the short gastrointestinal transit time, drug delivery systems having long gastric retention times have been studied extensively [55]. Sustained release in the stomach would result in improved bioavailability for many drugs with specific absorption windows. Gastric emptying of oral dosage forms is significantly dependent on two main parameters: the physical properties, such as size and density, of the oral dosage form and the presence of food in the stomach. These parameters have been exploited by various methods in the development of gastric retention devices. In intragastric floating systems, the device is designed to float on top of the gastric juice because of its low density. One example is a single-unit hydrodynamically balanced system made of gel-forming or highly swellable cellulose-type hydrocolloids and polysaccharides [56]. Another device is a mucoadhesive system, designed to stick to the mucosal surface of the stomach. One of the best mucoadhesives is cross-linked PAA [57], and it is highly mucoadhesive at pH (about 1 to 3) of the stomach. PAA interacts with mucins and other biomolecules through hydrogen bonding provided by carboxyl acid groups of PAA at acidic pH. Superporous hydrogels, which swell to a very large size, with a swelling ratio in the region of a few hundreds, were used to increase the gastric retention time. They also possess fast-swelling properties, which are important to avoid premature emptying by the housekeeper waves [58]. This was applied to develop a gastric retention device that can remain in the stomach owing to its large size after swelling. The mechanical strength of the swollen superporous hydrogels could be improved by adding composite materials [59]. One of the useful composite materials is Ac-Di-Sol, which is cross-linked carboxymethylcellulose sodium with a hollow microparticulate shape. The hollow microparticles provide physical entanglements of polymer chains around the particles. This increased the effective cross-linking density without making the superporous hydrogels too brittle. When tested in dogs, superporous hydrogel composites showed long-term gastric retention, ranging from several hours to a day [58,59].

5.4.5 HYDROTROPIC HYDROGELS FOR DELIVERY OF POORLY SOLUBLE DRUGS

For absorption of drugs into the body, drug molecules have to be first dissolved in the body fluid. Unfortunately, many drugs have been found to be poorly soluble in water, resulting in low absorption and low bioavailability. Designing clinically effective formulations for poorly soluble drugs has been one of the biggest challenges. Recently, hydrogels with hydrotropic properties have been developed [60]. Low-molecular-weight hydrotropes have been used to increase the aqueous solubility of poorly soluble drugs [61,62]. As the concentrations of hydrotropes used in the delivery of poorly soluble drugs are very high, there is an unfavorable absorption of significant amounts of hydrotropes by the body. To prevent the undesirable coabsorption of hydrotropes, polymeric forms of hydrotropes were developed [60]. The study showed that the cross-linked hydrotropic polymers (e.g., hydrotropic hydrogels) maintained the hydrotropic property. Paclitaxel solubility in hydrotropic hydrogels (e.g., hydrogels of poly(2-(4-vinylbenzyloxy)-N-picolylnicotinamide) was 5000 times higher than the paclitaxel solubility in pure water.

5.5 SUMMARY

Hydrogels have played a pivotal role in the development of various controlled-release formulations. Hydrogels are known to be highly biocompatible owing to their ability to absorb water into their structures. Recent advances in the synthesis of smart hydrogels have resulted in the development of modulated drug delivery systems. In addition, hydrogels with new properties, such as increasing the solubility of poorly soluble drugs, can be exploited to develop new controlled-release formulations. Hydrogels with novel properties will continue to play important roles in drug delivery applications.

ACKNOWLEDGMENT

This study was supported in part by National Institute of Health through grant GM65284.

REFERENCES

1. Hoffman, A.S., Hydrogels for biomedical application, *Adv. Drug Delivery Rev.,* 43, 3, 2002.
2. Bae, Y.H. and Kim, S.W., Hydrogel delivery systems based on polymer blends, block co-polymers or interpenetrating networks, *Adv. Drug Delivery Rev.,* 11, 109, 1993.
3. Wichterle, O. and Lim, D., Hydrophilic gels for biological use, *Nature,* 185, 117, 1960.
4. de la Torre, P.M., Torrado, S., and Torrado, S., Interpolymer complexes of poly(acrylic acid) and chitosan: influence of the ionoic hydrogel-forming medium, *Biomaterials,* 24, 1459, 2003.
5. Kumashiro, Y. et al., Modulatory factors on temperature-synchronized degradation of dextran grafted with thermoresponsive polymers and their hydrogels, *Biomacromolecules,* 2, 874, 2001.
6. Park, K., Shalaby, W. S. W., and Park, H., *Biodegradable Hydrogels for Drug Delivery,* Technomic Publishing, Lancaster, PA, 1993.
7. Kim, D. and Park, K., Swelling and mechanical properties of superporous hydrogels of poly(acrylamide-co-acrylic acid)/polyethylenimine interpenetrating polymer networks, *Polymer,* 45, 189, 2004.
8. Chen, J., Park, H., and Park, K., Synthesis of superporous hydrogels: Hydrogels with fast swelling and super-absorbent properties, *J. Biomed. Mater. Res.,* 44, 53, 1999.

9. Peppas, N.A. et al., Physicochemical foundations and structural design of hydrogels in medicine and biology, *Annu. Rev. Biomed. Eng.*, 2, 9, 2000.

10. Lee, K.Y. and Mooney, D.J., Hydrogels for tissue engineering, *Chem. Rev.*, 101, 1869, 2001.

11. Ikada, Y. and Tsuji, H., Biodegradable polyesters for medical and ecological applications, *Macromol. Rapid Commun.*, 21, 117, 2000.

12. Zhao, Z. et al., Polyphosphoesters in drug and gene delivery, *Adv. Drug Delivery Rev.*, 55, 483, 2003.

13. Markland, P. et al., A pH- and ionic strength-responsive polypeptide hydrogel: Synthesis, characterization, and preliminary protein release studies, *J. Biomed. Mater. Res.*, 47, 595, 1999.

14. Tanahashi, K., Jo, S., and Mikos, A.G., Synthesis and characterization of biodegradable cationic poly(propylene fumarate-co-ethylene glycol) copolymer hydrogels modified with agmatine for enhanced cell adhesion, *Biomacromolecules*, 3, 1030, 2002.

15. Yang, Z. et al., Poly(glutamic acid) poly(ethylene glycol) hydrogels prepared by photoinduced polymerization: synthesis, characterization, and preliminary release studies of protein drugs, *J. Biomed. Mater. Res.*, 62, 14, 2002.

16. Bos, G.W. et al., In situ crosslinked biodegradable hydrogels loaded with IL-2 are effective tools for local IL-2 therapy, *Eur. J. Pharm. Sci.*, 21, 561, 2004.

17. Berger, J. et al., Structure and interactions in covalently and ionically crosslinked chitosan hydrogels for biomedical applications, *Eur. J. Pharm. Biopharm.*, 57, 19, 2004.

18. Barbucci, R., Leone, G., and Vecchiullo, A., Novel carboxymethylcellulose-based microporous hydrogels suitable for drug delivery, *J. Biomater. Sci., Polym. Ed.*, 15, 607, 2004.

19. Martin, L. et al., Sustained buccal delivery of the hydrophobic drug denbufylline using physically cross-linked palmitoyl glycol chitosan hydrogels, *Eur. J. Pharm. Biopharm.*, 55, 35, 2003.

20. Hennink, W.E. and van Nostrum, C.F., Novel crosslinking methods to design hydrogels, *Adv. Drug Delivery Rev.*, 54, 13, 2002.

21. Miyata, T., Uragami, T., and Nakamae, K., Biomolecule-sensitive hydrogels, *Adv. Drug Delivery Rev.*, 54, 79, 2002.

22. Huh, K.M. et al., Supramolecular-structured hydrogels showing a reversible phase transition by inclusion complexation between poly(ethylene glycol) grafted dextran and α-cyclodextrin, *Macromolecules*, 34, 8657, 2001.

23. Bromberg, L.E. and Ron, E.S., Temperature-responsive gels and thermogelling polymer matrixes for protein and peptide delivery, *Adv. Drug Delivery Rev.*, 31, 197, 1998.

24. Bae, Y.H., Okano, T., and Kim, S.W., "On-off" thermocontrol of solute transport. II. Solute release from thermosensitive hydrogels, *Pharm. Res.*, 8, 624, 1991.

25. Bae, Y. H., Okano, T., and Kim, S.W., "On-off" thermocontrol of solute transport. I. Temperature dependence of swelling of N-isopropylacrylamide networks modified with hydrophobic components in water, *Pharm. Res.*, 8, 531, 1991.

26. Okano, T. et al., Thermally on-off switching polymers for drug permeation and release, *J. Controlled Release*, 11, 255, 1990.

27. Okuyama, Y. et al., Swelling controlled zero-order and sigmoidal drug release from thermo-responsive poly(N-isopropylacrylamide-co-butyl methacrylate) hydrogel, *J. Biomater. Sci., Polym. Ed.*, 4, 545, 1993.

28. Qiu, Y. and Park, K., Modulated drug delivery, in *Supramolecular Design for Biological Applications*, CRC Press, Boca Raton, FL, 2002, p. 227.

29. Katono, H. et al., Thermoresponsive swelling and drug release switching of interpenetrating polymer networks composed of poly(acrylamide-co-butyl methacrylate) and poly(acrylic acid), *J. Controlled Release*, 16, 215, 1991.

30. Jeong, B., Bae, Y.H., and Kim, S.W., Drug release from biodegradable injectable thermosensitive hydrogel of PEG-PLGA-PEG triblock copolymers, *J. Controlled Release*, 63, 155, 2000.

31. Firestone, B.A. and Siegel, R.A., Kinetics and mechanisms of water sorption in hydrophobic, ionizable copolymer gels, *J. Appl. Polym. Sci.*, 43, 901, 1991.

32. Yuk, S.H., Cho, S.H., and Lee, S.H., pH/temperature-responsive polymer composed of poly((N,N-dimethylamino)ethyl methacrylate-co-ethylacrylamide), *Macromolecules*, 30, 6856, 1997.

33. Ito, Y. et al., An insulin-releasing system that is responsive to glucose, *J. Controlled Release*, 10, 195, 1989.

34. Hassan, C.M., Doyle, F.J. III, and Peppas, N.A., Dynamic behavior of glucose-responsive poly(methacrylic acid-g-ethylene glycol) hydrogels, *Macromolecules*, 30, 6166, 1997.

35. Heller, J. et al., Release of insulin from pH-sensitive poly(ortho esters), *J. Controlled Release,* 13, 295, 1990.
36. Brownlee, M. and Cerami, A., A glucose-controlled insulin-delivery system: semisynthetic insulin bound to lectin, *Science,* 206, 1190, 1979.
37. Kim, J.J. and Park, K., Modulated insulin delivery from glucose-sensitive hydrogel dosage forms, *J. Controlled Release,* 77, 39, 2001.
38. Obaidat, A.A. and Park, K., Characterization of glucose dependent gel-sol phase transition of the polymeric glucose-concanavalin-A hydrogel system, *Pharm. Res.,* 13, 989, 1996.
39. Kitano, S. et al., A novel drug delivery system utilizing a glucose responsive polymer complex between poly(vinyl alcohol) and poly(N-vinyl-2-pyrrolidone) with a phenylboronic acid moiety, *J. Controlled Release,* 19, 161, 1992.
40. Qiu, Y. and Park, K., Environment-sensitive hydrogels for drug delivery, *Adv. Drug Delivery Rev.,* 53, 321, 2001.
41. Kamath, K. R. and Park, K., Biodegradable hydrogels in drug delivery, *Adv. Drug Delivery Rev.,* 11, 59, 1993.
42. Van den Mooter, G. et al., Use of azo polymers for colon-specific drug delivery, *J. Pharm. Sci.,* 86, 1321, 1997.
43. Kopecek, J. et al., Polymers for colon-specific drug delivery, *J. Controlled Release,* 19, 121, 1992.
44. Holland, T.A., Tabata, Y., and Mikos, A.G., In vitro release of transforming growth factor-b1 from gelatin microparticles encapsulated in biodegradable, injectable oligo(poly(ethylene glycol) fumarate) hydrogels, *J. Controlled Release,* 91, 299, 2003.
45. Jiang, G., Qiu, W., and DeLuca Patrick, P., Preparation and in vitro/in vivo evaluation of insulin-loaded poly(acryloyl-hydroxyethyl starch)-PLGA composite microspheres, *Pharm. Res.,* 20, 452, 2003.
46. Van de Weert, M., Hennink, W.E., and Jiskoot, W., Protein instability in poly(lactic-co-glycolic acid) microparticles, *Pharm. Res.,* 17, 1159, 2000.
47. Hennink, W.E. et al., Biodegradable dextran hydrogels crosslinked by stereocomplex formation for the controlled release of pharmaceutical proteins, *Int. J. Pharm.,* 277, 99, 2004.
48. Kissel, T., Li, Y., and Unger, F., ABA-triblock copolymers from biodegradable polyester A-blocks and hydrophilic poly(ethylene oxide) B-blocks as a candidate for in situ forming hydrogel delivery systems for proteins, *Adv. Drug Delivery Rev.,* 54, 99, 2002.
49. Li, Z. et al., Controlled gene delivery system based on thermosensitive biodegradable hydrogel, *Pharm. Res.,* 20, 884, 2003.
50. Yang, S. et al., Application of poly(acrylic acid) superporous hydrogel microparticles as a super-disintegrant in fast-disintegrating tablets, *J. Pharm. Pharmacol.,* 56, 429, 2004.
51. Veillard, M.M. et al., Preliminary studies of oral mucosal delivery of peptide drugs, *J. Controlled Release,* 6, 123, 1987.
52. Anders, R. and Merkle, H.P., Evaluation of laminated muco-adhesive patches for buccal drug delivery, *Int. J. Pharm.,* 49, 231, 1989.
53. Nagai, T. and Machida, Y., Buccal delivery systems using hydrogels, *Adv. Drug Delivery Rev.,* 11, 179, 1993.
54. Ishida, M. et al., New mucosal dosage form of insulin, *Chem. Pharm. Bull.,* 29, 810, 1981.
55. Hwang, S.-J., Park, H., and Park, K., Gastric retentive drug delivery systems, *CRC Crit. Rev. Ther. Drug Carrier Syst.,* 15, 243, 1998.
56. Singh, B.N. and Kim, K.H., Floating drug delivery systems: an approach to oral controlled drug delivery via gastric retention, *J. Controlled Release,* 63, 235, 2000.
57. Park, K. and Robinson, J.R., Bioadhesive polymers as platforms for oral-controlled drug delivery: method to study bioadhesion, *Int. J. Pharm.,* 19, 107, 1984.
58. Chen, J. et al., Gastric retention properties of superporous hydrogel composites, *J. Controlled Release,* 64, 39, 2000.
59. Chen, J. and Park, K., Synthesis and characterization of superporous hydrogel composites, *J. Controlled Release,* 65, 73, 2000.
60. Lee, S.C. et al., Hydrotropic polymers: synthesis and characterization of polymers containing picolylnicotinamide moieties, *Macromolecules,* 36, 2248, 2003.
61. Yalkowsky, S.H., Solubilization by complexation, in *Solubility and Solubilization in Aqueous Media,* Oxford University Press, New York, 1999, p. 321.

62. Coffman, R.E. and Kildsig, D.O., Effect of nicotinamide and urea on the solubility of riboflavin in various solvents, *J. Pharm. Sci.,* 85, 951, 1996.
63. Sawahata, K. et al., Electrically controlled drug delivery system using polyelectrolyte gels, *J. Controlled Release,* 14, 253, 1990.
64. Kwon, I.C. et al., Drug release from electric current sensitive polymers, *J. Controlled Release,* 17, 149, 1991.
65. Kwon, I.C., Bae, Y.H., and Kim, S.W., Electrically erodible polymer gel for controlled release of drugs, *Nature,* 354, 291, 1991.
66. Suzuki, A. and Tanaka, T., Phase transition in polymer gels induced by visible light, *Nature,* 346, 345, 1990.
67. Mamada, A. et al., Photoinduced phase transition of gels, *Macromolecules,* 23, 1517, 1990.
68. Yui, N., Okano, T., and Sakurai, Y., Photoresponsive degradation of heterogeneous hydrogels comprising crosslinked hyaluronic acid and lipid microspheres for temporal drug delivery, *J. Controlled Release,* 26, 141, 1993.
69. Miyata, T., Asami, N., and Uragami, T., A reversibly antigen-responsive hydrogel, *Nature,* 399, 766, 1999.

6 An Assessment of the Role of Polymers for Drug Delivery in Tissue Engineering

Patrick J. Ginty, Steven M. Howdle, Felicity R.A.J. Rose, and Kevin M. Shakesheff

CONTENTS

6.1 AN INTRODUCTION TO TISSUE ENGINEERING

The field of tissue engineering was born out of the need to reduce both the loss of life and debilitating effects resulting from the damage to, or malfunction of, human organs and tissues. It is still a relatively new field that involves the repair and regeneration of biological tissue that can be guided through the application and control of cells, materials, and growth factors [1,2]. Ultimately, it is envisaged that tissue engineering will drastically reduce the need and frequency of many painful and intrusive surgical procedures, which total approximately 34 million per year in the U.S. alone at an estimated at cost of $400 billion [3]. Since its inception, tissue engineering has embraced many scientific fields such as chemistry, drug delivery, cell biology, and biotechnology to help achieve this goal. This multidisciplinary approach has lead to the successful growth of many tissues such as skin [4], cartilage [5], and bone [6]. Furthermore, a number of tissue-engineering products are now on the market. Tissue-engineered skin substitutes, in particular, have been available for some time now (e.g., Epicel, Alloderm, and HSE [human-skin equivalents]).

In order to achieve realistic tissue reconstruction, it is important that cells receive both physical support and chemical direction during growth. For example, the cells that form cartilage, chondrocytes, produce collagen so that it can provide mechanical support and assist tissue growth. Collagen is a naturally occurring structural protein that binds to and surrounds the cells to form the extracellular matrix of cartilage (ECM). The role of the ECM is to provide the necessary physical and biological support to the cells during tissue formation [1]. A polymer scaffold or matrix can take on this role of physical and biological support, as will be discussed later. However, some degree of chemical direction is needed to supplement the support given by the ECM. Chemical direction is given by endogenous proteins known as *growth factors* and *cytokines*. Growth factors are molecules that stimulate the cellular processes that drive tissue growth, such as proliferation and differentiation. The term cytokine is generally used to describe chemical messengers secreted by cells of the immune system that mediate the immune response [7]. In order to deliver these molecules to the cells in question, some kind of controlled-release device is required that will allow sustained and effective delivery.

Such a device has to be capable of imitating the often complex release profile of endogenous growth factors, while providing localized delivery to promote tissue growth and maturation. This is where the fields of tissue engineering and drug delivery become intertwined, as both require the controlled release of bioactive molecules from polymer matrices.

6.1.1 Tissue-Engineering Strategies

Several strategies have been developed in order to regenerate functional tissue, the majority of which involve the use of polymer scaffolds specifically designed to direct tissue growth [8]. The cell transplantation method is one of the most commonly used in cartilage and bone formation [9,10]. Here, tissue is taken from the donor patient, and the desired cells are isolated from this tissue using enzymatic digestion to remove extracellular materials. The cells are then cultured outside of the body (*in vitro*) to achieve a large cell population and can either be "seeded" onto a biodegradable prefabricated polymer scaffold or directly implanted back into the patient. If a scaffold is used as a carrier, the seeded construct (as it is then known) can be transplanted into the patient. This method uses the inherent regenerative capabilities of the body to produce new tissue. An alternative approach that is commonly taken in cartilage engineering is where functional tissue is regenerated *in vitro* with the use of a bioreactor or alternative three-dimensional culture system [11]. A bioreactor mimics the physiological environment inside the body, providing the necessary nutrition and optimal conditions for tissue formation. It is of particular use in cartilage engineering, as it can also provide the mechanical forces often required to produce phenotypically correct cartilage, although this is not always the case. This use of bioreactors for the synthesis of cartilage tissue has been reviewed a number of times [12,13].

Other techniques that do not involve the transplantation of cells or tissues are used. Conduction, for example, is a passive method of engineering new tissue that involves the placement of a material, normally a synthetic polymer that simply occupies the tissue space left behind. This allows cells in the surrounding tissues to move into that space and regenerate the tissue, as reviewed by Alsberg [14]. There is also a more active method known as *induction* that involves the delivery of peptides and proteins to the defective site.

This has been used successfully in the formation of bone through the delivery of osteoblast stimulating factor-1 (OSF-1) [15,16] and bone morphogenetic protein-2 (BMP-2) [17], as reviewed by Rose et al. [18]. Such bioactive molecules are normally delivered by a polymeric device to a specific area where the molecules bind to cells and induce their migration to this area, encouraging tissue growth.

The purpose of this chapter is to introduce the fundamental aspects of tissue engineering and how polymeric devices have been used to deliver bioactive molecules to aid tissue reconstruction procedures.

6.1.2 THE IMPORTANCE OF POLYMER SCAFFOLDS IN TISSUE ENGINEERING

Scaffold technology is itself a field within a field. The purpose of the scaffold is to mimic the ECM by surrounding the cells and binding them into a tissue-like structure [1]. Therefore, any scaffold made for implantation into the body must fulfill a number of stringent criteria in order for it to receive medical approval (listed in Table 6.1). Some of these criteria include: little or no toxic effects, a large surface area (for adequate seeding densities), a high degree of porosity (for gas and nutrient exchange), and compatibility with the cells (allowing them to adhere). The scaffold, however, frequently has a dual role. In many emerging tissue-engineering strategies, the scaffold must be capable of the delivery of bioactive molecules such as growth factors, with the porous degradable properties of the polymer employed to achieve controlled release. Ideally, this release should mimic the body's own release kinetics in order to achieve the correct cellular response. This can be in addition to its role as a support for cellular attachment (*in vitro* tissue growth) or purely as a drug delivery device (induction method). The challenge, therefore, is to produce a scaffold that meets all of these criteria and is suitable for the desired application.

6.1.3 THE ROLE OF GROWTH FACTORS AND CYTOKINES IN TISSUE ENGINEERING

Growth factors are polypeptides that produce and transmit signals to control cellular activities. They can either stimulate or inhibit a number of cellular processes including proliferation and differentiation, as well as altering gene expression and triggering angiogenesis (the formation of blood vessels). As a result, they have a key role in the regeneration of both vascular tissue (e.g., skin) and nonvascular tissue (e.g., cartilage). Growth factors can initiate their action by binding to specific receptors on the surface of target cells. They can act locally (paracrine) or systemically (endocrine) and even upon the same cell from which they are released (autocrine) [7]. Each growth factor can have a specific role within the body to instigate specific processes. For example, transforming growth factor-β (TGF-β) is a protein that stimulates ECM production in cartilage and bone regeneration [19–21], whereas vascular endothelial growth factor (VEGF) stimulates endothelial cell proliferation during angiogenesis [22,23]. A summary of the growth factors commonly used in tissue engineering can be seen in Table 6.2.

6.1.4 THE COMPLEXITY OF GROWTH FACTOR RELEASE

There are a number of challenges that must be overcome in order to achieve tissue regeneration with the use of growth factors. One such challenge is to mimic the release profile of growth factors

---

TABLE 6.1
Desirable Properties for Tissue-Engineering Scaffolds

Desired Property or Criteria	Justification
Nontoxic	To prevent the release of toxic metabolites into the bloodstream
Large surface area	To allow sufficiently high seeding densities
Highly porous	For gas and nutrient exchange
Biocompatibility	To allow the cells to adhere to the scaffold without adverse reactions to the material
Biodegradability	To complement proliferation of cells and tissue formation
Good mechanical strength	To provide physical support to the growth of the new tissue
Economical	To retain feasibility on a large scale
Ease of processing (quickly and without toxic solvents)	To prevent residual toxic solvents in the final scaffold

TABLE 6.2
Growth Factors Commonly Used in Tissue Reconstruction Procedures

Factor	Action/Activity	Use in Tissue Engineering	References
Platelet-derived growth factor (PDGF)	Promotes proliferation of endothelial cells	Angiogenesis, bone and wound healing	24, 99, 100
Fibroblast growth factor (FGF)	Cell proliferation	Nerve growth, endothelial cell proliferation, angiogenesis	40, 95
Epidermal growth factor (EGF) and basic fibroblast growth factor (bFGF)	Cell proliferation	Wound healing, differentiation of neural stem cells	40, 51, 101–103
Nerve growth factor (NGF)	Axonal growth and cholinergic cell survival	Promotes neurite extension and neural cell survival	81, 95, 104
Transforming growth factor (TGF-β)	ECM protein production	Angiogenesis, bone and cartilage regeneration	19, 21, 66
Vascular endothelial growth factor (VEGF)	Endothelial cell proliferation	Angiogenesis	22, 23, 43
Bone morphogenetic protein-2 (BMP-2)	Cell proliferation	Bone regeneration	17, 105

in vivo, when the release of these molecules is intermittent, in response to the needs of the body. They may also have very short biological half-lives, sometimes of only a few minutes, leading to a rapid turnover. In addition, it may be that a number of growth factors are needed at different stages throughout the regeneration process, requiring the independent control of two or more growth factor types [24]. For example, for the regeneration of skin, fibroblastic growth factor (FGF) and keratinocyte growth factor (KGF) are required for cell proliferation, whereas interleukin 1α and VEGF are required for macrophage activation and angiogenesis, respectively [25]. In addition, the same growth factor can have different effects on different cells and even on the same cell at different concentrations. This complicates growth factor delivery, and it is for this reason that much work has been done to provide effective and efficient drug delivery systems in order to target cells and promote tissue growth.

When producing a protein growth factor delivery device, it is important to mimic the release profile, kinetics, dosage, duration, and cellular targeting found *in vivo* [26]. In addition to these factors, there is the question of maximizing the protein-loading capacity of the polymer. By incorporating these protein growth factors into polymeric devices (at the correct loading), it is hoped that controlled- and sustained-release profiles can be achieved. Moreover, by implanting the device into the area where regeneration is required, the delivery of the protein can be made more efficient. Such devices have been made from a number of synthetic polymers and biopolymers, in a variety of morphologies, dependent upon the processing method. Indeed, once the target cell is identified, the selection of the polymer or fabrication method is crucial to the successful controlled release of the protein. For example, adverse processing conditions such as the use of a toxic solvent can denature the conformation of a sensitive protein or may cause unwanted aggregation [27]. Similarly, a poor release mechanism resulting from an unsuitable choice of polymer may result in poor release kinetics or loss of efficacy. This is because, in most cases, the release mechanism for the protein is controlled by diffusion through a porous matrix or by degradation of the polymer.

6.2 POLYMERS USED IN THE DELIVERY OF PROTEINS AND GROWTH FACTORS

A number of polymers, both synthetic and natural, have been utilized as drug delivery devices. However, this section focuses upon those polymers that have been used most commonly in tissue-engineering applications. The molecular structures of all of the polymers mentioned here can be seen in Table 6.3 and Table 6.4.

6.2.1 SYNTHETIC POLYMERS

Synthetic polymers have featured in drug delivery devices more frequently than natural polymers or biopolymers. This is because these synthetic polymers offer several advantages over natural polymers such as low toxicity and tunable degradability [28]. Synthetic polymers used consist largely of the poly(α-hydroxyacids) and associated esters such as poly(lactic acid) (PLA), poly(glycolic acid) (PGA), the copolymer poly(lactic-co-glycolic acid) (PLGA), and poly(ε-caprolactone) (PCL).

TABLE 6.3
The Molecular Structures of Synthetic Polymers Commonly Used in Tissue-Engineering and Drug Delivery Applications

Polymer Name	Structure
Poly(lactic acid)	
Poly(D, L-lactic acid) ring structure (Note: The orientation of the methyl groups gives the largest possible distance between them, i.e., above and below the plane of the ring.)	
Poly(glycolic acid)	
Poly(lactic-co-glycolic acid)	
Poly(ε-caprolactone)	
Poly(ethylene glycol)	$OH(CH_2 - CH_2 - O)_n - H$

TABLE 6.4
The Molecular Structures of Biopolymers Commonly Used in Tissue-Engineering or Drug Delivery Applications

Polymer Name	Structure
Collagen (primary structure)	
Alginate	
Chitosan	

(a)   (b)

Note: The structure for alginate is composed of two sub-units; α-(1-4)-L-guluronic acid (a) and β-(1-4)-mannuronic acid (b).

To date, this is the only group of synthetic polymers that have been given approval by the U.S. Food and Drug Administration (FDA) for applications such as orthopedic implants, surgical sutures, and drug delivery devices. This is largely because of the manner in which these polymers degrade. This group of polymers degrades by hydrolysis of the ester bond rather than enzymatic attack (as part of a cellular response), so there is little in the way of toxic by-products that are released [29].

The variability in stereochemistry and copolymer ratios also makes this family of polymers a popular choice, as this can allow the degradation rate to be tailored to match the application. For example, poly(DL-lactic acid) ($P_{DL}LA$) is an amorphous polymer that undergoes hydrolysis more slowly than the rigid but hydrophilic PGA (a largely crystalline polymer). This is because the large number of methyl groups in the polymer structure and its highly hydrophobic nature combine to slow hydrolysis of the ester bonds and increase the degradation time when compared to PGA. In contrast poly(L-lactic acid) ($P_L LA$) is a rigid semi-crystalline polymer that has longer degradation times than the DL form, limiting its use in tissue engineering applications. However, it is still more popular than the D form, with respect to tissue engineering, as it yields the naturally occurring (L+)-lactic acid during hydrolysis [30]. In addition to changing the molecular weight and stereochemistry, degradation times for PLA can also be reduced or increased by varying the pore wall thickness and the pore surface-to-volume ratio of the polymer matrix [31]. Amorphous PLA finds more use in drug delivery applications, where it is important to have a homogenous dispersion of the bioactive species within a one-phase matrix. As a result, this amorphous form of PLA has been used successfully in the encapsulation and controlled release of model enzymes such as lysozyme [32] and ribonuclease A [33,34]. The more hydrophilic PGA is often used in tissue-engineering applications but almost exclusively for the reconstruction of hard tissues such as cartilage and bone as a result of its rigidity and improved mechanical strength [35–37].

When both lactic and glycolic acids are copolymerized to form PLGA, the degradation kinetics can be further tailored by altering the ratio of lactic acid to glycolic acid [38]. In addition, the increased mechanical strength and hydrophilicity provided by PGA improves the properties of the scaffold further. As a result, PLGA matrices have featured more often than any other drug delivery device in tissue-engineering research. This copolymer has been used to successfully demonstrate the controlled release of model proteins such as bovine serum albumin (BSA) [39]. More significantly, PLGA has been used for the controlled release of angiogenic growth factors such as VEGF, PDGF, and bFGF. A gas-foaming or particulate-leaching method was employed to deliver bFGF and VEGF from PLGA scaffolds by Hile et al. [40] and Peters et al. [41], respectively. The basis of this technique is to use CO_2 at high pressure to produce a porous foam with the pore size and, hence, release rate controlled by the use of salt (particulate) leaching. A 65:35 ratio of PLA to PGA was used by Hile et al. to deliver bFGF over 30 d and an 85:15 ratio was used by Peters et al. to deliver VEGF. The latter study also provided evidence of functional blood vessel formation within 7 d of the start of the study.

Similar studies with PLGA-release matrices provided further evidence for the controlled release of VEGF from these materials [42,43]. Perhaps most notable is the work carried out by Richardson et al. where dual-growth-factor release was achieved with VEGF and PDGF [24]. Both VEGF and PDGF are required for the generation of mature blood vessels, with PDGF playing a crucial role in maturation of blood vessels formed under the guidance of VEGF. An 85:15 ratio was used with the PLGA matrix formed by a gas-foaming or a double-emulsion method. The subsequent release of both growth factors from the same matrix mimicked the release of growth factors *in vivo*, where it is known that any number of growth factors can be involved in the generation of tissues and blood vessels. Poly(lactic-*co*-glycolic acid) microspheres have also been successfully used to encapsulate BSA (as a model protein) when coated with polyvinyl alcohol (PVA) [39]. More significantly, PLGA microspheres have been used to deliver insulin-like growth factor 1 (IGF-1), resulting in the induction of bone formation [44].

Poly(ε-caprolactone), or PCL, has also found use in polymeric drug delivery despite the fact that it has a very long degradation profile (up to one year). This semicrystalline polymer can be blended more easily and is generally more compatible with other polymers when compared to many others. A PCL–chitosan composite was fabricated by Im et al. to provide a controlled-release device to induce bone regeneration [45]. The controlled release of PDGF was observed over four weeks at a therapeutic concentration, with bone regeneration seen in rat calvarial defects. Another synthetic polymer, poly(ethylene glycol) (PEG), has been used in the form of a hydrogel for a number of applications. Frequently, PEG is modified with adhesion peptides (e.g., RGD) to promote cell adhesion [46]. However, it has been shown that the use of such peptides can cause ECM production to diminish [47]. Despite this, it has been shown that by incorporating TGF-β, ECM production can be significantly increased with chondrocytes but only if the growth factor is covalently attached to the hydrogel [21]. This covalent attachment allows localized delivery of the drug, resulting in a concentration at the target site higher than that otherwise achieved. A similar PEG-RGD-growth-factor matrix was used to promote angiogenesis in rats with VEGF attached to PEG-RGD matrices and the resultant constructs implanted into the animals subcutaneously [48]. These VEGF-containing matrices were remodeled into native vascularized tissue with the growth factor presented and released upon local cellular demand.

6.2.2 BIOPOLYMERS

Natural polymers such as collagen, alginate, and chitosan have featured frequently as drug delivery devices in the literature. Natural polymers such as these carry a number of advantages over the synthetic polymers already mentioned. One example is the reduced need for harsh processing conditions (e.g., high temperatures).

These natural macromolecules can be easily converted into physical or chemical gels that can entrap and release growth factors. Collagen is an abundant protein found in many tissues and structures in the body (hair, lips, fingernails, etc.). Because the natural function of collagen is that of physical support, it is a logical choice as a potential tissue-engineering device [49]. Because collagen is a protein, it has a structure completely different from polysaccharides such as chitosan and alginate.

Collagen has a primary, secondary, tertiary, and quaternary structure, with the primary structure (amino acid sequence) determining the function of the protein (shown in Table 6.4). As a result of variations in this structure, collagen comes in many forms (at least 19 types in humans) dependent upon the tissue in question. Type I collagen constitutes the main protein component of natural ECMs of skin and bone and has an important role in the conduit of tissue repair. In addition, type I collagen matrices can be produced as highly porous interconnecting networks and, as a result, have been used as scaffolds to grow skin, bone, and blood vessels [49]. Collagen matrices typically exhibit very poor loading capacities for growth factors. However, collagen can be modified by varying the cross-linking density with gluteraldehyde, thereby reducing the degradation rate and prolonging the delivery of VEGF [50].

Studies on the incorporation of several growth factors (VEGF, HGF, PDGF, and bFGF) into natural collagenous matrices made from pig and rat bladders were recently carried out by Kanematsu et al. [51]. Results indicated that growth factors could be carried and released by collagen-based materials, with bFGF release being the most sustained. However, collagen does have one major disadvantage in that it can be highly immunogenic as a result of differences between species or conformational changes during processing [52]. However, Gu et al. provided evidence for the use of a collagen scaffold capable of the delivery of PDGF without any immunologic response [53]. Collagen can be transformed into gelatin by a denaturing process known as *acidification*. Gelatin retains all of collagen's biological qualities, such as adhesiveness and proteolytic degradability, despite this harsh treatment. This form of collagen has been utilized successfully for the culture of chondrocytes with the aid of FGF-9 and for the delivery of FGF-2 [54,55].

Alginate is an anionic polysaccharide derived from brown algae. It comes in the form of a block copolymer composed of two subunits: β-D-mannuronic acid and α-L-glucoronic acid, otherwise known as M and G units or blocks. When complexed with divalent cations (Ca^{2+}), alginate forms a gel, almost independent of temperature, unlike many other biopolymers that require ~37°C. The gelation of alginates is based on their affinity towards specific ions, with the G blocks responsible for specific ionic binding.

This high level of binding gives the G blocks more rigidity and mechanical strength. Therefore, the ratio of G blocks to M blocks can be altered to change the properties of the gel, a useful tool when designing drug delivery devices [56]. Despite the fact that alginate has been shown to induce an inflammatory response [57,58] it is well tolerated and has been used to produce drug delivery matrices with some success. Alginate microspheres have been used to entrap angiogenic growth factors such as bFGF and VEGF [59,60]. However, studies of VEGF release from calcium–alginate microspheres under static conditions resulted in a large burst of growth factor release, followed by little or no release over the subsequent weeks. This been tackled by groups using heparinization of the alginate (see Subsection 6.3.4) to sustain the release of bFGF [61,62]. This technique has then been applied in the human and animal treatment of myocardial ischemia, with improved blood flow observed [63,64].

Chitosan is a linear glycosaminoglycan made up of *N*-acetyl-D-glucosamine units derived from chitin, a natural product found in the shells of crustaceans. This biopolymer has been used almost exclusively for the delivery of FGF and bFGF [65]. Chitosan delivery devices have been utilized as photo-cross-linked hydrogels to deliver growth factors such as FGF-1 and FGF-2 to promote angiogenesis [66]. Here, chitosan hydrogels incorporating growth factors, with and without heparin, were implanted into mice. Increased vascularization was observed within the hydrogels as they degraded, with prolonged vascularization observed with the addition of heparin. Chitosan has commonly been utilized alongside another polymer or in a different form. For example, methylpyrrolidinone chitosan, a water-soluble derivative, has been tested for the delivery of bFGF [65]. Chitosan–albumin fibers have also been used to demonstrate the release of FGF in rats and the resultant increase in vascularization [67]. Chitosan has also been used to deliver PDGF-BB for the repair of periodontal defects [68,69]. Chitosan sponges have been produced by a freeze-drying or a cross-linking method to incorporate and release PDGF. By varying the loading content, release kinetics could be tailored to reach therapeutic levels, and new bone formation was observed [68]. The same method was used make chitosan–PLA (semicrystalline) composites. The PLA was observed to provide the required mechanical strength, whereas chitosan acted as the release polymer and increased the wettability of the PLA scaffold. Once again, this type of matrix was able to induce osteogenesis [69].

6.3 IMPORTANT PROCESSING TECHNIQUES AND CONTROLLED-RELEASE SYSTEMS IN TISSUE ENGINEERING

There are many ways in which the polymers that have been mentioned can be processed to produce tissue-engineering scaffolds. A comprehensive list of these methods can be seen in Table 6.5. However, there are a number of processing techniques and controlled-release systems that have featured most frequently, both in this chapter and in the literature, that require further explanation.

6.3.1 ROLE OF SUPERCRITICAL CARBON DIOXIDE TECHNOLOGY AND THE DELIVERY OF PROTEINS AND DNA

When a substance such as CO_2 is raised above both its critical temperature ($31.1°C$) and pressure (73.8 bar), both the liquid and the gas phase form a single "supercritical phase." Once supercritical, CO_2 exhibits both gas-like properties such as high diffusivity and liquid-like properties such as high viscosity [70]. Traditionally, supercritical fluids have been used for extractions owing to their diffusive properties, one example being the extraction of caffeine from coffee [71]. However, the use of supercritical carbon dioxide in polymer processing has become increasingly common, resulting in the use of this technique for fabricating biomaterials and drug delivery devices as reviewed by Woods et al. [72]. Tissue-engineering scaffolds have been produced from a number of polymers using this technique, including $P_{DL}LA$, poly(methyl methacrylate) (PMMA) and PLGA (15,73,74). Once supercritical, CO_2 can act as a plasticizing agent for certain types of polymers, a result of the high solubility of the CO_2 in the polymer [75]. This reduces the glass transition temperature (Tg) of amorphous polymers or polymers with amorphous regions, allowing processing at ambient temperatures without the use of organic solvents [76]. Once the system is depressurized and the Tg of the polymer increases, gas bubble nucleation occurs as the CO_2 leaves the polymer. This nucleation becomes permanent as the polymer solidifies and results in the formation of permanent pores in the matrix. It is this type of porous matrix that facilitates cellular growth with the size and tortuosity of the pores controlling the release kinetics of the protein [33]. A gas-foaming or salt-leaching technique, utilizing supercritical and nonsupercritical CO_2, have been used to produce PLGA scaffolds with varying degrees of porosity for tissue-engineering purposes [8,40,41].

A similar gas-foaming or salt-leaching method has been used to entrap DNA plasmids encoding for PDGF into PLGA matrices [77]. The use of DNA delivery (gene therapy) to enhance endogenous growth factor production within the body is an exciting area of research. The theory is that DNA containing specific gene sequences encoding for protein growth factors could be delivered into the body. This would facilitate the production of growth factors inside the body and induce tissue regeneration and wound healing. However, poor transfection data, likely because of the minimal exposure of the DNA plasmids to the cells in question, has so far cast doubts over the use of this

TABLE 6.5
Methods Commonly Employed to Fabricate Polymer Scaffolds

Fabrication Technology (Processing Method)	Reproducibility	Pore Size Range (μm)	Porosity of Scaffold (%)	Advantages	Disadvantages	References
Solvent casting/particulate leaching (casting)	Dependent upon user and material	50–500	30–60	Pores were uniform, good interconnectivity	Uses toxic solvents; NaCl residues, time consuming	106
Supercritical fluid technology (casting)	Dependent upon user and material	10–600	60–70	No toxic solvents, minimal residues, pore size is controllable	Can result in poor interconnectivity	34
Supercritical fluid technology/particulate leaching (casting)	Dependent upon user and material	Not given	94	Good interconnectivity, controllable pore size, controlled release of DNA	NaCl residues in scaffold	79
Compression moulding/salt leaching (moulding)	Dependent upon user and material	~500	77	Very large pores, good interconnectivity	Very high temperatures and pressures required; NaCl residues in scaffold	107
Low-deposition moulding (moulding)	Computer controlled	5–400	90	Mechanically competent scaffolds, wide pore size range	Potentially harmful solvents used; cold temperatures required	108
Microsyringe deposition (solid free-form fabrication)	Computer controlled	~150	Not given	Low contamination, wide range of patterns and lateral dimensions can be microfabricated	Polymer must be soluble in a volatile solvent	109
Low-pressure injection moulding (moulding)	User, material and technique sensitive	Not given	Not given	No need for high pressure or temperature; no information given on scaffold microarchitecture	Acetic acid used as solvent, very low temperatures required	110

method [78]. Despite this, it has been shown that DNA plasmids can retain their integrity with controlled release over 21 d, leading to greater transfection rates of the target cells [77,79]. Supercritical CO_2 has also been used with some success for the controlled delivery of angiogenic growth factors. It has been shown that VEGF can be incorporated into foamed polymeric devices with 90% of the activity retained [23]. In addition, bFGF has been incorporated into such a scaffold but with use of methylene chloride. This resulted in a residual level of methylene chloride remaining in the scaffold that was above the safe limit imposed by the U.S. pharmacopoeia [40].

More recently, it has been proved that proteins can be incorporated into polymers using a novel one-step processing technique, with activity or controlled release achieved and without the use of toxic solvents, high temperatures, or sodium chloride. This involved the coprocessing of powdered protein with $P_{DL}LA$ at very high loadings (up to 70% w/w). It has been demonstrated that the enzyme ribonuclease can retain full activity after processing (despite the use of elevated pressures ~200 bar) with release measured over 80 d [33]. In a second study, it was shown that small quantities (in the nanogram scale) of the same protein could be incorporated and released, providing evidence for the possible incorporation of growth factors that are often released in parts per billion [34]. Because high temperatures are not required to plasticize the polymer and no toxic solvents are involved, the protein does not denature. In addition, the pore size is controllable by increasing or decreasing the depressurization time, facilitating controlled release. This technique was later used to encapsulate BMP-2 within $P_{DL}LA$ matrices for bone regeneration [80]. Controlled release of the BMP-2 was achieved, resulting in human osteoprogenitor bone formation on the $P_{DL}LA$ scaffolds.

6.3.2 MICROSPHERE TECHNOLOGY

Microspheres are polymer particles produced on a micron scale, capable of releasing a pre-loaded drug that has been incorporated into a central reservoir. These "spheres" can then release the drug via the surface or bulk degradation of the polymer, with release kinetics controlled by the type of polymer used and its properties. The most commonly employed method of producing drug-loaded microspheres is the use of a water-in-oil-in-water emulsion (w/o/w) to entrap the protein. Initially, the growth factor is dissolved in the water phase, and the polymer is dissolved in the oil phase (normally an organic solvent such as methylene chloride). The final water phase is the vehicle used to disperse this emulsion by using homogenization or sonication. The solvent is then removed by evaporation, and microspheres are formed, which can be harvested by filtration or centrifugation [81]. These spheres can then be incorporated into a porous synthetic scaffold or water-based hydrogel, which provides structural support and further control release (e.g., via diffusion through pores in the matrix). This technique has been used in the controlled release of VEGF from PLGA in order to promote angiogensis *in vivo* and *in vitro* [82,83]. In addition, PLGA and PCL microsphere systems have been used to deliver neuroactive molecules, such as recombinant NGF, using the w/o/w method [81,84]. However, the use of toxic solvents such as methylene chloride and dichloromethane can hamper the possible use of microspheres produced in this way as drug delivery systems [40]. In another example, the use of carbonic anhydrase led to the formation of aggregates at the oil–water interface resulting in a significant loss of activity [27]. A variation on this technique, whereby dichloromethane was used as the solvent, was used to entrap DNA in PLGA microspheres by Nof and Shea [85] and then again by Jang and Shea [79], without significant loss of activity. Controlled-release scaffolds were made by combining this technique with the gas-foaming technique (previously mentioned) but without the salt-leaching process, as reported by Harris et al. [86]. Microspheres were exposed to high-pressure CO_2 in order to encourage the formation of a porous matrix, in which the microspheres would be an integral part and ultimately control the release of the DNA. Greater control over the release kinetics of the DNA was seen in the second study, where manipulation of the processing conditions (e.g., pressure) and microsphere diameter was demonstrated [79].

Alternatively, biopolymers such as collagen have been utilized to produce microspheres for bFGF delivery [6]. The use of a novel gelatin–collagen sandwich, where the gelatin (acting as a stabilizer) is used to form the microspheres, has been used to deliver bEGF in beagle dogs for the repair of periodontal tissues. Vascularization and osteogenesis were active throughout a four-week period, with functional recovery of the periodontal ligament indicated by the orientation of the regenerated collagen fibres. Another method utilizing both a biopolymer (alginate) and a synthetic polymer (PLGA) was applied for the localized delivery of bFGF [87]. Here, the microspheres were produced from PLGA using the double emulsion method, and alginate was used to form the matrix by way of cross-linking. Enhanced localized vascularization was achieved on the mesenteric membrane in rat peritoneum, with the size of the microspheres and, hence, release kinetics controlled by the homogenization stage.

6.3.3 Hydrogel Systems

Hydrogels are defined as three-dimensional polymer networks that are swollen by water, the major component of the gel system. These swollen gels are cross-linked to form a porous matrix either by physical or chemical methods. Natural polymers such as chitosan, alginate, and agarose are favored when producing a hydrogel system because they are water-soluble macromolecules that produce physical gels. Other natural polymers such as collagen, gelatin, and fibrin form cross-linked gels when induced by chemical cross-linking agents such as transglutaminases. Natural hydrogels offer several advantages over synthetic systems, including increased hydrophilicity and increased porosity [48]. This increased porosity often results in a more rapid release profile, which may or may not be beneficial, depending upon the application. An example of such a system was demonstrated by Chenite et al. with a chitosan–polyol salt combination [88]. Because chitosan is water soluble, protein can be easily introduced when the polymer is in a liquid state. Once the temperature is increased to 37°C and the liquid turns into a gel, the protein becomes entrapped within the newly formed matrix. This was demonstrated after ectopic implantation with a bone-inducing growth factor derived from the BMP family, known simply as a *bone protein*.

Despite the benefits of using biopolymers, synthetic materials can also be used as hydrogels. Poly(ethylene glycol) has been used to produce hydrogels used in wound-healing applications [89,46] and to deliver TGF-β to induce ECM production, as previously mentioned [47]. PVA has also been used to produce synthetic hydrogels [90]. These release systems are often produced by ultraviolet-photo-cross-linking of the polymer. Using this method, growth factors such as PDGF-$\beta\beta$ have been incorporated into the resultant hydrogel and subsequently released over 3 d. Another method of producing controlled-release hydrogels is by entrapping the protein during polymerization. This has been demonstrated with PEG hydrogels that incorporate lactic acid units into the monomer, which allow the degradation of the hydrogel to be further tailored to meet specific requirements [91,92]. A further example of this method was provided by Burdick et al. when they entrapped TGF-β, bFGF, and BMP-2 within polymerized PLA-PEG-PLA hydrogels for bone tissue engineering [93].

This led to increased alkaline phosphatase production, mineralization, and other indicators of bone formation.

6.3.4 The Heparin–Fibrin Binding System

The heparin–fibrin delivery complex is an affinity-based system that behaves differently from the biodegradable matrices previously described. With this system, there is no diffusion of the growth factor out of a biodegradable polymer but a slow (passive) release of immobilized growth factors from heparin attached to binding sites within a fibrin matrix [94]. *Heparin* is an anticoagulant protein that inhibits the clotting of blood and production of fibrin. *Fibrin* is a nontoxic protein that is formed when fibrinogen is cleaved and is involved with the coagulation of blood and wound healing. Therefore, it can be created from the patients' blood supply and is already associated with the regeneration of tissue, making it a suitable candidate as a drug delivery matrix. The interaction between heparin and fibrin has been manipulated in recent years as a result of the affinity that specific growth factors have for heparin (e.g., bFGF) [94]. This drug delivery system consists of heparin-binding peptides that are covalently immobilized within the fibrin matrix, heparin (bound to the peptides), and growth factor (bFGF). A similar system was used to achieve the controlled release of NGF- and neurotrophin-3 from fibrin scaffolds to achieve neural outgrowth and nerve regeneration [95,96]. In both studies, it was shown that mobile (unbound) NGF did not enhance neurite extension or nerve regeneration, perfectly illustrating the necessity to immobilize the protein within the matrix. However, there is one major disadvantage to this system. Poor integration of the heparin–fibrin system at the site of the defect has led to poor release kinetics. The use of fibrin alone as a drug delivery matrix has also met with success in the controlled release of TGF-β1 from liposomes [97] and the induction of angiogenesis through the delivery of VEGF [98].

6.4 CONCLUDING REMARKS

Polymer matrices, both natural and synthetic, can play a vital role in the delivery of protein growth factors and cytokines to aid angiogenesis and tissue reconstruction procedures. These molecules are essential to tissue growth as they control a number of vital cellular processes including proliferation and differentiation. It has been shown that by careful selection of the polymer and the processing method, controlled-release matrices, incorporating proteins and growth factors, that induce and enhance tissue growth can be produced. It has also been shown that many of these polymers and techniques can achieve this without significant detriment to protein or growth factor activity. The future use of gene therapy as a way of regenerating tissue is an exciting area, and despite still being in its infancy, it may yet provide a solution to the challenge of delivering drugs and proteins more effectively in all areas of medicine.

REFERENCES

1. Langer, R. and Vacanti, J.P., Tissue engineering, *Science*, 260, 920, 1993.
2. Bonassar, L.J. and Vacanti, C.A., Tissue engineering: the first decade and beyond, *J. Cell. Biochem. Suppl.*, 30/31, 297, 1998.
3. Langer, R. and Vacanti, J.P., Tissue engineering: the challenges ahead, *Sci. Am.*, 280, 86, 1999.
4. Bell, F., Erlich, H.P., Buttle, D.J., and Nakatsuji, T., Living tissue formed *in vitro* and accepted as skin equivalent tissue of full thickness, *Science*, 211, 1052, 1981.
5. Cima, L.G., Langer, R., and Vacanti, J.P., Polymers for tissue and organ culture, *J. Bioact. Comp. Polym.*, 6, 232, 1991.
6. Nakahara, T., Nakamura, T., Kobayashi, E., Inoue, M., Shigeno, K., Tabata, Y., Eto, K., and Shimuzi, Y., Novel approach to regeneration of periodontal tissues based on *in situ* tissue engineering: effects of controlled release of basic fibroblast growth factor from a sandwich membrane, *Tissue Eng.*, 9, 153, 2003.
7. Mckay, I.A. and Leigh, I., *Growth Factors: A Practical Approach*, IRL Press, Oxford, 1993.
8. Mooney, D.J., Baldwin, D.F., Suh, N.P., Vacanti, L.P., and Langer, R., Novel approach to fabricate porous sponges of poly(D,L-lactic-co-glycolic acid) without the use of organic solvents, *Biomaterials*, 17, 1417, 1996.
9. Marler, J.J., Upton, J., Langer, R., and Vacanti, J.P., Transplantation of cells in matrices for tissue regeneration, *Adv. Drug Delivery Rev.*, 33, 165, 1998.
10. Brittberg, M., Tallheden, T., Sjoren-Jansson, B., and Peterson, L., Autologous chondrocytes used for articular cartilage repair — an update, *Clin. Orthopaed. Relat. Res.*, 391, S337, 2001.
11. Freed, L.E., Hollander, A.P., Martin, I., Barry, J.R., Langer, R., and Vunjak-Novakovic, G., Chondrogenesis in a cell-polymer-bioreactor system, *Exp. Cell Res.*, 240, 58, 1998.
12. LeBaron, R.G. and Athanasiou, K.A., Ex-vivo synthesis of articular cartilage, *Biomaterials*, 21, 2575, 2000.

13. Darling, E.M. and Athanasiou, K.A., Articular cartilage bioreactors and bioprocesses, *Tissue Eng.*, 9, 9, 2003.

14. Alsberg, E., Hill, E.E., and Mooney, D.J., Craniofacial tissue engineering, *Crit. Rev. Oral Biol. Med.*, 12, 65, 2001.

15. Yang, X.B., Roach, H.I., Clarke, N.M., Howdle, S.M., Shakesheff, K.M., and Oreffo, R.O., Induction of bone formation in vivo using human osteoprogenitor and osteoblast stimulating factor-1 adsorbed scaffold constructs, *J. Bone Miner. Res.*, 17, OC13, 2002.

16. Yang, X.B., Tare, R.S., Partridge, K.A., Roach, H.I., Clarke, N.M., Howdle, S.M., Shakesheff, K.M., and Oreffo, R.O., Induction of human osteoprogenitor chemotaxis, proliferation, differentiation, and bone formation by osteoblast stimulating factor-1/pleiotrophin: osteoconductive biomimetic scaffolds for tissue engineering, *J. Bone Miner. Res.*, 18, 47, 2003.

17. Yang, X.B., Whitaker, M.J., Clarke, N.M., Sebald, W., Howdle, S.M., Shakesheff, K.M., and Oreffo, R.O., In vivo human bone and cartilage formation using porous polymer scaffolds encapsulated with bone morphogenetic protein-2 (BMP-2), *J. Bone Miner. Res.*, 18, 1366, 2003.

18. Rose, F.R.A.J., Hou, Q-P., and Oreffo, R.O.C., Delivery systems for bone growth factors — the new players in skeletal regeneration, *J. Pharm. Pharmacol.*, 56, 415, 2004.

19. Nicoll, S.B., Denker, A.E., and Tuan, R.S., *In vitro* characterization of transforming growth factor-beta 1-loaded composites of biodegradable polymer and mesenchymal cells, *Cell. Mater.*, 5, 231, 1995.

20. Lind, M., Overgaard, S., Glerup, H., Soballe, K., and Bunger, C., Transforming growth factor-beta 1 adsorbed to tricalciumphosphate coated implants increases peri-implant bone remodelling, *Biomaterials*, 22, 189, 2001.

21. Mann, B.K., Schmedlen, R.H., and West, J.L., Tethered-TGF-beta increases extracellular matrix production of vascular smooth muscle cells, *Biomaterials*, 22, 439, 2001.

22. Weatherford, D.A., Sackman, J.E., Reddick, T.T., and Freeman, M.B., Stevens, S.L., and Goldman, M.H., Vascular endothelial growth factor and heparin in a biologic glue promotes human aortic endothelial cell proliferation with aortic smooth muscle cell inhibition, *Surgery*, 120, 433, 1996.

23. Sheridan, M.H., Shea, L.D., Peters, M.C., and Mooney, D.J., Bioabsorbable polymer scaffolds for tissue engineering capable of sustained growth factor delivery, *J. Controlled Release*, 64, 91, 2000.

24. Richardson, T.P., Peters, M.C., Ennet, A.B., and Mooney, D.J., Polymeric system for dual growth factor delivery, *Nat. Biotechnol.*, 19, 1029, 2001.

25. Eming, S.A., Smola, H., and Krieg, T., Treatment of chronic wounds: state of the art and future concepts, *Cell. Tissues, Organs,* 172, 105, 2002.

26. Maquet, V. and Jerome, R., Design of macroporous biodegradable polymer scaffolds for cell transplantation, *Mater. Sci.*, 250, 15, 1997.

27. Van de Weert, M., Hoechstetter, J., Hennink, W.E., and Crommelin, D.J.A., The effect of a water/organic solvent interface on the structural stability of lysozyme, *J. Controlled Release*, 68, 351, 2000.

28. Lu, L. and Mikos, A.G., The importance of new processing techniques in tissue engineering, *Mater. Res. Soc. Bull.*, 21, 28, 1996.

29. Athanasiou, K.A., Niederauer, G.G., and Agrawal, C.M., Sterilization, toxicity, biocompatibility and clinical applications of polylactic acid polyglycolic acid copolymer, *Biomaterials*, 17, 93, 1996.

30. Göpferich, A., Mechanisms of polymer degradation and erosion, *Biomaterials*, 17, 103, 1996.

31. Lu, L., Peter, S.J., Lyman, M.D., Lai, H-L., Leite, S.M., Tamada, J.A., Vacanti, J.P., Langer, R., and Mikos, A.G., *In vitro* degradation of porous poly(L-lactic acid) foams, *Biomaterials*, 21, 1595, 2000.

32. Young, T.J., Johnston, K.P., Mishima, K., and Tanaka, H., Encapsulation of lysozyme in a biodegradable polymer by precipitation with a vapor-over-liquid antisolvent, *J. Pharm. Sci.*, 88, 640, 1999.

33. Howdle, S.M., Watson, M.S., Whitaker, M.J., Popov, V.K., Davies, M.C., Mandel, F.S., Wang, J.D., and Shakesheff, K.M., Supercritical fluid mixing: preparation of thermally sensitive polymer composites containing bioactive materials, *Chem. Commun.*, 1, 109, 2001.

34. Watson, M.S., Whitaker, M.J., Howdle, S.M., and Shakesheff, K.M., Incorporation of proteins into polymer materials by a novel supercritical fluid processing method, *Adv. Mater.*, 14, 1802, 2002.

35. Dunkelman, N.S., Zimber, M.P., Lebaron, R.G., Pavelec, R., Kwan, M., and Purchio, A.F., Cartilage production by rabbit articular chondrocytes on PGA scaffolds in a closed bioreactor system, *Biotechnol. Bioeng.*, 46, 299, 1995.

36. Cao, Y.L., Rodriguez, A., Vacanti, M., Ibarra, C., Arevalo, C., and Vacanti, C.A., Comparative study of the use of poly(glycolic acid), calcium alginate and pluronics in the engineering of porcine cartilage, *J. Biomater. Sci. — Polym. Ed.*, 9, 475, 1998.

37. Kellner, K., Lang, K., Papadimitriou, A., Leser, U., Milz, S., Shulz, M.B., Blunk, T., and Göpferich, A., Effects of hedgehog proteins on tissue engineering of cartilage *in vitro*, *Tissue Eng.*, 8, 541, 2002.

38. Lu, L., Peter, S.J., Lyman, M.B., Lai, H-L., Leite, S.M., Tamada, J.A., Uyama, S., Vacanti, J.P., Langer, R., and Mikos, A.G., *In vitro* and in *vivo* degradation of porous poly(D,L-lactic-co-glycolic acid), *Biomaterials*, 21, 1837, 2000.

39. Hu, Y., Hollinger, J.O., and Marra, K.G., Controlled release from coated polymer microparticles embedded in tissue-engineered scaffolds, *J. Drug Targeting*, 9, 431, 2001.

40. Hile, D.D., Amirpour, M.L., Akgerman, A., and Pishko, M.V., Active growth factor delivery from poly(D,L-lactide-co-glycolide) foams prepared in supercritical CO_2, *J. Controlled Release*, 66, 177, 2000.

41. Peters, M.C., Polverini, P.J., and Mooney, D.J., Engineering vascular networks in porous polymer matrices, *J. Biomed. Mater. Res.*, 60, 668, 2002.

42. Faranesh, A.Z., Nastley, M.T., de la Cruz, C.P., Haller, M.F., Laquerriere, P., Leong, K.W., and McVeigh, E.R. In vitro release of vascular endothelial growth factor from gadolinium-doped biodegradable microspheres, *Magn. Resonance Med.*, 51, 1265, 2004.

43. Sun, Q.H., Chen, R., Mooney, D.J., Rajagopalan, S., and Grossman, P.M., Biodegradable scaffolds incorporating vascular endothelial factor as a novel sustained delivery platform to induce angiogenesis, *J. Am. College Cardiol.*, 43, 473A, 2004.

44. Meinel, L., Zoidis, E., Zapf, E., Hassa, P., Hottiger, M.O., Auer, J.A., Schneider, R., Gander, B., Luginbuehl, V., Bettschart-Wolfisberger, R., Illi, O.E., Merkle, H.P., and Von Rechenberg, B., Localized insulin-like growth factor I delivery to enhance new bone formation, *Bone*, 33, 660, 2003.

45. Im, S.Y., Cho, S.H., Hwang, J.H., and Lee, S.J., Growth factor releasing porous poly(epsilon-caprolactone)-chitosan matrices for enhanced bone regenerative therapy, *Arch. Pharmacol. Res.*, 26, 76, 2003.

46. Hern, D.L. and Hubbell, J.A., Incorporation of adhesion peptides into non-adhesive hydrogels useful for tissue resurfacing, *J. Biomed. Mater. Res.*, 39, 266, 1998.

47. Mann, B.K., Tsai, A.T., Scott-Burden, T., and West, J.L., Modification of surfaces with cell adhesion peptides alters extracellular matrix production, *Biomaterials*, 20, 2281, 1999.

48. Zisch, A.H., Lutolf, M.P., Ehrbar, M., Raeber, G.P., Rizzi, S.C., Davies, N., Schmokel, H., Bezuidenhout, D., Djonov, V., Zilla, P., and Hubbell, J.A., Cell-demanded release of VEGF from synthetic biointeractive cell in-growth matrices for vascularized tissue growth, *FASEB J*, 17, U374, 2003.

49. Auger, F.A., Lopez Valle, C.A., Guingard, R., Tremblay, N., Noel, B., Goulet, F., and Germain, L., Skin equivalent produced with human collagen, *In-Vitro Cell. Dev. Biol. — Animal*, 31, 432, 1995.

50. Tabata, Y., Miyao, M., Ozeki, M., and Ikada, Y., Controlled release of vascular endothelial growth factor by use of collagen hydrogels, *J. Biomater. Sci. — Polym. Ed.*, 11, 915, 2000.

51. Kanematsu, A., Yamamoto, S., Ozeki, M., Tetsuya, N., Kanatani, I., Ogawa, O., and Tabata, Y., Collagenous matrices as release carriers of exogenous growth factors, *Biomaterials*, 25, 4513, 2003.

52. Leonard, M.P., Decter, A., Hills, K., and Mix, L.W., Endoscopic subureteral collagen injection: are immunological concerns justified? *J. Urol.*, 160, 1012, 1998.

53. Gu, D.L., Nguyen, T., Gonzalez, A.M., Printz, M.A., Pierce, G.F., Sosnowski, B.A., Phillips, M.L., and Chandler, L.A., Adenovirus encoding human platelet-derived growth factor-B delivered in collagen exhibits safety, biodistribution, and immunogenicity profiles favourable for clinical use, *Mol. Ther.*, 9, 699, 2004.

54. Côté, M.F., Laroche, G., Gagnon, E., Chevallier, P., and Doillon, C.J., Denatured collagen as support for a FGF-2 delivery system: physiological characterizations and *in vitro* release kinetics and bioactivity, *Biomaterials*, 25, 3761, 2004.

55. Au, A., Polotsky, A., Krzyminski, K., Gutowska, A., Hungerford, D.S., and Frondoza, C.G., Evaluation of thermoreversible polymers containing fibroblast factor-9 (FGF-9) for chondrocyte culture, *J. Biomed. Mater. Res.*, 69A, 367, 2004.

56. Draget, K.I., Skjak-Braek, G., and Smidsrod, O., Alginate-based new materials, *Int. J. Biol. Macromol.*, 21, 47, 1997.

57. Smidsrod, O. and Skjak-Braek, G., Alginate as an immobilization matrix for cells, *Trend. Biotechnol.*, 8, 71, 1990.

58. Otterlei, M., Ostgaard, K., Skjak-Braek, G., Smidsrod, O., Soon-Shiong, T., Espevik, T., Induction of cytokine production from human monocytes stimulated with alginate, *J. Immunother.*, 10, 4, 286–291, 1991.

59. Peters, M.C., Isenberg, B.C., Rowley, J.A., and Mooney, D.J., Release from alginate enhances the biological activity of vascular endothelial growth factor, *J. Biomater. Sci. — Polym. Ed.*, 9, 1267, 1998.

60. Downs, E.C., Robertson, N.E., Riss, T.L., and Plunkett, M.L., Calcium alginate beads as a slow release system for delivering angiogenic molecules *in vivo* and *in vitro*, *J. Cell. Physiol.*, 152, 422, 1992.

61. Tanihara, M., Suzuki, Y., Yamamoto, E., Noguchi, A., and Mizushima, Y., Sustained release of basic fibroblast growth factor and angiogenesis in a novel covalently crosslinked gel of heparin and alginate, *J. Biomed. Mater. Res.*, 56, 216, 2001.

62. Edelman, E.R., Mathiowitz, E., Langer, R., and Klagsbrun, M., Controlled and modified release of basic fibroblast growth factor, *Biomaterials*, 12, 819, 1991.

63. Harada, K., Grossman, W., Friedman, M., Edelman, E.R., Prasad, P.V., Keighley, C.S., Manning, W.J., Sellke, F.W., and Simons, M., Basic fibroblast growth factor improves myocardial-function in chronically ischemic porcine hearts, *J. Clin. Invest.*, 94, 623, 1994.

64. Laham, R.J., Sellke, F.W., Edelman, E.R., Pearlman, J.D., Ware, J.A., Brown, D.L., Gold, J.P., and Simon, M., Local perivascular delivery of basic fibroblast growth factor in patients undergoing coronary bypass surgery — results of a phase I randomized, double-blind, placebo-controlled trial, *Circulation*, 100, 1865, 1999.

65. Berscht, P.C., Nies, B., Liebendorfer, A., and Kreuter, J., Incorporation of basic fibroblast growth factor into methylpyrrolidinone chitosan fleeces and determination of the in vitro release characteristics, *Biomaterials*, 15, 593, 1994.

66. Ishihara, M., Obara, K., Ishizuka, T., Fujita, M., Sato, M., Masuoka, K., Saito, Y., Yura, H., Matsui, T., Hattori, H., Kikuchi, M., and Kurita, A., Controlled release of fibroblast growth factors and heparin from photo-crosslinked chitosan hydrogels and subsequent effect on *in vivo* vascularization, *J. Biomed. Mater. Res. — Part A.*, 64A, 551, 2003.

67. Elcin, Y.M., Dixit, V., and Gitnick, G., Controlled release of endothelial cell growth factor from Chitosan-albumin microspheres for localized angiogenesis: in vitro and in vivo studies, *Artif. Cells Blood Substitutes Immobilization Biotechnol.*, 24, 257, 1996.

68. Park, Y.J., Lee, Y.M., Park, S.N., Sheen, S.Y., Chung, C.P., and Lee, S.J., Platelet derived growth factor releasing chitosan sponge for periodontal bone regeneration, *Biomaterials*, 21, 2, 153, 2000.

69. Lee, J.Y., Nam, S.H., Im, S.Y., Park, Y.J., Lee, Y.M., Seol, Y.J., and Lee, S.J., Enhanced bone formation by controlled growth factor delivery from chitosan-based materials, *J. Controlled Release*, 78, 187, 2002.

70. Darr, J.A. and Poliakoff, M., New directions in inorganic and metal-organic coordination chemistry in supercritical fluids, *Chem. Rev.*, 99, 495, 1999.

71. Mehr, C.B., Biswal, R.N., Collins, J.L., and Cochran, H.D., Supercritical carbon dioxide extraction of caffeine from Guarana, *J. Supercritical Fluids*, 9, 185, 1996.

72. Woods, H.M., Silva, M.M.C.G., Nouvel, C., Shakesheff, K.M., and Howdle, S.M., Materials processing in supercritical carbon dioxide: surfactants, polymers and biomaterials, *J. Mater. Chem.*, 14, 1663, 2004.

73. Barry, J.A., Gidda, H.S., Scotchford, C.A., and Howdle, S.M., Porous methacrylate scaffolds: supercritical fluid fabrication and in vitro chondrocyte responses, *Biomaterials*, 25, 3559, 2004.

74. Singh, L., Kumar, V., and Ratner, B.D., Generation of porous microcellular 85/15 poly(DL-lactide-co-glycolide) foams for biomedical applications, *Biomaterials*, 25, 2611, 2004.

75. Kazarian, S.G., Polymer processing with supercritical fluids, *Polym. Sci.*, 42, 78, 2000.

76. Cooper, A.I., Polymer synthesis and processing using supercritical carbon dioxide, *J. Mater. Chem.*, 10, 207, 2000.

77. Shea, L.D., Smiley, E., Bonadio, J., and Mooney, D.J., DNA delivery from polymer matrices for tissue engineering, *Nat. Biotechnol.*, 17, 551, 1999.

78. Ledley, F.D., Pharmaceutical approach to somatic gene therapy, *Pharm. Res.*, 13, 1595, 1996.

79. Jang, J-H. and Shea, L.D., Controllable delivery of non-viral DNA from porous scaffolds, *J. Controlled Release*, 86, 157, 2003.

80. Yang, B.B., Whitaker, M.J., Sebald, W., Clarke, N., Howdle, S.M., Shakesheff, K.M., and Oreffo, R.O.C., Human osteoprogenitor bone formation using encapsulated BMP-2 in porous polymer scaffolds, *Tissue Eng.*, 10, 1037, 2004.

81. Cao, X. and Shoichet, M.S., Delivering neuroactive molecules from biodegradable microspheres for application in central nervous system disorders, *Biomaterials*, 20, 329, 1999.
82. Cleland, J.L., Duenas, E.T., Park, A., Daugherty, A., Kahn, J., Kowalski, J., and Cuthbertson, A., Development of poly(D,L-lactide-co-glycolide) microsphere formulations containing recombinant human vascular endothelial growth factor to promote local angiogenesis, *J. Controlled Release*, 72, 13, 2001.
83. Kim, T.K. and Burgess, D.J., Pharmokinetic characterization C-14-vascular endothelial growth factor controlled release microspheres using a rat model, *J. Pharm. Pharmacol.*, 54, 897, 2002.
84. Saltzman, W.M., Mak, M.W., Mahoney, M.J., Duenas, E.T., and Cleland, J.L., Intracranial delivery of recombinant nerve growth factor: Release kinetics and protein distribution for three delivery systems, *Pharm. Res.*, 16, 232, 1999.
85. Nof, M. and Shea, L.D., Drug-releasing scaffolds fabricated from drug-loaded microspheres, *J. Biomed. Mater. Res.*, 59, 349, 2002.
86. Harris, L.D., Kim, B.S., and Mooney, D.J., Open pore biodegradable matrices formed with gas foaming, *J. Biomed. Mater. Res.*, 42, 396, 1998.
87. Perets, A., Baruch, Y., Weisbuch, F., Shoshany, G., Neufield, G., and Cohen, S., Enhancing the vascularization of three-dimensional porous alginate scaffolds by incorporating controlled release basic fibroblast growth factor microspheres, *J. Biomed. Mater. Res. — Part A*, 65A, 489, 2003.
88. Chenite, A., Chaput, C., Wang, D., Combes, C., Buschmann, M.D., Hoemann, C.D., Leroux, J.C., Atkinson, B.L., Binette, F., and Selmani, A., Novel injectable neutral solutions of chitosan form biodegradable gels in situ, *Biomaterials*, 21, 2155, 2000.
89. Slepian, M.J. and Hubbell, J.A., Polymeric endoluminal gel paving: hydrogel systems for local barrier creation and site-specific drug delivery, *Adv. Drug Delivery Rev.*, 24, 11, 1997.
90. Bourke, S.L., Al-Khalili, M., Briggs, T., Michniak, B.B., Kohn, J., and Poole-Warren, L.A., A photo-crosslinked poly(vinyl alcohol) hydrogel growth factor release vehicle for wound healing applications, *AAPS PharmSci.*, 5, Article No. 33, 2003.
91. Han, D.K. and Hubbell, J.A., Lactide-based poly(ethylene glycol) polymer networks for scaffolds in tissue engineering, *Macromolecules*, 29, 523, 1996.
92. Han, D.K. and Hubbell, J.A., Synthesis of polymer network scaffolds from L-lactide and poly(ethylene glycol) and their interaction with cells, *Macromolecules*, 30, 6077, 1997.
93. Burdick, J.A., Mason, M.N., Hinman, A.D., Thorpe, K., and Anseth, K.S., Delivery of osteoinductive growth factors from degradable PEG hydrogels influences osteoblast differentiation and mineralization, *J. Controlled Release*, 83, 53, 2002.
94. Sakiyama-Elbert, S.E. and Hubbell, J.A., Development of fibrin derivatives for controlled release of heparin-binding growth factors, *J. Controlled Release*, 65, 389, 2000.
95. Sakiyama-Elbert, S.E. and Hubbell, J.A., Controlled release of nerve growth factor from a heparin-containing fibrin-based cell in-growth matrix, *J. Controlled Release*, 69, 149, 2000.
96. Lee, A.C., Yu, V.M., Lowe, J.B., Brenner, M.J., Hunter, D.A., Mackinnon, S.F., and Sakiyama-Elbert, S.E., Controlled release of nerve growth factor enhances sciatic nerve regeneration, *Exp. Neurol.*, 184, 295, 2003.
97. Giannoni, P. and Hunziker, E.B., Release kinetics of transforming growth factor-beta 1 from fibrin clots, *Biotechnol. Bioeng.*, 83, 1, 121, 2003.
98. Ehrbar, M., Djonov, V.G., Schnell, C., Tschanz, S.A., Martiny-Baron, G., Schenk, U., Wood, J., Burri, P.H., Hubbell, J.H., and Zisch, A.H., Cell-demanded liberation of VEGF(121) from fibrin implants induces local and controlled blood vessel growth, *Circ. Res.*, 94, 1124, 2004.
99. Lohmann, C.H., Schwartz, Z., Niederauer, G.G., Carnes, D.L., Dean, D.D., and Boyan, B.B., Pre-treatment with platelet derived growth factor-BB modulates the ability of costochondral resting zone chondrocytes incorporated into PLA/PGA scaffolds to form new cartilage in vivo, *Biomaterials*, 21, 49, 2000.
100. Park, Y.J., Lee, Y.M., Lee, J.Y., Seol, Y.J., Chung, C.P., and Lee, S.J., Controlled release of platelet-derived growth factor-BB from chondroitin sulfate-chitosan sponge for guided bone regeneration, *J. Controlled Release*, 67, 385, 2000.
101. Chen, G.P., Ito, Y., and Imanishi, Y., Photo-immobilization of epidermal growth factor enhances its mitogenic effect by artificial juxtacrine signalling, *Biochem. et Biophys. Acta —Mol. Cell Res.*, 1358, 200, 1997.

102. Von recum, H., Kikuchi, A., Yamato, M., Sakurai, Y., Okano, T., and Kim, S.W., Growth factor and matrix molecules preserve cell function on thermally responsive culture surfaces, *Tissue Eng.*, 5, 251, 1999.

103. Mooney, D.J., Kaufmann, P.M., Sano, K., Schwendeman, S.P., Majahod, K., Schloo, B., Vacanti, J.P., and Langer, R., Localized delivery of epidermal growth factor improves the survival of transplanted hepatocytes, *Biotechnol. Bioeng.*, 50, 422, 1996.

104. Krewson, C.E. and Saltzman, W.M., Transport and elimination of recombinant human NGF during long-term delivery to the brain, *Brain Res.*, 727, 169, 1996.

105. Partridge, K., Yang, X., Clarke, N.M.P., Okubu, Y., Bessho, K., Sebald, W., Howdle, S.M., Shakesheff, K.M., and Oreffo, R.O.C., Adenoviral BMP-2 gene transfer in mesenchymal stem cells: *in vitro* and *in vivo* bone formation on biodegradable polymer scaffolds, *Biochem. Biophys. Res. Commun.*, 292, 144, 2002.

106. Khang, G., Rhee, J.M., Shin, P., Kim, I.Y., Lee, B., Lee, S.J., Lee, Y.M., Lee, H.B., and Lee, I., Preparation and characterization of small intestine submucosa powder impregnated poly(L-lactide) scaffolds: The application for tissue engineered bone and cartilage, *Macromol. Res.*, 10, 158, 2002.

107. Sohier, J., Haan, R.E., de Groot, K., and Bezemer, J.M., A novel method to obtain protein release from porous polymer scaffolds: emulsion coating, *J. Controlled Release*, 87, 57, 2003.

108. Xiong, Z., Yan, Y., Wang, S., Zhang, R., and Zhang, C., Fabrication of porous scaffolds for bone tissue engineering via low-temperature deposition, *Scripta Mater.*, 46, 771, 2001.

109. Vozzi, G., Flaim, C.J., Bianchi, F., Ahluwalia, A., and Bhatia, S., Microfabricated PLGA scaffolds: a comparative study for application to tissue engineering, *Mater. Sci. Eng. C*, 20, 43, 2002.

110. Sundback, C., Hadlock, T., Cheney, M., and Vacanti, J., Manufacture of porous polymer nerve conduits by a novel low-pressure injection moulding process, *Biomaterials*, 24, 819, 2002.

7 Poly(lactic-*co*-glycolic acid) Microspheres

Camille Bouissou and Chris van der Walle

CONTENTS

7.1 INTRODUCTION

Poly(lactic-*co*-glycolic acid) microspheres have increasingly become the focus of research efforts in the scientific community and pharmaceutical industry. Their application as drug delivery vehicles has risen in line with the expanding biotechnology sector and the promise of new drugs discovered in the wake of the human genome project and proteomics. Commercial formulations employing poly(lactic acid) or poly(lactic-*co*-glycolic acid) matrices for drug delivery are growing in number, and this is expected to continue (Table 7.1). In this chapter we will focus on the encapsulation of recombinant DNA and protein drugs, although it should be borne in mind that there are many formulations of small organic molecules encapsulated in polyester microspheres.

The term *microsphere* as used in the following text refers to a small sphere with a porous inner matrix and variable surface — from smooth and porous to irregular and nonporous. The drug, when encapsulated, is dispersed throughout the inner matrix. The size range of microspheres is typically 1 to 500 μm in diameter. Alternative terms such as *microcapsules* and *microparticles* are also encountered in the literature, with *nanospheres* or *nanoparticles* referring to particles around 10 to 1000 nm in size.

7.2 CHEMISTRY AND PHYSICAL CHARACTERISTICS OF POLY(LACTIC-*CO*-GLYCOLIC ACID)

Many polymers have been utilized for the encapsulation and controlled release of various drugs. Examples of naturally-derived polymers include chitosan and alginate [1–3]. Synthetic examples include poly(alkylcyanoacrylates) [4], poly(anhydrides) [5], and polyesters. The polyesters

TABLE 7.1
Current Microsphere Formulations Encapsulating Polypeptides Approved for Use in Humans

Active Ingredient	Product Name	Polymer	Dosage/Drug Release (Months)
Leuprorelin acetate	Lupron Depot®	PLGA	3
Leuprorelin acetate	Prostap® 3	PLGA	3
Octreotide acetate	Sandostatin LAR®	PLGA-glucose	1
Somatropin (hGH)	Neutropin® Depot	PLGA	0.5
Somatropin (hGH)	Ascentra™	PLGA-PEG[a]	1
Triptorelin pamoate	Trelstar™ Depot	PLGA	1
Triptorelin pamoate	Decapeptyl®	PLGA	1
Lanreotide acetate	Somatuline® LA	PLGA	0.5

[a] Polyethylene glycol

include poly(e-caprolactone) [6], poly(lactic acid) or poly(lactide) (PLA), and poly(lactic-*co*-glycolic acid) or poly(lactide-*co*-glycolide) (PLGA or PLG, respectively). PLA and especially PLGA are most commonly employed in the fabrication of microspheres and will be the focus of the discussion here. The important characteristic of these polymers is that they are biodegradable and biocompatible, having low immunogenicity and toxicity [7]. The attraction of PLGA in particular is its established use in humans (Table 7.1 and Reference 8), thereby minimizing acceptance procedures by the regulatory bodies. PLGA is also finding an expanded role in tissue engineering because it has good mechanical properties and predictable biodegradation kinetics [9–11].

A wide range of molecular weights of PLGA are described for the fabrication of microspheres. For a certain batch of PLGA obtained or synthesized, this can either be determined by gel-permeation chromatography or derived from the inherent viscosity. PLGA is synthesized by ring-opening of lactic acid and glycolic acid monomers and linkage via ester bonds (Figure 7.1). The molar ratio and

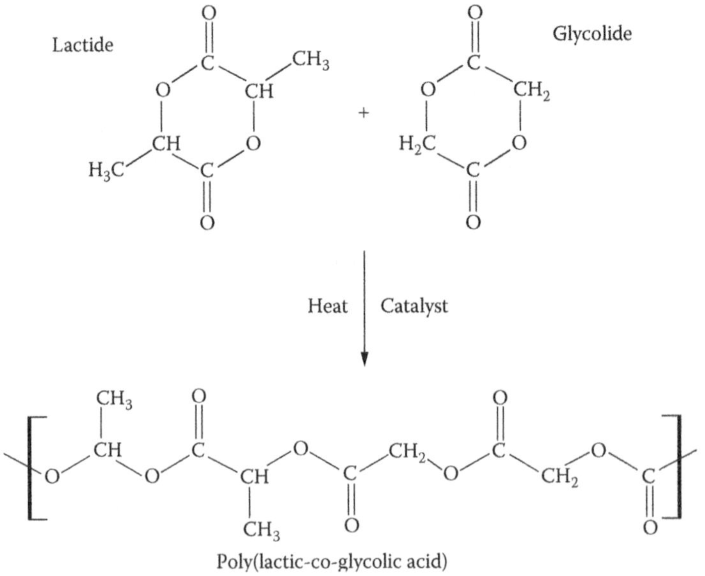

FIGURE 7.1 Synthesis of poly(lactic-*co*-glycolic acid).

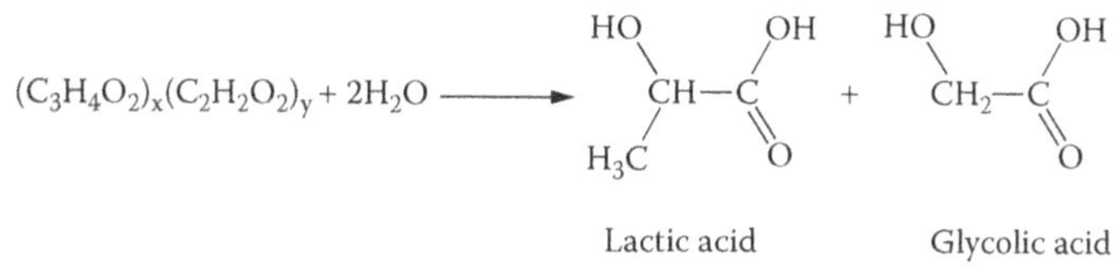

$$(C_3H_4O_2)_x(C_2H_2O_2)_y + 2H_2O \longrightarrow$$

Lactic acid   Glycolic acid

FIGURE 7.2 Hydrolytic degradation of the poly(lactic-*co*-glycolic acid) chain.

sequential arrangement of lactide–glycolide units determine the physicochemical properties of the copolymer. Lactic acid can exist in both L and D stereoisomers, and whereas the L isomer occurs *in vivo*, D,L-lactic acid is often used in synthesis. The packing arrangement of the D,L-lactic acid chains is disordered with respect to L-lactic acid and is further perturbed on introduction of glycolic acid [11]. Poly(D,L-lactic acid) and PLGA containing less than 85% glycolide (with D,L lactide) are amorphous, whereas poly(glycolic acid) and poly(L-lactic acid) are crystalline. Solvation in organic solvent is also dependent on the lactide:glycolide ratio because the lactide is more hydrophobic than glycolide [12]; a 50:50 ratio is commonly used in microsphere fabrication.

On exposure of PLGA microspheres to an aqueous environment, degradation of PLGA occurs through hydrolysis of the ester linkages (Figure 7.2) [13]. Lactic acid and glycolic acid are freed and eliminated from the body solely by metabolism and exhalation as carbon dioxide and water in the case of lactic acid or in combination with direct excretion via the kidneys in the case of glycolic acid [14,15]. In respect of the internal environment of the microsphere during degradation, the entrapped drug experiences a considerable drop in pH, which may result in chemical and/or physical instability [16]. Degradation also occurs during γ radiation, which may be used as a method of terminal sterilization of the product, and this influences drug release rates [17]. It is easy to assume that the release of drug from the matrix can be controlled simply by changing the rate of bulk erosion, but, for reasons outlined in the following sections, this is generally not the case.

PLGA hydrolysis increases as the amorphous content of the copolymer increases [18]. If the temperature to which the microspheres are exposed is greater than the glass transition temperature (Tg) of the amorphous copolymer, then degradation is further increased [19]. Tg is an important property of all amorphous polymers such as PLGA and needs to be considered in the context of product storage, transportation, and drug release mechanisms. For PLGA, Tg increases with increasing molecular weight and lactide content (around 40 to 50°C), and so low-molecular-weight PLGA (14 kDa, 50:50 lactide:glycolide) has a Tg around body temperature. Tg can be observed as a transition in the heat capacity of a polymer during heating and is distinct from melting, which is exhibited by crystalline substances. Physically, the polymer chains exist in a "glassy state" below the Tg and in a "rubbery state" above. The mechanical strength of the microsphere therefore falls abruptly above the Tg, and the same consideration also needs to be given to the structure of its internal porous matrix. As water penetrates the microsphere, the Tg of the polymer gradually decreases, initiating a rapid increase in chain mobility, water uptake, and drug release [20]. Similarly, residual water within the microspheres remaining after freeze-drying or acquired during storage lowers the Tg of PLGA [21].

7.3 FABRICATION OF PLGA MICROSPHERES

A number of encapsulation techniques have been developed, and selection of one over the other depends on the nature of the polymer and the properties of the drug. With respect to proteins and DNA, the two following criteria must be observed whatever the technique: (1) the biological activity must not be altered and (2) the size of the spheres has to support the intended administration route: this may be from 3 μm for inhalation to submicron sizes for intravenous injection, including sizes below 100 nm if the particles are intended to be taken up by the cell via the process of endocytosis.

There are four key fabrication techniques, which are described in the following subsections.

7.3.1 EMULSION–SOLVENT EVAPORATION

For single oil-in-water (o/w) emulsions or solid-in-oil-in-water (s/o/w) emulsions, the solvent evaporation from the continuous (aqueous) phase results in PLGA precipitation and microsphere hardening, simultaneously encapsulating the drug in the internal matrix [22,23]. In the case of water-in-oil-in-water (w/o/w) double emulsions (Figure 7.3), extraction of the dichloromethane into the second aqueous phase leads to rapid formation of microspheres, the secondary emulsion being transient [24]. In these emulsions, dichloromethane (methylene chloride) is generally used in preference to ethyl acetate as the oil phase on account of its better solubilization of PLGA 50:50 lactide:glycolide, higher volatility, and better compatibility with steel (homogenizer parts). PLGA is dissolved in the oil phase at a concentration typically around 5 to 10% w/v, and the drug may either be dissolved in dichloromethane, in aqueous solution, or micronized and suspended in either phase. Double-walled microspheres, wherein two distinct polyesters form the inner core and outer layer, respectively, have been fabricated [25,26]. An elegant "one-pot" approach has been utilization of the differential phase separation behaviour of PLA and PLGA during the solvent evaporation step [27].

Stability of the primary emulsion prior to solvent extraction and evaporation is critical to the successful encapsulation of drug in microspheres [28]. The stabilizer polyvinyl alcohol (PVA) is most commonly used, although nonionic surfactants and triblock copolymers may be more useful for certain protein formulations [29]. Solvent extraction and evaporation (microsphere hardening) is continued for 4 to 16 h to ensure near-complete removal of the toxic organic solvent. Hardened microspheres are then harvested by centrifugation or filtration and washed. Protein-loaded or DNA-loaded microspheres are generally dried to minimize degradation of both the polymer and drug.

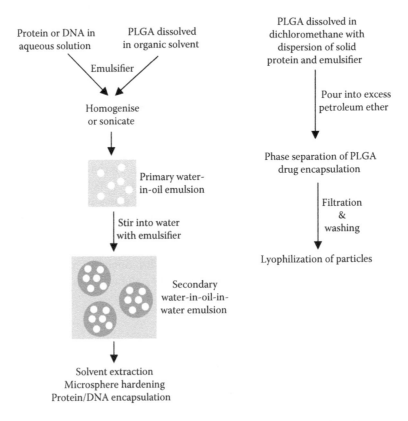

FIGURE 7.3 Overview of w/o/w emulsion solvent extraction (left) and phase inversion nanoencapsulation protocols (right) commonly used in PLGA microsphere fabrication.

However, it should not be automatically assumed that lyophilized proteins are more stable than when in aqueous solution [30]. Drying is most commonly achieved by snap-freezing in liquid nitrogen and lyophilizing overnight.

Although this is the most commonly reported technique, probably because of its apparent simplicity, one needs to be aware that there is often little consensus between published protocols. Nevertheless, the physical and chemical processes underlying microsphere morphology are becoming apparent and these are discussed in Section 7.4.

7.3.2 Coacervation and Phase Inversion Nanoencapsulation

Coacervation starts with a solid dispersed-in-oil or water-in-oil emulsion, the drug being in the dispersed phase and the polymer dissolved in the continuous phase (dichloromethane or ethyl acetate). A nonsolvent such as silicone oil is then added to extract the dichloromethane from the polymer phase, causing precipitation of the polymer. The nonsolvent is then removed by addition of a second volatile solvent such as heptane or petroleum ether, which facilitates microsphere hardening. Microspheres are harvested and dried after removal of excess solvent [31]. Phase inversion nanoencapsulation is similar to coacervation but with the primary dispersion or emulsion being simply poured into petroleum ether without stirring, causing phase separation of the polymer and microparticle formation (Figure 7.3) [6].

7.3.3 Spray-Drying

Spray-drying requires fine control of air flow and inlet and outlet air temperatures. Quite simply, the drug is emulsified or dispersed in a solution of polymer in volatile solvent (e.g., dichloromethane) and then spray-dried through a small nozzle [32].

7.3.4 The Use of Supercritical Carbon Dioxide

This is an interesting, emerging technique wherein microspheres can be formed via the following: (1) solution-enhanced dispersion by supercritical fluids (SEDS), which still requires initial solubilization of PLGA in dichloromethane before spraying through a nozzle [33], (2) rapid expansion from supercritical solution with a nonsolvent (RESS-N), in which drug and polymer are dissolved in supercritical CO_2 with the aid of a low-molecular-weight alcohol as cosolvent and then sprayed through a nozzle [34], and (3) liquefied PLGA in supercritical CO_2 at room temperature mixed with drug and then sprayed into a chamber to form particles, the reduced temperatures attenuating thermally induced protein unfolding [35]. The latter method is likely to gain wider acceptance because there is no need to use a toxic solvent and the technique is also applicable for the production of three-dimensional foams [36].

7.4 MORPHOLOGICAL CHARACTERISTICS OF MICROSPHERES

During the microsphere fabrication process, even slight changes in the protocol can have radical effects on the morphology of the resulting spheres. Indeed, reproducibility is hard to achieve when working at small (milligram) scales. External morphology is defined by the size, external porosity, and surface roughness, whereas internal morphology is defined by the matrix porosity and connectivity. Morphological studies aid our comprehension of the fabrication process (e.g., emulsion stability) and also impinge on the intended medical application (e.g., aerosols). Several techniques are used for analysis of microsphere morphology (Table 7.2). These techniques are commonly reported in the literature, particularly for manufacture of emulsion extraction, which will be the focus here. Other manufacturing techniques result in somewhat different morphologies on comparison [37].

TABLE 7.2
Techniques Commonly Used for the Visualization of Microsphere Morphology and Measurement of Porosity

External Morphology		Internal Morphology	
Overall shape	Scanning electron microscopy (SEM)	Overall shape	SEM and cryo-SEM (freeze-fracture)
Size	SEM and light scattering	Pore size	TEM and cryo-SEM
Surface topography	Atomic force microscopy (AFM)	Drug (fluorescent) distribution	Confocal laser scanning microscopy (CLSM)
External porosity	SEM or dye encapsulation	Porosity (for pores of radius <10 μm)	Mercury porosimetry

Both the primary and secondary emulsion steps determine microsphere size, as well as drug loading and release. The ternary composition (oil, water, and stabilizer) of the primary emulsion is of key importance with regard to viscosity and stability. For instance, high oil-phase volumes, the addition of gelatin, or increasing the PLGA concentration lead to more viscous emulsions that are less easy to break by homogenization, thus producing bigger spheres [38,39]. On the contrary, low-molecular-weight PLGA diminishes the oil-phase or emulsion viscosity and reduces microsphere size [40]. However, increasing the drug-to-PLGA ratio only slightly increases microsphere size, whereas use of nonionic surfactants within the inner aqueous phase, rather than PVA (at equivalent concentrations), has a negligible effect on microsphere size [29,41,42]. In respect of the secondary emulsion, microsphere size reduces significantly when the PVA concentration is increased, higher stirring speeds (or sonication) are used, or the volume of the outer water phase is reduced [43]. Solvent extraction is further influenced by temperature: high temperatures (>40°C) promote solvent evaporation from the embryonic microspheres such that PLGA precipitates almost instantaneously without shrinking [44].

External (surface) porosity regulates water inflow and outflow and drug release during incubation, although it is less clear whether the drug entrapment is affected [44,45]. It has been determined that the formation of the surface pores originates from water mobility between inner and outer phases under osmotic pressure, pore size and number increasing with increasing osmotic potential of the inner water phase, e.g., with increasing drug-to-PLGA ratios [37]. External porosity is further influenced by the PLGA concentration, the volume of the inner water phase, and substitution of nonionic surfactants for PVA [46] (cf. Figures 7.4a and 7.4b). The same parameters also influence surface roughness, which has application to aerosol delivery (corrugated particles having lower powder cohesiveness), and the adhesion of microspheres to the intestine's Peyer's patches [47,48]. In particular, the addition of nonionic surfactants to the primary emulsion changes surface roughness according to the hydrophile–lipophile balance [29].

Internal porosity is defined by the spherical cavities dispersed in the polymeric matrix and their connectivity (Figure 7.4c). A more homogeneous pore network also allows the drug to be more evenly dispersed across the matrix, and in turn this appears to cause a weaker initial burst release [39,44]. It is not clear if the internal morphology influences the escape of PLGA fragments during hydrolysis, even though this would naturally determine the extent of the pH drop within the matrix [49,50]. Internal pores are created during solvent evaporation and PLGA precipitation, and their size and homogeneity are dependent on the stability of the primary emulsion: the larger the water droplet size, the larger the internal cavities [28,51]. High shear, the addition of surfactant, low oil phase volume, and low-molecular-weight PLGA during the primary emulsion tend to decrease the size of the internal pores while improving their homogeneity. However, if fabrication occurs at low temperatures, the solvent evaporates slowly and the outer shell of the embryonic microspheres pushes the inner water droplets toward the soft core as it hardens, facilitating droplet coalescence [44].

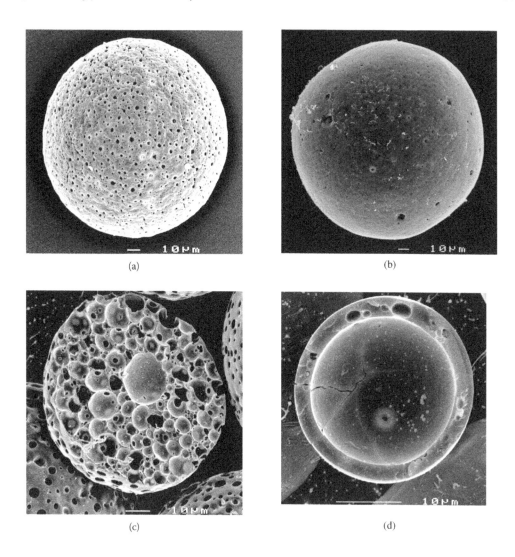

FIGURE 7.4 Scanning electron microscope images of the external morphology for microspheres fabricated using (a) PVA and (b) Pluronic F68 in the primary emulsion; and the internal morphology for microspheres fabricated from stable (c) and unstable (d) primary emulsions.

Pore connectivity regulates drug diffusion, a low density of interconnecting channels resulting in a slower drug release. The origin of the connecting channels is less clear, but the partial coalescence of very small droplets may evolve into cylinders during solvent removal and may also be influenced by the drug itself [46]. Encapsulation of proteins complicates interpretation of data because proteins are themselves surface-active molecules. However, one report suggests that high-molecular-weight proteins (> 200 kDa) are distributed at the surface of the microsphere, whereas low-molecular-weight proteins are more evenly spread throughout the sphere. Further, a more homogeneous porous network is created throughout the matrix when small proteins are loaded [52].

7.5 DEGRADATION AND EROSION OF MICROSPHERES

Degradation of microspheres and drug release are interdependent [53]. There exist two possibilities regarding the rate of degradation of the polymer; either this is faster than the water uptake into the matrix, which then dilapidates only at the surface (surface erosion), or the water rapidly penetrates the whole structure before surface erosion begins (bulk erosion) [54]. In the case of surface erosion, the slow ingress of the water results in its heterogeneous dispersion throughout the matrix during which erosion operates at a constant velocity, leading to a reduction in the diameter size. In the case of bulk erosion, the water homogeneously disperses throughout the matrix such that the sphere tends to maintain its original size for longer while eroding from within, the erosion kinetics being biphasic (Figure 7.5) [20,55]. It has been determined that in the case of PLGA, surface erosion occurs only above pH 13 or with extremely large spheres or discs [54]. Therefore, an understanding of the bulk erosion process would appear to be more relevant than surface erosion to drug delivery scenarios employing microspheres at physiological pHs. Further, although it may be assumed that chain hydrolysis leads to an immediate loss of mass, this is not the case despite an instantaneous loss in PLGA molecular weight. Two concepts were introduced to explain this: "degradation," which is a loss in the molecular weight of the PLGA chains, and "erosion," which is a loss in mass of the microsphere [56].

Degradation occurs via random hydrolysis, cutting the polymeric chain into segments of various sizes and solubility. At this stage, the molecular weight of the PLGA decreases while the microsphere's

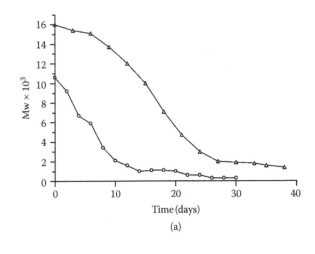

(a)

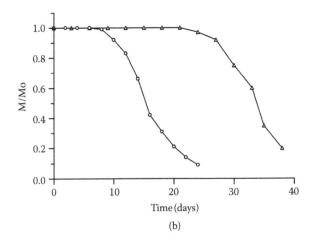

(b)

FIGURE 7.5 Degradation (a) vs. erosion (b) of poly(α-hydroxy esters) at pH 2 ($\bigcirc$ = PLGA 8000 Mw, $\triangle$ = PLGA 14000 Mw end capped; M/Mo = mass/mass at time 0; PLGA lactide:glycolide molar ratio = 1:1). (From von Burkersroda, F., Schedl, L., and Gopferich, A., Why degradable polymers undergo surface erosion or bulk erosion, *Biomaterials*, 23, 4221–4231, 2002.)

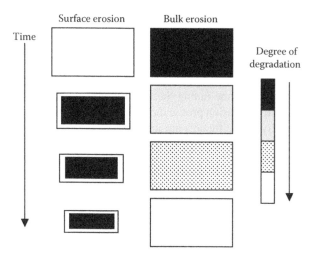

FIGURE 7.6 Schematic illustration of the changes a polymer matrix undergoes during surface erosion and bulk erosion. (From von Burkersroda, F., Schedl, L., and Gopferich, A., Why degradable polymers undergo surface erosion or bulk erosion, *Biomaterials*, 23, 4221–4231, 2002.)

mass remains unchanged. The diffusion of these segments out of the matrix is limited by their size relative to the pore diameter and tortuosity [45]. However, it is assumed that segmentation leads to the expansion of the inner cavities and accumulation of acidic products, reducing the pH and enhancing hydrolysis further by a phenomenon known as *autocatalysis*. Eventually, when the inner cavities become connected to the outer pores and the water-soluble polymers are small enough, diffusion drives the fragments to the external medium. Only then does the sphere demonstrate a mass loss, i.e., it erodes (Figure 7.6).

Data acquired for microsphere erosion and degradation must be analyzed bearing in mind the limitations and inaccuracy of the methodology employed. Similarly, protein-release data, generally produced by the same method of incubation, do not entirely reflect reality [41,57]. In general, microspheres are incubated into a predefined volume of release medium (e.g., phosphate-buffered saline with a preservative such as sodium azide and occasionally a surfactant), which may itself enhance autocatalysis. Even if the buffer is replenished frequently, the enclosed conditions do not allow the rapid removal of the acidic products released by erosion, and in this case the pH values vary according to the size of the spheres [50]. Unfortunately, the complexity of the parameters involved makes it difficult to find an appropriate protocol.

Control and prediction of the degradation–erosion mechanism is important if we are to be able to influence the "burst release" of drug from microspheres, an issue which is under investigation in the field. Approaches aimed at controlling release generally focus on the polymer itself: stability of the ester bond, hydrophobicity, steric effects, autocatalysis, and Tg (discussed earlier) [56,58,59]. All these variables are essentially determined by the PLA:PGA molecular ratio and sequential arrangement, chain length, and capping of the terminal carboxyl groups. Undoubtedly, one must choose the best type of PLGA in accordance with the expected profile. For instance, a PLGA with a lactic acid:glycolic acid ratio of 75:25 exhibits a longer degradation than a PLGA with a lactic acid:glycolic acid ratio of 50:50 because of ester bonds neighboring glycolic acid units have a high hydrolytic reactivity. Similarly, it is known that the scission of the chain end is faster than the degradation of the internal bonds. Consequently, end-capping the polymer with a lactic acid ethyl ester in contrast to the free COOH terminal delays degradation. Direct conjugation of the polymeric backbone to a drug via covalent bonds has been studied, wherein the drug–PLGA conjugate is processed into microspheres and drug release controlled by polymer degradation [60]. Similarly, drugs encapsulated into microspheres fabricated from PLGA conjugated to polyvinyl alcohol (PVA) or polyethylene glycol (PEG) have a lower initial burst release [61,62].

Ideally, given certain factors such as the microsphere morphology, the molecular weight and composition of the polymer, it should be possible to simulate the degradation–erosion mechanism and achieve the desired profile by fine-tuning these parameters. Several mathematical models for the prediction of the degradation–erosion profile have been proposed [53–56,63–65]. Unfortunately, the accuracy and applicability of the models are unreliable. This may be not so much through the fault of the model *per se* but rather due to experimental difficulties in acquiring unambiguous data for the multitude of parameters that must be taken into account. So far, no mathematical model has succeeded in conforming closely to the observed data, although work on this continues.

7.6 PROTEIN AND DNA ENCAPSULATION AND RELEASE

Microspheres encapsulating oligonucleotides, proteins, and DNA are often fabricated via w/o/w double emulsions [66–68]. However, there does appear to be a trend towards using s/o/w emulsions or phase inversion nanoencapsulation for lyophilized proteins suspended in the oil phase on grounds of reduced "stress" and loss of activity [69,70]. Whatever the method employed, optimization will be required, which can be time consuming given the number of variables. Drug loss occurs mainly during emulsion, particularly for w/o/w emulsions, but also during microsphere hardening and washing [71]. Protein or DNA loss may be quite severe, although encapsulation efficiencies of around 90% have been reported for model proteins such as lysozyme and bovine serum albumin (BSA) [72]. Emulsification is the primary driving force behind peptide backbone unfolding because proteins are essentially amphipathic and migrate to water–air or water–solvent interfaces [73–75]. Loss of structural integrity of labile proteins can be exacerbated by local rises in temperature during homogenization, particularly by sonication. Protein aggregation may occur during emulsification, concomitant with structural changes in the solid state seen by infrared spectroscopy [76,77]. The DNA or protein may further suffer subtle physical and chemical changes, resulting in loss of biological activity [29,78]; this is especially true for proteins given their exquisite structure–activity relationships. Also, there is a need to avoid an immune response to nonnative folding of polypeptide chains.

Much of our understanding of protein encapsulation rests with the use of BSA or lysozyme as "model proteins." However, it is often overlooked that lysozyme has an unusually stable three-dimensional conformation and high isoelectric point of pH 11 [79], and BSA is itself a protein emulsifier owing to its amphipathic alpha helical structure [80]. In both cases this is somewhat unfortunate because neither is especially characteristic of labile proteins such as immunoglobulins, which are particularly targeted in drug development. Nevertheless, fluorescent labeling of such model proteins has been particularly useful for the visualization of drug distribution within the microsphere. Images are acquired using confocal laser scanning microscopy (CLSM), which effectively scans the microsphere in the z axis ("slicing" across) such that the images are complementary to those acquired for the internal porous matrix by scanning electron microscopy (Figure 7.7) [39,42].

To develop an efficacious drug formulation, knowledge of the release profile of the drug from the polymeric matrix is critical. Although PLGA microspheres are purported to facilitate a steady, prolonged release of protein, this is generally not the case. The biggest problem in this respect is the so-called "burst release," wherein around 60 to 80% of the protein load is released within the first 24 h [45]. With reference to the CSLM images for fluorescent protein in microspheres, the majority of the protein is seen to be dispersed within the pores of the matrix with the remainder within the PLGA matrix itself. The burst release is therefore thought to arise from proteins loosely associated within the porous network of the microsphere matrix. However, this has not been unequivocally proven despite studies aiming to mathematically model the erosion, pore tortuosity, water diffusivity, and, ultimately, drug release [55,81]. Following burst release, the rate of drug release drops dramatically, which continues for 4 to

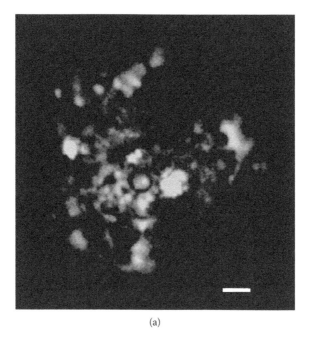

(a)

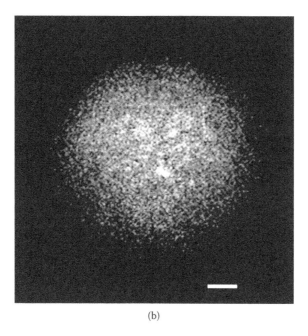

(b)

FIGURE 7.7 An equatorial "slice" of two PLGA microsphere (~100-mm diameter) formulations encapsulating (a) FITC-labeled FIII9'-10 (From Bouissou, C., Potter, U., Altroff, H., Mardon, H., and van der Walle, C., Controlled release of the fibronectin central cell binding domain from polymeric microspheres, *J. Controlled Release*, 95, 557–566, 2004.) and (b) FITC-labeled lysozyme as imaged by CLSM. Light-shaded areas indicate distribution of labeled protein, showing outlines of, and deposition within, the internal pores. Bar = 10 μm.

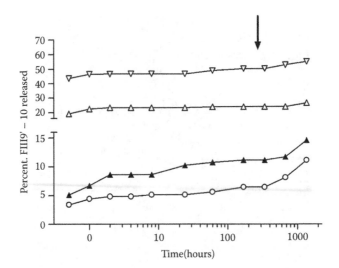

FIGURE 7.8 Cumulative *in vitro* release profiles for FIII9'-10 over an eight-week period, expressed as the percentage of the theoretical load. The curves represent the means of four microsphere preparations but standard error bars are omitted for clarity. Symbols relate to the surfactant added to the primary emulsion: ▲ = Tween 20, ○ = Tween 80, ∇ = Igepal CA-630, △ = PVA. Arrow indicates general onset of the second phase of protein release. (From Bouissou, C., Potter, U., Altroff, H., Mardon, H., and van der Walle, C., Controlled release of the fibronectin central cell binding domain from polymeric microspheres, *J. Controlled Release*, 95, 557–566, 2004.)

8 weeks before a small second release phase is observed, which is common (Figure 7.8). The influence of protein charge, shape, and molecular weight is not clear and difficult to deconvolute experimentally. The release rate has also been demonstrated to depend on the molecular weight of PLGA, which appears to correlate with the Tg and degradation rate of the polymer [52]. The rationale in the fabrication of double-walled microspheres has primarily been to attenuate the burst release and/or allow a pulsatile release profile [26]. Essentially, this is achieved by differential erosion of the outer coating relative to the inner core, although this is of course dependent on the distribution of protein [27]. Nominally, it may be possible to have some control of this process and thus design double-walled microspheres with a pulsatile release that may be of use in vaccine formulation.

There are fewer studies of DNA encapsulation in PLGA microspheres, probably because gene delivery has focused on the development of cationic polymers and lipids. Although there are reports of effective gene delivery via microspheres [82], the focus has turned to the development of DNA vaccines [83]. DNA appears to be less efficiently encapsulated than protein, particularly naked DNA, and condensation of DNA with polyamine prior to encapsulation is favorable [68]. Nevertheless, DNA can be encapsulated in PLGA nanospheres (preferably around 100-nm diameter or less) in quantities sufficient to facilitate protein expression subsequent to cellular uptake of PLGA nano-particles via endocytosis, at least *in vitro* [84].

If the intention is to release DNA within the cell for protein vaccine synthesis, then the nucleus is the target site. Release profiles determined for near-sink conditions in aqueous solution are of little relevance. Rather, the migration of the microsphere within the cell following endocytosis is of as much importance as the migration of DNA in the crowded intracellular environment [85]. Uptake via clathrin- or calveolin-mediated endocytosis generally leads to processing via various stages of endosomes and finally the lysosome [86]. The increasing acidic and lytic environments would be deleterious to entrapped DNA; however, it appears that PLGA microspheres escape the endosome rapidly [87]. This is of advantage if the DNA can then escape the microsphere and enter the nucleus for transcription.

7.7 CLINICAL APPLICATIONS EMPLOYING PLGA-ENCAPSULATED PROTEIN OR DNA

Much of this work aims at the development of vaccines or formulations aiding cancer therapy. For example, the cytokine interleukin-12 has been encapsulated and injected intratumorally to tumor-bearing mice [88]. This treatment resulted in tumor regression and metastatic suppression, and of note was that a subsequent systemic immunity arose as a consequence of the formulation (Table 7.3). Improved immune responses to antibody vaccines have also been observed with a breast cancer antibody encapsulated with monophosphoryl lipid A in microspheres [89]. Although this formulation showed promise as a breast cancer treatment, repeated administration in mice was required before tumor regression was observed. Advantages in coencapsulating antigens currently in clinical use in PLGA microspheres have also been observed [90]. Whereas this was attributed in part to a mutual stabilization between the antigens, the microspheres themselves are suggested to be an effective, alternative vaccine adjuvant [91]. The application of such vaccines to immunization against malaria has not gone unnoticed but is unlikely to provide a solution by itself. SPf66 malaria vaccines, encapsulated in PLGA microspheres as single-dose immunizations, have been employed in studies using monkeys and mice. These yielded strong immune responses and offered some protection against blood parasites after repeated clinical challenges [92].

As a demonstration of DNA encapsulation into PLGA nanoparticles, delivery of plasmid DNA encoding the p53 tumor suppressor gene resulted in marked reduction in the proliferation of breast cancer cells [93]. The formulation was shown to be superior to DNA complexation with a cationic polymer, and this may be as a result of favorable release kinetics from the endosome following cell uptake. An exciting use of DNA-loaded PLGA microspheres remains in genetic vaccination, and this work has been steadily gaining momentum. To this aim, poly(ortho ester) (POE) substitutes for PLGA have been synthesized, which predominantly undergo surface erosion (to minimize acidic products) and degrade most rapidly below pH 7 (as in the lysosome). Uptake of DNA-POE particles by antigen-presenting cells in mice stimulated primary and secondary humoral and cellular immune responses, wherein the polymer type used allowed DNA to be released in synchrony with these

---

TABLE 7.3
The Potency of the Protective Antitumor Immunity Induced by the Il-12-Loaded Microspheres Is Dependent on the Vaccination Method

Method of Vaccination	Percentage of Tumors Rejected after Challenge[a]
Established tumor + IL-12 microspheres[b]	80 (12 of 15)
Live line-1 cells[c] + IL-12 microspheres[d]	57 (8 of 14)
Irradiated line-1 cells + IL-12 microspheres[e]	10 (1 of 10)
Irradiated line-1 cells alone	10 (1 of 10)
No treatment	0 (0 of 5)

[a]Mice challenged with 1×10^4 tumor cells injected subcutaneously
[b]Tumor injected with 2 mg of microspheres
[c]Lung alveola cell carcinoma cell line
[d]1×10^6 tumor cells + 50 μg of microspheres
[e]2×10^6 tumor cells + 50 μg of microspheres

Source: From Egilmez, N.K., Jong, Y.S., Sabel, M.S., Jacob, J.S., Mathiowitz, E., Bankert, R.B., In situ tumor vaccination with interleukin-12-encapsulated biodegradable microspheres: induction of tumor regression and potent antitumor immunity, *Cancer Res.*, 60, 3832–3837, 2000.

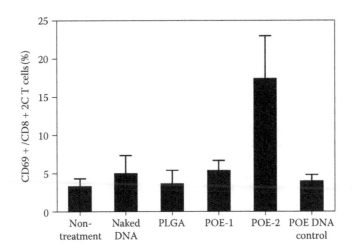

FIGURE 7.9 Secondary T-cell response assayed three days after challenging mice with the peptide antigen SIYRYYGL (single-letter amino acid notation, specific for CD8 + T cells expressing a T-cell receptor called 2C). Each error bar represents the standard error between two mice. POEs were composed from 3,9-diethylidene-2,4,8,10-tetraoxaspiro[5.5]undecane (DETOSU) with various diols and a small amount of triethylene glygol glycolide. POE-2 differed from POE-1 by the addition of *N*-methyldiethanolamine to impart a positive charge at pH 5. (From Wang, C., Ge, Q., Ting, D., Nguyen, D., Shen, H.R., Chen, J.Z., Eisen, H.N., Heller, J., Langer, R., and Putnam, D., Molecularly engineered poly(ortho ester) microspheres for enhanced delivery of DNA vaccines, *Nat. Mater.*, 3, 190–196, 2004.)

events (Figure 7.9) [94]. Characterization of microspheres encapsulating an antisense oligonucleotide against the transforming growth factor beta-1 has also been made, although clinical evaluation of the formulation is yet to be performed [95].

PLGA microspheres have further been applied as ultrasound contrast agents [96]. With the surface of the microspheres appropriately modified to target cancer cells, it should be possible to highlight either benign or malignant cancerous tissue. The critical component in this case is the surface moiety that targets, say, a characteristic cell membrane receptor, and so far only peptides have been investigated. However, the surface of microspheres can be derivatized in various manners with proteins; therefore, in principle, this method could be applied to immunoglobulins [97].

7.8 CONCLUDING REMARKS

In summary, the continued study of the underlying mechanisms of PLGA encapsulation of drugs into microspheres is likely to lead to this formulation route becoming routinely employed for drug delivery. The potential applications are broad-ranging, and in some cases may replace the more established liposomal and microemulsion systems. Of particular promise is the use of PLGA microspheres for the formulation of therapeutic proteins and vaccines.

REFERENCES

1. Yoshino, T., Machida, Y., Onishi, H., and Nagai, T., Preparation and characterization of chitosan microspheres containing doxifluridine, *Drug Dev. Ind. Pharm.*, 29, 417–427, 2003.
2. Gombotz, W.R. and Wee, S.F., Protein release from alginate matrices, *Adv. Drug Delivery Rev.*, 31, 267–285, 1998.
3. Berthold, A., Cremer, K., and Kreuter, J., Preparation and characterization of chitosan microspheres as drug carrier for prednisolone sodium phosphate as model for antiinflammatory drugs, *J. Controlled Release*, 39, 17–25, 1996.

4. Couvreur, P., Polyalkylcyanoacrylates as colloidal drug carriers, *CRC Crit. Rev. Ther. Drug Carrier Syst.*, 5, 1–20, 1988.
5. Shen, E., Kipper, M.J., Dziadul, B., Lim, M.K., and Narasimhan, B., Mechanistic relationships between polymer microstructure and drug release kinetics in bioerodible polyanhydrides, *J. Controlled Release*, 82, 115–125, 2002.
6. Mathiowitz, E., Jacob, J.S., Jong, Y.S., Carino, G.P., Chickering, D.E., Chaturvedi, P., Santos, C.A., Vija-yaraghavan, K., Montgomery, S., Bassett, M., and Morrell, C., Biologically erodable microspheres as potential oral drug delivery systems, *Nature*, 386, 410–414, 1997.
7. Anderson, J.M. and Shive, M.S., Biodegradation and biocompatibility of PLA and PLGA micro-spheres, *Adv. Drug Delivery Rev.*, 28, 5–24, 1997.
8. Reed, A.M. and Gilding, D.K., Biodegradable polymers for use in surgery: poly(glycolic)/poly(lactic acid) homo and co-polymers. 2. Invitro degradation, *Polymer*, 22, 494–498, 1981.
9. Karp, J.M., Shoichet, M.S., and Davies, J.E., Bone formation on two-dimensional (D,L-lactide-co-glycolide) (PLGA) films and three-dimensional PLGA tissue engineering scaffolds in vitro, *J. Biomed. Mater. Res.*, Part A, 64A, 388–396, 2003.
10. Beumer, G.J., Vanblitterswijk, C.A., and Ponec, M., Degradative behavior of polymeric matrices in (sub)dermal and muscle-tissue of the rat — a quantitative study, *Biomaterials*, 15, 551–559, 1994.
11. Engelberg, I. and Kohn, J., Physicomechanical properties of degradable polymers used in medical applications — a comparative-study, *Biomaterials*, 12, 292–304, 1991.
12. Bodmeier, R. and Mcginity, J.W., Solvent selection in the preparation of poly(D,L-Lactide) micro-spheres prepared by the solvent evaporation method, *Int. J. Pharm.*, 43, 179–186, 1988.
13. Spenlehauer, G., Vert, M., Benoit, J.P., and Boddaert, A., Invitro and invivo degradation of poly(D,L-lactide glycolide) type microspheres made by solvent evaporation method, *Biomaterials*, 10, 557–563, 1989.
14. Brady, J.M., Cutright, D.E., Miller, R.A., and Barristone, G.C., Resorption rate, route of elimination and ultrastructure of the implant site of polylactic acid in the abdominal wall of the rat, *J. Biomed. Mater. Res.*, 7, 155–166, 1973.
15. Thanoo, B.C., Doll, W.J., Mehta, R.C., Digenis, G.A., and DeLuca, P.P., Biodegradable indium-111 labeled microspheres for in vivo evaluation of distribution and elimination, *Pharm. Res.*, 12, 2060–2064, 1995.
16. Zhu, G., Mallery, S.R., and Schwendeman, S.P., Stabilization of proteins encapsulated in injectable poly (lactide-co-glycolide), *Nat. Biotechnol.*, 18, 52–57, 2000.
17. Yoshioka, S., Aso, Y., and Kojima, S., Drug release from poly(dl-lactide) microspheres controlled by gamma-irradiation, *J. Controlled Release*, 37, 263–267, 1995.
18. Pistner, H., Bendix, D.R., Muhling, J., and Reuther, J.F., Poly(L-lactide) — a long-term degradation study invivo. 3. Analytical characterization, *Biomaterials*, 14, 291–298, 1993.
19. Aso, Y., Yoshioka, S., Po, A.L.W., and Terao, T., Effect of temperature on mechanisms of drug-release and matrix degradation of poly(D,L-lactide) microspheres, *J. Controlled Release*, 31, 33–39, 1994.
20. Deng, M. and Uhrich, K.E., Effects of in vitro degradation on properties of poly(D,L-lactide-co-glycolide) pertinent to its biological performance, *J. Mater. Sci. — Mater. Med.*, 13, 1091–1096, 2002.
21. Passerini, N. and Craig, D.Q.M., An investigation into the effects of residual water on the glass transition temperature of polylactide microspheres using modulated temperature DSC, *J. Controlled Release*, 73, 111–115, 2001.
22. Arshady, R., Microspheres and microcapsules, a survey of manufacturing techniques. 3. Solvent evaporation, *Polym. Eng. Sci.*, 30, 915–924, 1990.
23. Morita, T., Horikiri, Y., Suzuki, T., and Yoshino, H., Applicability of various amphiphilic polymers to the modification of protein release kinetics from biodegradable reservoir-type microspheres, *Eur. J. Pharm. Biopharm.*, 51, 45–53, 2001.
24. Sah, H.K., Toddywala, R., and Chien, Y.W., Biodegradable microcapsules prepared by a W/O/W technique — effects of shear force to make a primary W/O emulsion on their morphology and protein release, *J. Microencapsul.*, 12, 59–69, 1995.
25. Leach, K., Noh, K., and Mathiowitz, E., Effect of manufacturing conditions on the formation of double-walled polymer microspheres, *J. Microencapsul.*, 16, 153–167, 1999.
26. Pekarek, K.J., Jacob, J.S., and Mathiowitz, E., Double-walled polymer microspheres for controlled drug release, *Nature*, 367, 258–260, 1994.

27. Rahman, N.A. and Mathiowitz, E., Localization of bovine serum albumin in double-walled microspheres, *J. Controlled Release*, 94, 163–175, 2004.

28. Schugens, C., Laruelle, N., Nihant, N., Grandfils, C., Jerome, R., and Teyssie, P., Effect of the emulsion stability on the morphology and porosity of semicrystalline poly L-lactide microparticles prepared by W/O/W double emulsion-evaporation, *J. Controlled Release*, 32, 161–176, 1994.

29. Bouissou, C., Potter, U., Altroff, H., Mardon, H., and van der Walle, C., Controlled release of the fibronectin central cell binding domain from polymeric microspheres, *J. Controlled Release*, 95, 557–566, 2004.

30. Wang, W., Lyophilization and development of solid protein pharmaceuticals, *Int. J. Pharm.*, 203, 1–60, 2000.

31. Arshady, R., Microspheres and microcapsules, a survey of manufacturing techniques. 2. Coacervation, *Polym. Eng. Sci.*, 30, 905–914, 1990.

32. Bittner, B., Morlock, M., Koll, H., Winter, G., and Kissel, T., Recombinant human erythropoietin (rhEPO) loaded poly(lactide-co-glycolide) microspheres: influence of the encapsulation technique and polymer purity on microsphere characteristics, *Eur. J. Pharm. Biopharm.*, 45, 295–305, 1998.

33. Ghaderi, R., Artursson, P., and Carlfors, J., Preparation of biodegradable microparticles using solution-enhanced dispersion by supercritical fluids (SEDS), *Pharm. Res.*, 16, 676–681, 1999.

34. Mishima, K., Matsuyama, K., Tanabe, D., Yamauchi, S., Young, T.J., and Johnston, K.P., Microencapsulation of proteins by rapid expansion of supercritical solution with a nonsolvent, *AIchE J.*, 46, 857–865, 2000.

35. Hao, J.Y., Whitaker, M.J., Wong, B., and Serhatkulu, G., Shakesheff, K.M., and Howdle, S.M., Plasticization and spraying of poly (D,L-lactic acid) using supercritical carbon dioxide: control of particle size, *J. Pharm. Sci.*, 93, 1083–1090, 2004.

36. Singh, L., Kumar, V., and Ratner, B.D., Generation of porous microcellular 85/15 poly (D,L-lactide-co-glycolide) foams for biomedical applications, *Biomaterials*, 25, 2611–2617, 2004.

37. Witschi, C. and Doelker, E., Influence of the microencapsulation method and peptide loading on poly(lactic acid) and poly(lactic-co-glycolic acid) degradation during in vitro testing, *J. Controlled Release*, 51 327–341, 1998.

38. Jeffery, H., Davis, S.S., and Ohagan, D.T., The preparation and characterization of poly(lactide-co-glycolide) microparticles. 2. The entrapment of a model protein using a (water-in-oil)-in-water emulsion solvent evaporation technique, *Pharm. Res.*, 10, 362–368, 1993.

39. Yang, Y.Y., Chung, T.S., and Ng, N.P., Morphology, drug distribution, and in vitro release profiles of biodegradable polymeric microspheres containing protein fabricated by double-emulsion solvent extraction/evaporation method, *Biomaterials*, 22, 231–241, 2001.

40. Mehta, R.C., Thanoo, B.C., and DeLuca, P.P., Peptide containing microspheres from low molecular weight and hydrophilic poly(D,L-lactide-co-glycolide), *J. Controlled Release*, 41, 249–257, 1996.

41. Park, T.G., Lu, W.Q., and Crotts, G., Importance of in-vitro experimental conditions on protein release kinetics, stability and polymer degradation in protein encapsulated poly(D,L-lactic acid-co-glycolic acid) microspheres, *J. Controlled Release*, 33, 211–222, 1995.

42. Rojas, J., Pinto-Alphandary, H., Leo, E., Pecquet, S., Couvreur, P., Gulik, A., and Fattal, E., A polysorbate-based non-ionic surfactant can modulate loading and release of beta-lactoglobulin entrapped in multiphase poly(D,L-lactide-co-glycolide) microspheres, *Pharm. Res.*, 16, 255–260, 1999.

43. Jeyanthi, R., Thanoo, B.C., Metha, R.C., and DeLuca, P.P., Effect of solvent removal technique on the matrix characteristics of polylactide/glycolide microspheres for peptide delivery, *J. Controlled Release*, 38, 235–244, 1996.

44. Yang, Y.Y., Chia, H.H., and Chung, T.S., Effect of preparation temperature on the characteristics and release profiles of PLGA microspheres containing protein fabricated by double-emulsion solvent extraction/evaporation method, *J. Controlled Release*, 69, 81–96, 2000.

45. Wang, J., Wang, B.M., and Schwendeman, S.P., Characterization of the initial burst release of a model peptide from poly(D,L-lactide-co-glycolide) microspheres, *J. Controlled Release*, 82, 289–307, 2002.

46. Crotts, G. and Park, T.G., Preparation of porous and nonporous biodegradable polymeric hollow microspheres, *J. Controlled Release*, 35, 91–105, 1995.

47. Chew, N.Y.K. and Chan, H.K., Use of solid corrugated particles to enhance powder aerosol performance, *Pharm. Res.*, 18, 1570–1577, 2001.

48. Florence, A.T., The oral absorption of micro- and nanoparticulates: neither exceptional nor unusual, *Pharm. Res.*, 14, 259–266, 1997.

49. Crotts, G., Sah, H., and Park, T.G., Adsorption determines in-vitro protein release rate from biodegradable microspheres: Quantitative analysis of surface area during degradation, *J. Controlled Release*, 47, 101–111, 1997.

50. Fu, K., Pack, D.W., Klibanov, A.M., and Langer, R., Visual evidence of acidic environment within degrading poly(lactic-co-glycolic acid) (PLGA) microspheres, *Pharm. Res.*, 17, 100–106, 2000.

51. Nihant, N., Schugens, C., Grandfils, C., Jerome, R., and Teyssie, P., Polylactide microparticles prepared by double emulsion/evaporation technique. 1. Effect of primary emulsion stability, *Pharm. Res.*, 11, 1479–1484, 1994.

52. Sandor, M., Enscore, D., Weston, P., and Mathiowitz, E., Effect of protein molecular weight on release from micron-sized PLGA microspheres, *J. Controlled Release*, 76, 297–311, 2001.

53. Lemaire, V., Belair, J., and Hildgen, P., Structural modeling of drug release from biodegradable porous matrices based on a combined diffusion/erosion process, *Int. J. Pharm.*, 258, 95–107, 2003.

54. von Burkersroda, F., Schedl, L., and Gopferich, A., Why degradable polymers undergo surface erosion or bulk erosion, *Biomaterials*, 23, 4221–4231, 2002.

55. Batycky, R.P., Hanes, J., Langer, R., and Edwards, D.A., A theoretical model of erosion and macromolecular drug release from biodegrading microspheres, *J. Pharm. Sci.*, 86, 1464–1477, 1997.

56. Gopferich, A., Mechanisms of polymer degradation and erosion, *Biomaterials*, 17, 103–114, 1996.

57. Blanco-Prieto, M.J., Besseghir, K., Orsolini, P., Heimgartner, F., Deuschel, C., Merkle, H.P., Ho, N.T., and Gander, B., Importance of the test medium for the release kinetics of a somatostatin analogue from poly(D,L-lactide-co-glycolide) microspheres, *Int. J. Pharm.*, 184, 243–250, 1999.

58. Shih, C., Waldron, N., and Zentner, G.M., Quantitative analysis of ester linkages in poly(D,L-lactide) and poly(D,L-lactide-co-glycolide), *J. Controlled Release*, 38, 69–73, 1996.

59. Park, T.G., Degradation of poly(lactic-co-glycolic acid) microspheres — effect of copolymer composition, *Biomaterials*, 16, 1123–1130, 1995.

60. Yoo, H.S., Oh, J.E., Lee, K.H., and Park, T.G., Biodegradable nanoparticles containing doxorubicin-PLGA conjugate for sustained release, *Pharm. Res.*, 16, 1114–1118, 1999.

61. Pistel, K.F., Breitenbach, A., Zange-Volland, R., and Kissel, T., Brush-like branched biodegradable polyesters, part III — protein release from microspheres of poly(vinyl alcohol)-graft- poly(D,L-lactic-co-glycolic acid), *J. Controlled Release*, 73, 7–20, 2001.

62. Pean, J.M., Boury, F., Venier-Julienne, M.C., Menei, P., Proust, J.E., and Benoit, J.P., Why does PEG 400 co-encapsulation improve NGF stability and release from PLGA biodegradable microspheres?, *Pharm. Res.*, 16, 1294–1299, 1999.

63. Zhang, M.P., Yang, Z.C., Chow, L.L., and Wang, C.H., Simulation of drug release from biodegradable polymeric microspheres with bulk and surface erosions, *J. Pharm. Sci.*, 92, 2040–2056, 2003.

64. Siepmann, J., Faisant, N., and Benoit, J.P., A new mathematical model quantifying drug release from bioerodible microparticles using Monte Carlo simulations, *Pharm. Res.*, 19, 1885–1893, 2002.

65. Faisant, N., Siepmann, J., Richard, J., and Benoit, J.P., Mathematical modeling of drug release from bioerodible microparticles: effect of gamma-irradiation, *Eur. J. Pharm. Biopharm.*, 56, 271–279, 2003.

66. Hussain, M., Beale, G., Hughes, M., and Akhtar, S., Co-delivery of an antisense oligonucleotide and 5-fluorouracil using sustained release poly (lactide-co-glycolide) microsphere formulations for potential combination therapy in cancer, *Int. J. Pharm.*, 234, 129–138, 2002.

67. Alonso, M.J., Cohen, S., Park, T.G., Gupta, R.K., Siber, G.R., and Langer, R., Determinants of release rate of tetanus vaccine from polyester microspheres, *Pharm. Res.*, 10, 945–953, 1993.

68. Dunne, M., Bibby, D.C., Jones, J.C., and Cudmore, S., Encapsulation of protamine sulphate compacted DNA in polylactide and polylactide-co-glycolide microparticles, *J. Controlled Release*, 92, 209–219, 2003.

69. Carino, G.P., Jacob, J.S., Mathiowitz, E., Nanosphere based oral insulin delivery, *J. Controlled Release*, 65, 261–269, 2000.

70. Perez, C., Castellanos, I.J., Costantino, H.R., Al-Azzam, W., and Griebenow, K., Recent trends in stabilizing protein structure upon encapsulation and release from bioerodible polymers, *J. Pharm. Pharmacol.*, 54, 301–313, 2002.

71. Pays, K., Giermanska-Kahn, J., Pouligny, B., Bibette, J., Leal-Calderon, F., Double emulsions: how does release occur? *J. Controlled Release,* 79, 193–205, 2002.

72. Sah, H., A new strategy to determine the actual protein content of poly(lactide-co-glycolide) microspheres, *J. Pharm. Sci.,* 86, 1315–1318, 1997.

73. Sah, H., Stabilization of proteins against methylene chloride/water interface-induced denaturation and aggregation, *J. Controlled Release,* 58, 143–151, 1999.

74. Sah, H., Protein behavior at the water/methylene chloride interface, *J. Pharm. Sci.,* 88, 1320–1325, 1999.

75. van de Weert, M., Hoechstetter, J., Hennink, W.E., Crommelin, D.J., The effect of a water/organic solvent interface on the structural stability of lysozyme, *J. Controlled Release,* 68, 351–359, 2000.

76. van de Weert, M., van't Hof, R., van der Weerd, J., Heeren, R.M., Posthuma, G., Hennink, W.E., Crommelin, D.J., Lysozyme distribution and conformation in a biodegradable polymer matrix as determined by FTIR techniques, *J. Controlled Release,* 68, 31–40, 2000.

77. Kwon, Y.M., Baudys, M., Knutson, K., and Kim, S.W., In situ study of insulin aggregation induced by water-organic solvent interface, *Pharm. Res.,* 18, 1754–1759, 2001.

78. van de Weert, M., Hennink, W.E., and Jiskoot, W., Protein instability in poly(lactic-co-glycolic acid) microparticles, *Pharm. Res.,* 17, 1159–1167, 2000.

79. Green, R. and Pace, N., Urea and guanidine hydrochloride denaturation of ribonuclease, lysozyme, alpha-chymotrypsin and beta-lactoglobulin, *J. Biol. Chem.,* 249, 5388–5393, 1974.

80. Poon, S., Clarke, A., Currie, G., and Schultz, C., Influence of alpha-helices on the emulsifying properties of proteins, *Biosci. Biotechnol. Biochem.,* 65, 1713–1723, 2001.

81. Faisant, N., Siepmann, J., and Benoit, J.P., PLGA-based microparticles: elucidation of mechanisms and a new, simple mathematical model quantifying drug release, *Eur. J. Pharm. Sci.,* 15, 355–366, 2002.

82. Cohen, H., Levy, R.J., Gao, J., Fishbein, I., Kousaev, V., Sosnowski, S., Slomkowski, S., Golomb, G., Sustained delivery and expression of DNA encapsulated in polymeric nanoparticles, *Gene Ther.,* 7, 1896–1905, 2000.

83. Benoit, M.A., Ribet, C., Distexhe, J., Hermand, D., Letesson, J.J., Vandenhaute, J., and Gillard, J., Studies on the potential of microparticles entrapping pDNA-poly(Aminoacids) complexes as vaccine delivery systems, *J. Drug Targeting,* 9, 253–266, 2001.

84. Prabha, S. and Labhasetwar, V., Critical determinants in PLGA/PLA nanoparticle-mediated gene expression, *Pharm. Res.,* 21, 354–364, 2004.

85. Lukacs, G.L., Haggie, P., Seksek, O., Lechardeur, D., Freedman, N., Verkman, A.S., Size-dependent DNA mobility in cytoplasm and nucleus, *J. Biol. Chem.,* 275, 1625–1629, 2000.

86. Qaddoumi, M.G., Gukasyan, H.J., Davda, J., Labhasetwar, V., Kim, K.J., and Lee, V.H.L., Clathrin and caveolin-1 expression in primary pigmented rabbit conjunctival epithelial cells: role in PLGA nanoparticle endocytosis, *Mol. Vision,* 9, 559–568, 2003.

87. Panyam, J., Zhou, W.Z., Prabha, S., Sahoo, S.K., and Labhasetwar, V., Rapid endo-lysosomal escape of poly(D,L-lactide-co-glycolide) nanoparticles: implications for drug and gene delivery, *FASEB J.,* 16, 1217–1226, 2002.

88. Egilmez, N.K., Jong, Y.S., Sabel, M.S., Jacob, J.S., Mathiowitz, E., Bankert, R.B., In situ tumor vaccination with interleukin-12-encapsulated biodegradable microspheres: induction of tumor regression and potent antitumor immunity, *Cancer Res.,* 60, 3832–3837, 2000.

89. Ma, J., Luo, D., Qi, W.M., and Cao, L.R., Antitumor effect of the idiotypic cascade induced by an antibody encapsulated in poly(D,L-lactide-co-glycolide) microspheres, *Jpn. J. Cancer Res.,* 92, 1110–1115, 2001.

90. Boehm, G., Peyre, M., Sesardic, D., Huskisson, R.J., Mawas, F., Douglas, A., Xing, D., Merkle, H.P., Gander, B., Johansen, P., On technological and immunological benefits of multivalent single-injection microsphere vaccines, *Pharm. Res.,* 19, 1330–1336, 2002.

91. Vajdy, M. and O'Hagan, D.T., Microparticles for intranasal immunization, *Adv. Drug Delivery Rev.,* 51, 127–141, 2001.

92. Rosas, J.E., Pedraz, J.L., Hernandez, R.M., Gascon, A.R., Igartua, M., Guzman, F., Rodriguez, R., Cortes, J., Patarroyo, M.E., Remarkably high antibody levels and protection against P- falciparum malaria in Aotus monkeys after a single immunisation of SPf66 encapsulated in PLGA microspheres, *Vaccine,* 20, 1707–1710, 2002.

93. Prabha, S. and Labhasetwar, V., Nanoparticle-mediated wild-type p53 gene delivery results in sustained antiproliferative activity in breast cancer cells, *Mol. Pharm.*, 1, 211–219, 2004.

94. Wang, C., Ge, Q., Ting, D., Nguyen, D., Shen, H.R., Chen, J.Z., Eisen, H.N., Heller, J., Langer, R., and Putnam, D., Molecularly engineered poly(ortho ester) microspheres for enhanced delivery of DNA vaccines, *Nat. Mater.*, 3, 190–196, 2004.

95. De Rosa, G., Bochot, A., Quaglia, F., Besnard, M., and Fattal, E., A new delivery system for antisense therapy: PLGA microspheres encapsulating oligonucleotide/polyethyleneimine solid complexes, *Int. J. Pharm.*, 254, 89–93, 2003.

96. Lathia, J.D., Leodore, L., and Wheatley, M.A., Polymeric contrast agent with targeting potential, *Ultrasonics*, 42, 763–768, 2004.

97. Muller, M., Voros, J., Csucs, G., Walter, E., Danuser, G., Merkle, H.P., Spencer, N.D., and Textor, M., Surface modification of PLGA microspheres, *J. Biomed. Mater. Res.*, Part A, 66A, 55–61, 2003.

8 Polymeric Nanoparticles as Drug Carriers

Hervé Hillaireau and Patrick Couvreur

CONTENTS

8.1 INTRODUCTION

One of the major obstacles to drug efficacy is the nonspecific distribution of the biologically active compound after administration. This is generally due to the fact that the drug distributes according to its physicochemical properties, which means that diffusion through biological barriers may be limited. Also, certain chemical entities are either rapidly degraded and/or metabolized after administration (peptides, proteins, and nucleic acids). This is the reason the idea that nanotechnologies may be employed to modify or even to control the drug distribution at the tissue, cellular, or subcellular levels (Figure 8.1) has emerged. Among the technologies utilized for drug targeting are polymer-based nanoparticles, which have been developed since the early 1980s, when progress in polymer chemistry allowed the design of biodegradable and biocompatible materials. Nanoparticles may be defined as being submicron (<1 μm) colloidal systems generally composed of polymers. Thus, nanoparticles are colloidal systems with a size 7 to 70 times smaller than the red cells (Figure 8.2). They may be administered intravenously without any risk of embolization. Depending on the method used in the preparation of nanoparticles, either nanospheres or nanocapsules can be obtained. Nanospheres are matrix systems in which the drug is dispersed within the polymer throughout the particle. On the contrary, nanocapsules are vesicular systems, which are formed by a drug-containing liquid core (aqueous or lipophilic) surrounded by a single polymeric membrane. Nanocapsules may thus be considered as a "reservoir" system (Figure 8.3). This chapter will review the application of nanoparticles as drug carriers.

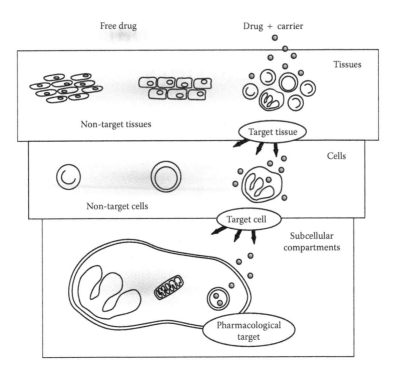

FIGURE 8.1 Nanoparticles as specific drug delivery systems to tissues, cells, and subcellular compartments (black circles). For comparison, a free drug is nonspecific (diffuse gray).

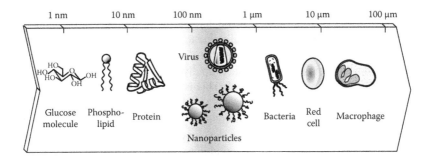

FIGURE 8.2 Sizes of nanoparticles compared with other biological entities.

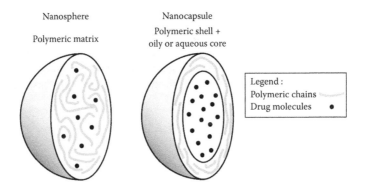

FIGURE 8.3 Morphology of nanospheres and nanocapsules.

8.2 INTRAVENOUS ROUTE OF ADMINISTRATION

8.2.1 THE FIRST GENERATION OF NANOPARTICLES FOR LIVER TARGETING

Upon intravenous injection, nanoparticles are rapidly cleared from the bloodstream by the normal reticuloendothelial defence mechanism [1], irrespective of their composition (nature of the polymer used in their preparation) or morphology (nanospheres or nanocapsules). As shown by tissue distribution data, nanoparticles concentrate mainly in the liver, spleen, and bone marrow [2]. Thus, the liver acts as a reservoir for nanoparticles, conditioning their rapid first-phase disappearance from the blood and their expected second-phase release in the body (in a degraded and excretable form). Additional studies have shown that, in the liver, Kupffer cells are the major sites for cell accumulation of the nanoparticles [1]. Endothelial and especially parenchymal cells have a very low cell association with nanoparticles. One application that takes advantage of the concentration of nanoparticles in the liver is the treatment of liver metastasis using biodegradable polyalkylcyanoacrylate nanoparticles loaded with doxorubicin. The specific delivery of this compound to the liver induces a dramatic reduction in the number of metastasis in the histiosarcoma M5076 experimental cancer; it was found that the Kupffer cells were able to play the role of a drug reservoir allowing the slow diffusion of doxorubicin toward the tumor cells as the result of the nanoparticles biodegradation [3]. On the other hand, the nanoparticle formulation resulted in a reduced cardiac concentration of doxorubicin when compared to the free drug; this, in turn, reduced the cardiac toxicity of the drug [4].

It was found that endocytosis plays a major role in the cell uptake process [5]. This opens possibilities for the treatment of intracellular infections. These infections are often resistant to commonly used antibiotics because of low intracellular uptake or reduced activity at the acidic pH of lysosomes. An alternative strategy to the development of new antibiotics would be the use of polymer-based nanotechnologies, thereby improving the efficiency of existing drugs. In particular, the need for antibiotics with intracellular efficacy led to the development of colloidal antibiotic systems, which can be endocytosed by the infected cells. As an illustration of that concept, it has been shown that linking of ampicillin to polyisohexylcyanoacrylate (PIHCA) nanospheres increased by 120 the efficacy in treating *Salmonella typhimurium* infection in mice [6]. This was attributable to the combined effect of two types of targeting: firstly, the linkage of ampicillin to nanospheres led to the concentration of the drug in the liver and the spleen; secondly, the uptake of ampicillin by infected macrophages was higher when the drug was bound to nanospheres than when it was in the free form [7,8]. Ampicillin bound to PIHCA nanospheres was also effective against experimental listeriosis in athymic nude mice, a model involving a chronic infection of both liver and spleen macrophages [9,10].

8.2.2 THE SECOND GENERATION OF NANOPARTICLES FOR LONG BLOOD CIRCULATION ("STEALTH™" NANOPARTICLES) AND PASSIVE TARGETING

Despite the promising results with the "first-generation" nanoparticles, their usefulness is limited by their rapid and massive recognition by the mononuclear phagocyte system (liver, spleen, and bone marrow). A great deal of work has been devoted to developing so-called nanoparticles that are "invisible" to macrophages ("Stealth™" nanoparticles). A major breakthrough in the field has been the coating of nanoparticles with poly(ethyleneglycol) (PEG), also known as poly(oxyethylene) (Figure 8.4). This provides a "cloud" of hydrophilic chains at the particle surface, which repels plasma proteins. These "sterically stabilized" nanoparticles have circulating half-lives of several hours, as opposed to a few minutes for conventional nanoparticles (Figure 8.5). They have been shown to function as reservoir systems and can penetrate into sites such as solid tumors. There are two strategies to preparing sterically stabilized nanoparticles: they either adsorb copolymers of polyoxypropylene-polyoxyethylene (pluronics) to already prepared nanoparticles [11], or they perform the chemical synthesis of a copolymer composed of the hydrophilic PEG and the hydrophobic biodegradable moiety (polyester, cyanoacrylate, etc.) before preparing the nanoparticles (by usual methods of nanoprecipitation or solvent evaporation) [12–14].

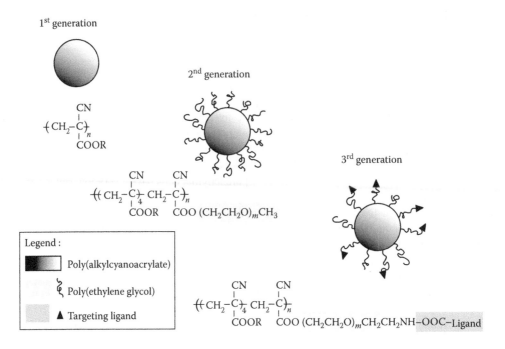

FIGURE 8.4 Three generations of nanoparticles for drug delivery.

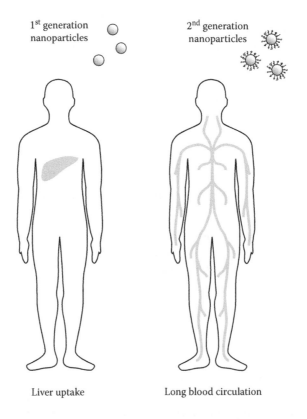

Liver uptake   Long blood circulation

FIGURE 8.5 Biodistribution of first- and second-generation nanoparticles.

As an illustration of the first strategy, coating the nanoparticles with poloxamine 908 was found to decrease the combined liver–spleen uptake to about 8% (instead of 90% without coating) and allowed a major fraction (65%) of the nanoparticles to remain in the circulation for an extended period [11]. Physicochemical studies carried out on these systems have shown that coating colloidal particles with block copolymers induces a steric repulsion towards opsonins (fibronectin, Fc fragment of the immunoglobulins, proteins of the complement cascade, etc.). Therefore, the relative phagocytic uptake was found to decrease with increasing adsorbed layer thickness, which corresponds, in case of the steric stabilization effect, in an increase in the surface hydrophilicity [15]. However, when performed through a single adsorption procedure, the surface-adsorbed polymers (i.e., poloxamers, PEG, etc.), depending on their physicochemical characteristics, may be displaced by blood proteins. The situation is further complicated when using biodegradable polymers for the design of the nanoparticle matrix because the nanoparticle is often eroded from the surface to the core. Therefore, the single adsorption procedure may lead to the premature release of the coating layer, thus decreasing the steric shielding and making nanoparticles prone to phagocytoses. This is the reason a chemical linkage strategy is preferable for the decoration of nanoparticles' surfaces. This has been performed by the synthesis of copolymers containing at least one PEG block. As such, PEG-coated nanoparticles with biodegradable cores made of polyesters such as polylactide (PLA), poly(lactide-*co*-glycolide) (PLGA), poly(ε-caprolactone) (PCL), polyanhydride, and poly(alkylcyanoacrylate) have been prepared. In general, these nanoassemblies were able to prolong the blood circulation time when compared to the particles made with the non-PEGylated polymer counterparts [12]. Apart from the nature of the nanoparticle coating, size is another important parameter for keeping the particles longer in the blood circulation. Indeed, the smaller the particles are, the more important is the radius of curvature in keeping the particle in circulation and thus the less efficient is the opsonization process.

There are several reasons why mononuclear phagocyte system (MPS) evading nanoparticles may be interesting for drug targeting and delivery. The more obvious one is to provide a long-circulating drug reservoir for compounds that have short elimination half-lives, due, for instance, to instability or rapid metabolic degradation of the active (peptides or proteins, such as cytokines or growth factors, and nucleic acids). Another reason is that various physiopathological disorders are associated with structural changes of the vasculature, thus providing unique opportunities for long-circulating nanoparticles to escape from the blood circulation selectively into the diseased tissues. This is generally the case when the endothelial barrier is perturbed by inflammatory processes due to infections, tumors, or autoimmune diseases. In other words, it is expected that when having a longer blood circulation time, the nanoparticles will have a better chance of reaching the diseased tissue, resulting in improved treatment. This was clearly observed with nanospheres prepared from poly(ethyleneglycol-*co*-hexadecylcyanoacrylate), which were observed to selectively extravasate across the blood–brain barrier in the experimental 9L gliosarcoma [16]. The maximal tumor-to-brain ratio, measured 4 h after intravenous injection, was found to be 11. Similar results were obtained with the experimental allergic encephalomyelitis model for which the concentration of PEGylated nanoparticles in the central nervous system (CNS), especially in white matter, was greatly increased in comparison to conventional non-PEGylated nanoparticles [17]. In addition, this increase was significantly higher in pathological situations in which blood–brain barrier (BBB) permeability was perturbed and/or to which macrophages had infiltrated. Passive diffusion and macrophage uptake in inflammatory lesions seem to be the mechanisms underlying such brain penetration by particles.

Apart from the surface modification of nanoparticles using poly(ethyleneglycol) polymers or copolymers, an interesting and unexpected observation was that the polysorbate 80 coating allowed nanoparticles to enter the brain. Drugs that have successfully been transported using this type of carrier include the hexapeptide dalargin, dipeptide kytorphin, loperamide, tubocurarine, and doxorubicin. The mechanism by which polysorbate 80 induces nanoparticle-mediated transport is not fully elucidated. The most likely mechanism is endocytosis by the endothelial cells lining the blood capillaries of the brain. It is suspected that polysorbate 80 is able to modify the blood protein adsorption profile at the surface of the particles in favour of the adsorption of significant amounts of apolipoprotein E, which have specific receptors at the surface of the brain endothelial cells [18].

8.2.3 The Third Generation of Nanoparticles with Molecular Recognition (Active Targeting)

Efforts have been made to achieve molecular addressing of nanoparticles. This approach consists of the decoration of the nanoparticle surface with the aid of molecules able to recognize a biological target (receptor, antigen, etc.) (Figure 8.4). The molecules used for targeting purposes are of a varied nature: they may be macromolecules (such as antibodies, peptides, or poly/oligosaccharides) or small molecules (such as hormones or vitamins). It is without question that this strategy will have an increased interest in the near future because of the progress made in genomics and postgenomics in the discovery of new biological targets.

As an illustration of this approach, the vitamin folic acid (molecular weight = 441 Da) may be exploited to actively target cancer cells. Indeed, the folic acid receptor (folate-binding protein, FBP) is frequently overexpressed on the surface of human cancer cells [19], although it is highly restricted in most normal tissues, so that this receptor has been identified as a tumor marker, especially in ovarian carcinomas [20]. In addition, the folate receptor is efficiently cell internalized after binding with its ligand (folic acid) with a very high affinity (Kd~1 nM), and then it moves into the cell cytoplasm [21], which is an advantage for more efficient intracellular delivery of anticancer agents than using a cell membrane marker that is not cell internalized. Thus, folic acid has been coupled onto PEG-coated biodegradable nanoparticles [22]. Interestingly, surface plasmon resonance revealed that folate grafted to PEGylated cyanoacrylate nanoparticles had a tenfold higher apparent affinity for the FBP than free folate did. Indeed, the particles represent a multivalent form of the ligand folic acid, and folate receptors often present as clusters [22]. As a result, conjugated nanoparticles display a multivalent and hence stronger interaction with the surface of the malignant cells. Moreover, confocal microscopy demonstrated that folate nanoparticles, when compared to nonconjugated nanoparticles, were selectively taken up by the folate-receptor-bearing cells but not by the cells devoid of folate receptors.

8.2.4 Polymer Nanoparticles and Cell Internalization and Trafficking

In fact, nanospheres are able to interact with cells in different ways, the most common cell internalization pathway being through endocytosis with the cell lines displaying some endocytotic or phagocytotic activity. After cell membrane invagination, particles are cell internalized into early endosomes, which will then become more acidic before fusing with cell lysosomes. Then, the nanospheres will be in an enzyme-rich environment, allowing the polymer to be degraded or metabolized and the drug to be released (Figure 8.6a). Depending on its physicochemical characteristics, the biologically active molecule will or will not diffuse through the lysosomal membrane, thus inducing an extra- or intralysosomal effect. It is noteworthy that in some cases the polymer can induce the disruption of the lysosomal membrane by different mechanisms and this can lead to an extralysosomal effect, even if the encapsulated drug is not naturally diffusible through the lysosomal membrane (Figure 8.6b).

Cell capture through endocytosis is, however, not the only mechanism for nanospheres to interact with cancer cells, especially if those cells have no or low endocytic capacity. Indeed, it has been demonstrated that *in vitro* resistance of tumor cells to doxorubicin can be fully circumvented using biodegradable polyisohexylcyanoacrylate nanoparticles [23,24]. The mechanism behind this important observation is not fully understood, although it was found that polyisobutylcyanoacrylate nanoparticles produced higher intracellular concentrations of doxorubicin, which was correlated with a higher cytotoxicity compared to the free drug. However, the fact that drug incorporation by the cells was not influenced by cytochalasin B (a blocker of the endocytotic process) suggests that endocytosis is clearly not the main mechanism of nanoparticle–cell association in this case [25].

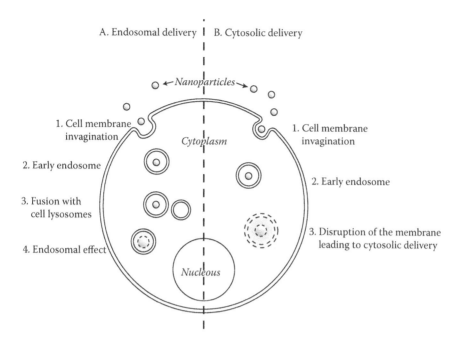

FIGURE 8.6 Cell internalization of nanoparticles can lead to (a) endosomal or (b) cytosolic drug delivery.

It has been hypothesized that the rapid drug release of doxorubicin from nanoparticles adhering to the cell membrane could lead to an overflow and saturation of the P-glycoprotein (P-gp) efflux pump, resulting in the observed increase of drug diffusion in the intracellular compartment.

It was observed that such a mechanism of P-gp saturation was associated with the formation of an ion pair between the positively charged doxorubicin and negatively charged polycyanoacrylic acid (which is a metabolite of the cyanoacrylate polymer) [24]. Such a complex between the (degraded) polymer and the drug improves greatly the diffusion of doxorubicin into cells. Finally, doxorubicin nanoparticles have been tested in doxorubicin-resistant C6 rat glioblastoma lines differing by their degree and mechanism of resistance [26]. The key finding of this study was that the reversal of doxorubicin resistance by nanoparticles was closely dependent on the nature of the resistance: nanoparticles were only efficient in pure multidrug resistance (MDR) phenotype cells and not when there were additional mechanisms underlying the resistance to doxorubicin. This observation comes in line with the above-mentioned mechanism of interaction between cancer cells and polyalkylcyanoacrylate and acryl nanospheres.

8.3 ORAL ROUTE OF ADMINISTRATION

The main problems encountered in the oral administration of drugs are: (1) the drug must be dissolved before absorption occurs, (2) some drugs are only absorbed through certain portions of the gastrointestinal tract ("window of absorption"), and (3) a lot of compounds, especially those arising from biotechnologies, are degraded in the gastrointestinal tract. In the light of these facts, nanotechnologies may be useful transporters for improving the oral bioavailability of drugs. For instance, it is obvious that for poorly-water-soluble compounds, the kinetics of dissolution in the gastrointestinal tract is proportional to the specific surface area; therefore, the formulation of these compounds as submicroscopic colloidal systems may help to accelerate the dissolution process, thus improving bioavailability. On the other hand, after oral administration, the absorption efficacy directly depends on the residence time of the drug in front of the window of absorption. However, intestinal transit results in reducing the drug residence time, which also limits the drug's bioavailability.

This is the reason the concept of bioadhesion has emerged to allow the immobilization of a drug at the surface of the intestinal epithelium [27]. It has been shown that, owing to their very small size, nanoparticles are able to diffuse into the mucus layer, which allows their immobilization in close contact with the epithelium absorptive membrane. For example, the bioavailability of reverse-transcriptase inhibitors may be improved after their administration as nanoparticles [28]. The bioadhesion process of nanoparticles may be improved by controlling particle surfaces (i.e., charges and hydrophilicity or hydrophobicity). Other approaches involve the development of biomimetic strategies such as decorating the nanoparticles with the adhesion proteins that normally allow bacteria to infect the intestinal mucosa.

Oral administration of peptides is another important challenge for nanotechnologies. Nanocapsules were shown 15 years ago to be able to encapsulate a peptide-like insulin and to increase its activity as assessed by the induction of hypoglycemia [29,30]. It was suggested that nanocapsules could protect insulin from proteolytic degradation in intestinal fluids. It was suggested that nanocapsules could protect insulin from proteolytic degradation in intestinal fluids. The capacity of insulin nanocapsules to reduce glycemia could be explained by their translocation through the intestinal barrier by the paracellular pathway or via M cells in Peyer's patches [30]. Incorporation of other peptides such as octreotide, a somatostatin analog, in nanocapsules also improved and prolonged the therapeutic effect of this peptide after administration by the oral route. However, capture of nanoparticles by M cells in Peyer's patches and further translocation of the particles is rate- and quantity-limited, making this strategy less attractive for the oral administration of therapeutic peptides.

The development of new vaccines is another application of nanotechnologies by the oral route; indeed, the processing by Peyer's patches of small amounts of antigen may induce mucosal immunity with IgA production. The encapsulation of antigens into microparticles and nanoparticles allows the protection of the antigen after oral administration as well as its delivery to the M cells of Peyer's patches. This approach has been shown to be feasible with different model antigens for which mucosal immunity with protection against at least two types of infections has been obtained [31,32]. This opens new perspectives for the development of oral vaccines [33].

8.4 CONCLUSIONS

From the research done at the interface of physics, chemistry, and life sciences has emerged the concept of using nanotechnologies for the administration, transport, and targeting of drugs at the tissue, cellular, and subcellular levels. These innovations are no longer mere laboratory curiosities because they have already led to new medicines for the treatment of cancer and infectious diseases.

REFERENCES

1. Lenaerts, V., Nagelkerke, J.F., Van Berkel, T.J., Couvreur, P., Grislain, L., Roland, M., and Speiser, P., In vivo uptake of polyisobutyl cyanoacrylate nanoparticles by rat liver Kupffer, endothelial, and parenchymal cells, *J. Pharm. Sci.*, 73(7), 980–982, 1984.
2. Grislain, L., Couvreur, P., Lenaerts, V., Roland, M., Deprez-Decampeneere, D., and Speiser, P., Pharmacokinetics and distribution of a biodegradable drug-carrier, *Int. J. Pharm.*, 15(3), 335–345, 1983.
3. Chiannilkulchai, N., Ammoury, N., Caillou, B., Devissaguet, J.P., and Couvreur, P., Hepatic tissue distribution of doxorubicin-loaded nanoparticles after i.v. administration in reticulosarcoma M 5076 metastasis-bearing mice, *Cancer Chemother. Pharmacol.*, 26(2), 122–126, 1990.
4. Verdun, C., Brasseur, F., Vranckx, H., Couvreur, P., and Roland, M., Tissue distribution of doxorubicin associated with polyisohexylcyanoacrylate nanoparticles, *Cancer Chemother. Pharmacol.*, 26(1), 13–18, 1990.
5. Couvreur, P., Tulkens, P., Roland, M., Trouet, A., and Speiser, P., Nanocapsules: a new type of lysosomotropic carrier, *FEBS Lett.*, 84(2), 323–326, 1977.

6. Fattal, E., Youssef, M., Couvreur, P., and Andremont, A., Treatment of experimental salmonellosis in mice with ampicillin-bound nanoparticles, *Antimicrob. Agents Chemother.,* 33(9), 1540–1543, 1989.

7. Balland, O., Pinto-Alphandary, H., Pecquet, S., Andremont, A., and Couvreur, P., The uptake of ampicillin-loaded nanoparticles by murine macrophages infected with Salmonella typhimurium, *J. Antimicrob. Chemother.,* 33(3), 509–522, 1994.

8. Balland, O., Pinto-Alphandary, H., Viron, A., Puvion, E., Andremont, A., and Couvreur, P., Intracellular distribution of ampicillin in murine macrophages infected with Salmonella typhimurium and treated with (3H)ampicillin-loaded nanoparticles, *J. Antimicrob. Chemother.,* 37(1), 105–115, 1996.

9. Forestier, F., Gerrier, P., Chaumard, C., Quero, A.M., Couvreur, P., and Labarre, C., Effect of nanoparticle-bound ampicillin on the survival of Listeria monocytogenes in mouse peritoneal macrophages, *J. Antimicrob. Chemother.,* 30(2), 173–179, 1992.

10. Youssef, M., Fattal, E., Alonso, M. J., Roblot-Treupel, L., Sauzieres, J., Tancrede, C., Omnes, A., Couvreur, P., and Andremont, A., Effectiveness of nanoparticle-bound ampicillin in the treatment of Listeria monocytogenes infection in athymic nude mice, *Antimicrob. Agents Chemother.,* 32(8), 1204–1207, 1988.

11. Illum, L., Davis, S.S., Muller, R.H., Mak, E., and West, P., The organ distribution and circulation time of intravenously injected colloidal carriers sterically stabilized with a block copolymer — poloxamine 908, *Life Sci.,* 40(4), 367–374, 1987.

12. Gref, R., Minamitake, Y., Peracchia, M.T., Trubetskoy, V., Torchilin, V., and Langer, R., Biodegradable long-circulating polymeric nanospheres, *Science* 263(5153), 1600–1603, 1994.

13. Peracchia, M.T., Vauthier, C., Desmaele, D., Gulik, A., Dedieu, J.C., Demoy, M., D'Angelo, J., and Couvreur, P., Pegylated nanoparticles from a novel methoxypolyethylene glycol cyanoacrylate-hexadecyl cyanoacrylate amphiphilic copolymer, *Pharm. Res.,* 15(4), 550–556, 1998.

14. Peracchia, M.T., Fattal, E., Desmaele, D., Besnard, M., Noel, J.P., Gomis, J.M., Appel, M., d'Angelo, J., and Couvreur, P., Stealth PEGylated polycyanoacrylate nanoparticles for intravenous administration and splenic targeting, *J. Controlled Release,* 60(1), 121–128, 1999.

15. Muller, R.H., *Colloidal Carriers for Controlled Drug Delivery and Targeting,* CRC Press, Boca Raton, FL, 1991.

16. Brigger, I., Morizet, J., Aubert, G., Chacun, H., Terrier-Lacombe, M.J., Couvreur, P., and Vassal, G., Poly(ethylene glycol)-coated hexadecylcyanoacrylate nanospheres display a combined effect for brain tumor targeting, *J. Pharmacol. Exp. Ther.,* 303(3), 928–936, 2002.

17. Calvo, P., Gouritin, B., Villarroya, H., Eclancher, F., Giannavola, C., Klein, C., Andreux, J.P., and Couvreur, P., Quantification and localization of PEGylated polycyanoacrylate nanoparticles in brain and spinal cord during experimental allergic encephalomyelitis in the rat, *Eur. J. Neurosci.,* 15(8), 1317–1326, 2002.

18. Kreuter, J., Ramge, P., Petrov, V., Hamm, S., Gelperina, S.E., Engelhardt, B., Alyautdin, R., von Briesen, H., and Begley, D.J., Direct evidence that polysorbate-80-coated poly(butylcyanoacrylate) nanoparticles deliver drugs to the CNS via specific mechanisms requiring prior binding of drug to the nanoparticles, *Pharm. Res.,* 20(3), 409–416, 2003.

19. Weitman, S.D., Lark, R.H., Coney, L.R., Fort, D.W., Frasca, V., Zurawski, V.R., Jr., and Kamen, B.A., Distribution of the folate receptor GP38 in normal and malignant cell lines and tissues, *Cancer Res.,* 52(12), 3396–3401, 1992.

20. Campbell, I.G., Jones, T.A., Foulkes, W.D., and Trowsdale, J., Folate-binding protein is a marker for ovarian cancer, *Cancer Res.,* 51(19), 5329–5338, 1991.

21. Rothberg, K.G., Ying, Y.S., Kolhouse, J.F., Kamen, B.A., and Anderson, R.G., The glycophospholipid-linked folate receptor internalizes folate without entering the clathrin-coated pit endocytic pathway, *J. Cell Biol.,* 110(3), 637–649, 1990.

22. Stella, B., Arpicco, S., Peracchia, M.T., Desmaele, D., Hoebeke, J., Renoir, M., D'Angelo, J., Cattel, L., and Couvreur, P., Design of folic acid-conjugated nanoparticles for drug targeting, *J. Pharm. Sci.,* 89(11), 1452–1464, 2000.

23. Cuvier, C., Roblot-Treupel, L., Millot, J.M., Lizard, G., Chevillard, S., Manfait, M., Couvreur, P., and Poupon, M.F., Doxorubicin-loaded nanospheres bypass tumor cell multidrug resistance, *Biochem. Pharmacol.,* 44(3), 509–517, 1992.

24. de Verdiere, A.C., Dubernet, C., Nemati, F., Soma, E., Appel, M., Ferte, J., Bernard, S., Puisieux, F., and Couvreur, P., Reversion of multidrug resistance with polyalkylcyanoacrylate nanoparticles: towards a mechanism of action, *Br. J. Cancer,* 76(2), 198–205, 1997.

25. Colin de Verdiere, A., Dubernet, C., Nemati, F., Poupon, M.F., Puisieux, F., and Couvreur, P., Uptake of doxorubicin from loaded nanoparticles in multidrug-resistant leukemic murine cells, *Cancer Chemother. Pharmacol.*, 33(6), 504–508, 1994.

26. Bennis, S., Chapey, C., Couvreur, P., and Robert, J., Enhanced cytotoxicity of doxorubicin encapsulated in polyisohexylcyanoacrylate nanospheres against multidrug-resistant tumour cells in culture, *Eur. J. Cancer*, 30A(1), 89–93, 1994.

27. Ponchel, G. and Irache, J., Specific and non-specific bioadhesive particulate systems for oral delivery to the gastrointestinal tract, *Adv. Drug Delivery Rev.*, 34(2–3), 191–219, 1998.

28. Dembri, A., Montisci, M.J., Gantier, J.C., Chacun, H., and Ponchel, G., Targeting of 3-azido 3-deoxythymidine (AZT)-loaded poly(isohexylcyanoacrylate) nanospheres to the gastrointestinal mucosa and associated lymphoid tissues, *Pharm. Res.*, 18(4), 467–473, 2001.

29. Damge, C., Michel, C., Aprahamian, M., and Couvreur, P., New approach for oral administration of insulin with polyalkylcyanoacrylate nanocapsules as drug carrier, *Diabetes*, 37(2), 246–251, 1988.

30. Damge, C., Michel, C., Aprahamian, M., Couvreur, P., and Devissaguet, J.P., Nanocapsules as carriers for oral peptide delivery, *J. Controlled Release*, 13(2–3), 233–239, 1990.

31. Allaoui-Attarki, K., Fattal, E., Pecquet, S., Trolle, S., Chachaty, E., Couvreur, P., and Andremont, A., Mucosal immunogenicity elicited in mice by oral vaccination with phosphorylcholine encapsulated in poly (D,L-lactide-co-glycolide) microspheres, *Vaccine*, 16(7), 685–691, 1998.

32. Pecquet, S., Leo, E., Fritsche, R., Pfeifer, A., Couvreur, P., and Fattal, E., Oral tolerance elicited in mice by beta-lactoglobulin entrapped in biodegradable microspheres, *Vaccine*, 18(13), 1196–1202, 2000.

33. Trolle, S., Chachaty, E., Kassis-Chikhani, N., Wang, C., Fattal, E., Couvreur, P., Diamond, B., Alonso, J., and Andremont, A., Intranasal immunization with protein-linked phosphorylcholine protects mice against a lethal intranasal challenge with streptococcus pneumoniae, *Vaccine*, 18(26), 2991–2998, 2000.

9 Polymeric Micelles as Pharmaceutical Carriers

Vladimir P. Torchilin

CONTENTS

9.1 INTRODUCTION

One can name a variety of soluble polymers, microparticles made of insoluble or biodegradable natural and synthetic polymers, microcapsules, cells, cell ghosts, lipoproteins, liposomes, and micelles among the drug carriers suggested to minimize drug degradation and loss, prevent harmful side effects, and increase drug bioavailability. Each of these carriers offers its own advantages and has its own shortcomings, therefore the choice of a certain carrier for each given case can be made only by taking into account all of relevant considerations.

Low solubility in water appears to be an intrinsic property of many drugs and anticancer agents, in particular, because many of them are bulky polycyclic compounds [1]. If the molecular target of a drug is located inside the cell, a drug molecule must have a certain degree of hydrophobicity in order to cross the cell membrane [2,3]. It has also been observed that a drug or drug candidate often needs a lipophilic group to show an affinity toward the target receptor [4,5]. On the other hand, therapeutic application of hydrophobic, poorly-water-soluble agents is associated with serious problems. Low solubility in water is usually associated with poor absorption and bioavailability upon oral administration [5]. Intravenous administration of aggregates formed by an insoluble drug can cause embolization of blood vessels resulting in side effects as severe as respiratory system failure [6]. The formation of drug aggregates can also result in high localized concentrations at the sites of deposition associated with local toxicity and/or lowered systemic bioavailability [7]. By some estimates, almost a half of the potentially valuable drug candidates identified by high-throughput screening are rejected because of their poor water solubility [8]. The ways to address the poor solubility of drugs in order to increase their bioavailability is to use excipients such as ethanol and some other organic solvents [7]. The administration of many cosolvents, however, causes toxic or other undesirable side effects [9]. Formation of salts or adjusting pH can facilitate the dissolution of poorly soluble drugs if they contain ionizable groups [10]. More recent approaches include the use of liposomes [11], microemulsions [12], and cyclodextrins [8]; however, the solubilization capacity of these systems varies with the nature of the drug.

When one deals with poorly-water-soluble pharmaceuticals, micelles as drug carriers provide a set of evident advantages. First, they can efficiently solubilize water-insoluble drugs, increasing their bioavailability and protecting the incorporated drug from the inactivation in biological surroundings. Second, they can stay in the circulation long enough providing gradual accumulation in body regions with leaky vasculature via the enhanced permeability and retention effect, EPR, known also as a "passive" targeting or accumulation via an impaired filtration mechanism, and enhance drug delivery in those areas [13–15]. Third, they can be targeted by attaching a specific ligand to their outer surface.

Micelles represent colloidal dispersions with particle sizes between 5 and 50 to 100 nm. Among colloidal dispersions, micelles belong to a group of association or amphiphilic colloids, which, under certain conditions (concentration and temperature), are spontaneously formed by amphiphilic or surface-active agents (surfactants), which are molecules that consist of two clearly distinct regions with opposite affinities towards water [16]. At low concentrations, these amphiphilic molecules exist separately; however, as their concentration is increased, aggregation takes place within a rather narrow concentration interval. Those aggregates, micelles, consist of several dozens of amphiphilic molecules and usually have a spherical shape. The concentration of a monomeric amphiphile at which micelles appear is called the *critical micelle concentration* (CMC), whereas the number of individual molecules forming a micelle is called the *aggregation number of the micelle*.

An important pharmacy-related property of micelles is their ability to increase the solubility of sparingly soluble substances. This phenomenon was extensively investigated and reviewed in many publications (for example, Reference 17 and Reference 18). Micelles made of nonionic surfactants (the most frequently used pharmaceutical micelles) are known to have the anisotropic water distribution within their structure — water concentration decreases from the surface toward the core of the micelle. Because of this anisotropy, such micelles demonstrate a polarity gradient from the highly hydrated surface to the hydrophobic core. As a result, the spatial position of a certain solubilized substance (drug) within a micelle will depend on its polarity. In aqueous systems, nonpolar molecules will be solubilized within the micelle core, polar molecules will be adsorbed on the micelle surface, and substances with intermediate polarity will be distributed along surfactant molecules in certain intermediate positions. The capacity of surfactants for drugs depends on various factors, such as chemical structure of a drug and surfactant, polarity of a drug, the location of a drug within the micelles, temperature, pH, etc. Thus, an increase in the length of a hydrophobic region of a surfactant facilitates the solubilization of a hydrophobic drug inside the micelle core.

Micellization of biologically-active substances is a general phenomenon believed, for example, to increase the bioavailability of lipophilic drugs upon oral administration via drug solubilization in the gut by naturally occurring biliary lipid or fatty-acid-containing mixed micelles produced by an organism. Surfactant micelles are also widely used as adjuvant and drug carrier systems in many areas of pharmaceutical technology and research on controlled drug delivery. As it is evident from the numerous publications, for example, Reference 19 and Reference 20 and references therein, almost every possible drug administration route has benefited from the use of micellar forms of drugs in terms of either a reduction of adverse effects or an increased bioavailability due to enhanced permeability across the physiological barrier and/or substantial changes in drug biodistribution. Even the blood–brain barrier can be considered as a potential penetration target for micelle-incorporated drugs [21,22].

Amid other micelle-forming amphiphilic substances, low-molecular-weight oligoethyleneglycol-based surfactants are widely used in pharmaceutical technology as solubilizers for poorly-water-soluble drugs, for example, polysorbate 80, for parenteral and oral routes of drug delivery [23–25]. The main advantage of oligoethyleneglycol-based surfactants for pharmacological applications is their low toxicity [26–29]. The definite drawback of many micellar systems prepared from low-molecular-weight surfactants is their instability in aqueous media and dissociation upon the dilution. CMC values of these surfactants are usually in the millimolar range. *In vivo*, this results in micelle collapse in the blood upon administration because of instant dilution with the entire blood volume, with subsequent precipitation of the incorporated drug or its transfer to plasma proteins. Hence, in terms of drug delivery carrier development, there is a need to use more stable micelles with lower CMC values. Amphiphilic polymers known to form stable, low-CMC polymeric micelles in aqueous solutions have been proposed as drug carriers [30].

9.2 POLYMERIC MICELLES

Polymeric micelles represent a separate class of micelles and are formed from copolymers consisting of both hydrophilic and hydrophobic monomer units. Amphiphilic diblock AB-type or triblock ABA-type copolymers with the length of a hydrophilic block exceeding to some extent that of a hydrophobic one can form spherical micelles in aqueous solutions (Figure 9.1). The particulates are composed of the core of the hydrophobic blocks stabilized by the corona of hydrophilic polymeric chains. If the length of a hydrophilic block is too large, copolymers exist in water as unimers (individual molecules), whereas molecules with very long hydrophobic blocks form structures

A. *Structures of micelle-forming copolymers*

Block copolymers

| A - hydrophilic unit |
| B - hydrophobic unit |

di - block   AAAAAAABBBBBB

tri - block   AAAABBBBBAAAA

Graft copolymer   AAAAAAAAAAAAA
                        B   B
                        B   B
                        B   B
                                       B

B. *Examples of block copolymers*

C. *Micelle formation from di-block and tri-block co-polymers*

Di-block copolymers

1.   HO–(CH$_2$CH$_2$O)–(CH$_2$CH)$_m$–H

Poly(ethylene oxide)-*b*-poly (styrene) block copolymer

2.   H$_3$O–(CH$_2$CH$_2$O)$_n$–(CH$_2$CH)$_m$–H
                                    |
                                    CH$_3$

Poly(ethylene oxide)-*b*-poly(D, L-lactide) block copolymer

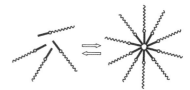

Tri-block copolymers

3.   HO–(CH$_2$CH$_2$O)$_n$–(CH$_2$CH)$_m$–H
                              |
                              CH$_3$

Poly(ethylene oxide)-b-poly(propylene oxide)-*b*-
poly(ethylene oxide)tri-block copolymer

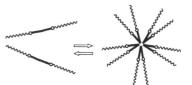

FIGURE 9.1 Micelle-forming copolymers (A and B) and micelle assembly (C).

with nonmicellar morphology, such as rods and lamellae [31]. The major driving force behind micellization is the decrease in the free energy of the system because of the removal of hydrophobic fragments from the aqueous surroundings with the formation of the micelle core stabilized with hydrophilic blocks exposed to water [32,33]. Polymeric micelles often are more stable compared to micelles prepared from conventional detergents, and some amphiphilic copolymers have CMC values as low as 10^6 M [34,35]. In addition to the high thermodynamic stability (determined by low CMC), micelles from certain copolymers have high kinetic stability (retarded disintegration at concentrations lower than the CMC) [36], apparently because of the presence of multiple sites capable of hydrophobic interaction within each polymer molecule. The lower the CMC value of a given amphiphilic polymer, the more stable are the micelles even at a low net concentration of an amphiphile in the medium [37]. This is especially important from a practical point of view because, upon dilution with a large volume of blood, micelles with high CMC values may dissociate into unimers and their contents may precipitate in the blood.

From the practical point of view, the size of unimers formed upon micelle dissociation plays an important physiological role in the efficacy of its kidney filtration. In an optimal case, the unimer molecular size should not exceed 20 to 30 kDa, which roughly corresponds to the renal filtration limit [38]. Although both hydrophilic and hydrophobic blocks influence the micelle CMC value, the hydrophobic block plays a more crucial role [39,40]. The following general principles can be applied to characterize the role of the different structural blocks in maintaining micelle stability: (1) an increase in the length of a hydrophobic block at a given length of a hydrophilic block causes a noticeable decrease in the CMC value and an increase in micelle stability, (2) an increase in the length of a hydrophilic block at a given length of a hydrophobic block results in only a small rise of the CMC value, (3) an increase in the molecular weight of the unimer at a given hydrophilic: hydrophobic ratio causes some decrease in the CMC value, and (4) in general, CMC values for triblock copolymers are higher than those for diblock copolymers at the same molecular weight and hydrophilic:hydrophobic ratio [39–43]. The stability of micelles is also strongly influenced by properties of the micelle core, such as its microviscosity, and the core microviscosity can be experimentally determined using fluorescent probes [44,45] or proton magnetic resonance [46].

The "ideal" pharmaceutical micelle [47] should possess a suitable size (from 10 to 100 nm), demonstrate sufficiently high stability both *in vitro* and *in vivo*, i.e., have a good combination of a low CMC value and high kinetic stability, be long-circulating and still able to eventually disintegrate into bioinert and nontoxic unimers that should be easily cleared from the body, and carry a substantial quantity of a micelle-incorporated pharmaceutical agent. The core compartment of the pharmaceutical polymeric micelle should demonstrate a high loading capacity, controlled-release profile for the incorporated drug, and good compatibility between the core-forming block and incorporated drug. The micelle corona should provide an effective steric protection for the micelle. It also determines micelle hydrophilicity, micelle charge, the presence of reactive groups suitable for further micelle derivatization, such as an attachment of targeting moieties, and is itself determined by the length and density of hydrophilic blocks [22,48–51]. The micellar corona properties control important biological characteristics of a micellar carrier, such as its pharmacokinetics, biodistribution, biocompatibility, longevity, surface adsorption of biomacromolecules, adhesion to biosurfaces, and targetability [22,48–53]. Numerous studies have been published on the theory of micelle formation and on micelle properties. Reference 20, Reference 37, and Reference 54 represent a few examples.

The hydrophilic blocks in diblock and triblock copolymers frequently contain polyethylene glycol (PEG) chains, because this polymer is known to be highly hydrated and is able to serve as an efficient steric protector for various particulates (micelles, liposomes, nanoparticles, and nanocapsules) in biological media [55,56]. Triple copolymers of hydrophilic ethylene oxide units with hydrophobic propylene oxide units (such polymers are known as *pluronics*) are the most common examples of pharmaceutical triblock copolymers. Some structures of pharmaceutical di- and triblock copolymers are presented in Figure 9.1. In the case of grafted copolymers, multiple hydrophobic chains are distributed along the main chain composed of hydrophilic units [45,57].

Whatever route of micelle formation is envisioned, in the majority of cases, the structure of amphiphilic unimers still follows some simple rules: PEG blocks with a molecular weight from 1 to 15 kDa are usually corona-forming blocks, and the length of a hydrophobic core-forming block is close to or somewhat lower than that of a hydrophilic block [38]. Although some other hydrophilic polymers may be used to make corona blocks [58,59], PEG still remains the hydrophilic block of choice. At the same time, a variety of polymers may be used to build hydrophobic core-forming blocks. The list includes polymers of propylene oxide [22,60], aspartic acid [61,62], β-benzoyl-L-aspartate [34,63], γ-benzyl-L-glutamate [64], caprolactone [65,66], D,L-lactic acid [67,68], and spermine [69]. Phospholipid residues — short, but extremely hydrophobic due to the presence of two long-chain fatty acyl groups — can also be successfully used as hydrophobic core-forming groups [13]. In certain cases, the starting copolymers can be prepared from two hydrophilic blocks and then one of those blocks may be modified by the attachment of a hydrophobic pharmaceutical agent (such as paclitaxel, cisplatin, anthracycline antibiotics, hydrophobic diagnostic units, etc.) yielding amphiphilic micelle-forming copolymers [20,70,71].

The stability of micelles significantly depends on the strength of van der Waals interactions between hydrophobic blocks forming the core of the particle and the molecular size of the hydrophilic block counterbalancing the non-water-soluble part of the macromolecule. As mentioned previously, phospholipid residues can be successfully used as hydrophobic core-forming groups [19]. Diacyllipid-PEG conjugates, such as PEG-phosphatidylethanolamine (PEG-PE), initially introduced as polymeric surface modifiers for liposomes [72], by themselves represent amphiphilic polymers and form very stable micelles in an aqueous environment [19,73]. PEG-PEs with a molecular weight of PEG chains from 750 to 5000 Da form micelles spontaneously upon simply shaking a dry PEG-PE film in the presence of an aqueous medium or by a detergent or water-miscible solvent removal method. All versions of PEG-PE conjugates form micelles with sizes of 7 to 35 nm. Micelles formed from conjugates with PEG blocks of higher molecular weight have a slightly larger size, indicating that the micelle size may be tailored for a particular application by varying the length of PEG. Normally, PEG-PE micelles have a spherical shape and uniform size distribution [74]. CMCs of all PEG-PE conjugates studied are in a 10^5 M range, which is at least 100-fold lower than those of conventional detergents [75]. Such low CMC values of PEG-PE conjugates indicate that micelles prepared from these polymers will maintain their integrity even upon strong dilution (for example, in the blood during a therapeutic application). For parenteral therapeutic applications, it is important that a delivery system is not affected by biological fluids. PEG$_{2000}$-DSPE and PEG$_{5000}$-DSPE micelles retain their size and integrity even after a 48-h incubation in the blood plasma [76].

PEG-PE micelles can efficiently incorporate some sparingly soluble and amphiphilic substances [19,77]. Radiolabeled PEG-PE micelles were found to have sufficiently long half-lives, from 1.5 to 2.5 h in mice, depending on the molecular size of PEG block (though somewhat shorter than those for PEG-containing liposomes). The shorter micelle half-life compared to PEG-liposomes may be explained by the faster micelles extravasation from the vasculature owing to their considerably smaller size [76]. As with long-circulating liposomes, the exposure of PEG residues on the surface prevents rapid uptake of the particles by the reticuloendothelial system, making them long circulating. PEG-PE has very low toxicity, and it is currently approved for clinical use as a component of Doxil® — long-circulating liposomes loaded with doxorubicin [78].

Quite a few amphiphilic polymers have been shown to possess properties similar to that of PEG-PE [55,58,79,80]. Such polymers can be incorporated into liposomes; they can provide liposomes with efficient steric protection [55] and form micelles [19]. Polymers of vinyl pyrrolidone (PVP) are of special interest because of their high biocompatibility. Various amphiphilic PVP derivatives have been synthesized using long-chain acyls (such as palmitoyl and stearoyl) or phospholipid residues as hydrophobic blocks [81]. Fast, spontaneous micellization and low CMC values (in a low μM range) were found for an amphiphilic PVP with the PVP block of molecular weight less than 15 kDa. This means that stable micelles may be prepared from the whole variety of different amphiphilic polymers, which broadens the possibility of preparing micelles with the required physicochemical and biological properties for each particular purpose.

9.3 LOADING POLYMERIC MICELLES WITH DRUGS

Similar to micelles formed by conventional detergents, polymeric micelles solubilize poorly-water-soluble drugs by incorporating them into their hydrophobic core, thus allowing for an increased bioavailability [20,32,82]. The high stability of polymeric micelles ensures the retention of encapsulated drugs in the solubilized form upon parenteral administration. Moreover, the use of polymeric micelles often allows the achievement of an extended circulation time, favorable biodistribution, and lower toxicity of a drug. The process of solubilization of water-insoluble drugs by micelle-forming amphiphilic block copolymers strongly depends on the interactions between a solubilized drug and micelle core-forming hydrophobic block of a copolymer [41]. Mathematical simulation of the solubilization process [83] demonstrated that the initial solubilization proceeds via the displacement of solvent (water) molecules from the micelle core, and later a solubilized drug begins to accumulate in the very center of the micelle core, "pushing" the hydrophobic blocks away from this area. Extensive solubilization may result in some increase of micelle size because of the expansion of its core with a solubilized drug. The size of both core-forming and corona-forming blocks, among other factors, influence the efficacy of drug loading into the micelle [47]. The larger the hydrophobic block, the bigger the core size and its ability to entrap hydrophobic drugs. On the other hand, an increase in the length of the hydrophilic block increases the CMC value and decreases the quantity of the micelle-associated drug. The hydrophobic–hydrophilic balance of the drug molecule itself will also influence load efficacy, because, depending on this balance, the drug molecule will be located in different micellar compartments and, hence, will associate with the micelle with varying affinities. Molecules that are located within the corona area can be released from the micelle pretty rapidly, providing the "fast release" component of the net release [84]. The phase state of the drug can also be important for its association with a micelle because, in some cases, the drug is not dissolved in the core compartment and exists as a separate phase inside the core, which may hinder its release [85]. An excessive stabilization of drug-bearing polymeric micelles may thus negatively influence drug efficacy and bioavailability [86].

The drug can be incorporated into the micelle by simple physical entrapment in the micelle core or via preliminary covalent or electrostatic binding with a hydrophobic block of a micelle-forming amphiphilic block copolymer. Because the hydrophobic interactions constitute the main driving force behind micellar solubilization of water-insoluble drugs, the increase in the hydrophobic block content within the polymer molecule was shown to enhance insoluble drug incorporation into micelles [87]. The successful incorporation of charged drugs (such as DNA) into micelles requires the presence of the opposite charge on the hydrophobic block of a micelle-forming copolymer. If a drug is chemically or electrostatically attached to a hydrophobic block of a micelle-forming copolymer, its incorporation into the micelle core proceeds simultaneously with micelle formation. To physically entrap a drug into a micelle, several techniques have been offered, such as the direct dissolution protocol, in which a copolymer solution in water is added to a drug dried from a solution in an organic solvent. Solutions of PEG-PE and a drug of interest in miscible volatile organic solvents are mixed, and organic solvents are evaporated to form a PEG-PE–drug film. The film obtained is then hydrated in the presence of an aqueous buffer, and the micelles are formed by intensive shaking. If the amount of a drug exceeds the solubilization capacity of micelles, the excess drug precipitates in a crystalline form and the precipitated crystals are removed by filtration. Alternatively, the drug dissolved in a volatile organic solvent is added to the water solution of preformed micelles with a subsequent solvent evaporation from the system [82]. In the case of a dialysis method [34,68,88], a drug to be incorporated is simply dissolved together with micelle-forming copolymers in an organic solvent with further dialysis against water. In some cases, to improve drug solubilization, additional micelle-forming compounds may be added to PEG-PE micelles. Thus, to increase the encapsulation efficiency of paclitaxel, egg phosphatidyl-choline (ePC) was added to the micelle composition. The addition of ePC into the micelle composition approximately doubles the paclitaxel encapsulation efficiency [88]. The increased efficiency of paclitaxel encapsulation into PEG-PE or ePC may be explained by the fact that ePC, unlike PEG-PE, does not have a bulky hydrophilic PEG domain and its addition to micelle dispersions results in particles with a higher hydrophobic content [89].

Whatever the exact protocol used, Pluronic®-based micelles were shown to effectively solubilize drugs such as diazepam, indomethacin [90,91], adriamycin [63,92,93], anthracycline antibiotics [94], and polynucleotides [95]. Doxorubicin incorporated into Pluronic® micelles was superior, when compared to the free drug, in the experimental treatment of murine tumors (leukemia P388, myeloma, Lewis lung carcinoma) and human tumors (breast carcinoma MCF-7) in mice [86]. In addition, a reduction of the side effects of the drug was observed in many cases. For example, a decrease in toxicity was found for the polymeric micelle-incorporated antitumor drug KRN5500 [96].

Early detailed studies of the *in vivo* behavior and biodistribution of therapeutic polymeric micelles using the micelles formed by a copolymer of poly(ethylene glycol) and poly(aspartic acid) (PEG-*b*-PAA) with covalently bound adriamycin [PEG-*b*-PAA(ADR)] have been performed by Kataoka et al. [20,61]. Micelles formed from this conjugate are rather stable *in vivo,* and their disintegration takes hours. It has been found that upon intravenous injection, the circulation time and biodistribution of micelles depend on the relative size of the copolymer blocks. PEG-*b*-PAA(ADR) micelles with a PEG block of 12 kDa and PAA(ADR) with 20 aspartyl adriamycin units has a half-life (t_f) of approximately 7 h in mice; similar micelles with 5 kDa PEG block have a t_f of approximately 1.5 h, and micelles with 1 kDa PEG block have a t_f substantially lower than 1 h. It seems that longer PEG blocks and shorter PAA segments favor longer circulation times and lower uptake by the reticuloendothelial system [97].

A set of micelle-forming copolymers of PEG with poly(L-aminoacids) was used to prepare drug-loaded micelles by direct entrapment of a drug into the micelle core without covalent attachment of drug molecules to core-forming blocks [61,98–100]. The most vivid example is the micellar form of indomethacin [87]. A similar "noncovalent" approach was used for the successful solubilization of paclitaxel by micelle-forming copolymers of PEG and poly(D,L-lactic acid) (PEG-*b*-PLA) [74,111]. The use of micelles increased paclitaxel solubility from less than 0.1 to 20 mg/ml. In addition, the micelles decrease the toxicity of paclitaxel in normal organs and tissues. Also PEG-*b*-poly(caprolactone) copolymer micelles have been successfully used as delivery vehicles for dihydrotestosterone [101].

Similar to other polymeric micelles, PEG-PE micelles can also efficiently incorporate some sparingly soluble and amphiphilic substances. A variety of sparingly soluble and amphiphilic substances including paclitaxel, tamoxifen, camptothecin, porphyrine, and vitamin K_3 have been successfully solubilized by PEG-PE micelles [102,103]. It is conceivable that the most successful therapeutic applications of PEG-lipid polymeric micelles as drug carriers would be those involving the use of the appropriately hydrophobized prodrugs. The hydrophobized prodrug approach is not a new one in the area of drug delivery systems as it has been successfully used to increase the permeation of peptides across intestinal membranes and to increase the loading of anticancer drug derivatives into reconstituted low-density lipoproteins by covalent coupling of the lipophilic anchor directly to the drug [104].

An important area of polymeric micelle-mediated drug delivery is gene therapy, because both plasmid DNA and antisense oligonucleotides can assemble into micelle-like particles in the presence of various amphiphilic block copolymers, such as PEG-*b*-poly(L-lysine) (i.e., PEG-*b*-PLL) or PEG-*b*-polyspermine, primarily via electrostatic interactions [105–107] (the formation of a tight electrostatic complex between oppositely charged DNA and PLL block). Table 9.1 presents some

TABLE 9.1

Some Examples of the Block Copolymers Used to Prepare Drug-Loaded Micelles

Block Copolymers	Drugs Incorporated
Pluronics®	Doxorubicin, cisplatin–doxorubicin, epirubicin–doxorubicin, haloperidol, ATP
Polycaprolactone-*b*-PEG	FK506, L-685,818
Polycaprolactone-*b*-methoxy-PEG	Indomethacin
Poly(*N*-isopropylacrylamide)-*b*-PEG	Miscellaneous
Poly(aspartic acid)-*b*-PEG	Doxorubicin, cisplatin, lysozyme
Poly(*γ*-benzyl-L-glutamate)-*b*-PEG	Clonazepam
Poly(D,L-lactide)-*b*-methoxy-PEG	Paclitaxel, testosterone
Poly(*β*-benzyl-L-aspartate)-*b*- poly(*α*-hydroxy-ethylene oxide)	Doxorubicin
Poly(*β*-benzyl-L-aspartate)-*b*-PEG	Doxorubicin, Indomethacin, KRN, amphotericin B
Poly(L-lysine)-*b*-PEG	DNA
Oligo(methyl methacrylate)-*b*-poly(acrylic acid)	Doxorubicin
PEG-PE	Dequalinium, soya bean trypsin inhibitor, paclitaxel, camptothecin, tamoxifen, porphyrine, vitamin K_3

examples of various amphiphilic micelle-forming polymers that have been used for the preparation of micellar drugs.

Micelle-incorporated drugs may be slowly released from an intact micelle, especially if those drugs are not too hydrophobic (log P value is not too high). Still, in some cases a micellar drug demonstrates lower activity than a free drug, and such low activity has been specifically attributed to the retarded release of the drug from the micelle [102,108]. When the drug is covalently attached to a hydrophobic block, the drug-to-polymer bond must be cleaved to facilitate drug release. The rate of drug release from the micelle can be controlled by a wide variety of parameters such as micelle structure, the size of a hydrophobic block, phase state of the micelle core, pH value of the external medium, and temperature. Manipulating pH from acidic to neutral, for example, results in an accelerated release of indomethacin from micelles made of PEG-poly(*β*-benzyl-L-aspartate) copolymer [34].

9.4 TARGETED POLYMERIC MICELLES

Making micelles capable of specific (preferential) accumulation in desired body compartments or pathological zones (i.e., making targeted micelles) can further increase the efficiency of micelle-encapsulated pharmaceuticals. There are several approaches to micelle targeting. One of them is based on the preferential accumulation of drug-loaded micelles in areas with "leaky" vasculature (such as tumors and infarcts) via the enhanced permeability and retention (EPR) effect [13–15]. The EPR effect is based on the spontaneous penetration (extravasation) of long-circulating macromolecules, molecular aggregates, and nanoparticulate drug carriers into the interstitium through the compromised vasculature in certain pathological sites in the body. It has been shown that the EPR effect is typical for solid tumors and infarcts [13–15]. Thus, micelle formulations from PEG_{750}-PE, PEG_{2000}-PE, and PEG_{5000}-PE conjugates demonstrated much higher accumulation in tumors compared to normal tissue (muscle) in experimental Lewis lung carcinoma (tumors with a relatively small vasculature cutoff size [109,110]) in mice. The largest total tumor uptake of the injected dose within the observation period area under the curve (AUC) was found for micelles formed by PEG_{5000}-PE. This was explained by the fact that these micelles had the longest circulation time and suffered little extravasation into the normal tissue compared to micelles prepared from the shorter

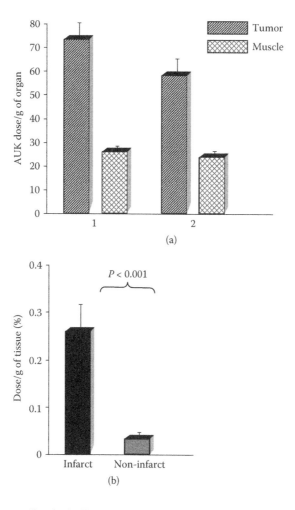

FIGURE 9.2 EPR-effect-mediated micelle accumulation *in vivo* in pathological areas with increased vascular permeability: (a) accumulation of PEG-PE micelles (as AUC) in murine Lewis lung carcinoma tumor (1) and in EL4 T cell lymphoma tumor (2) compared to adjacent normal tissue, (b) accumulation of PEG-PE micelles in the area of experimental myocardial infarction in rabbit (as dose per gram of tissue).

PEG-PE conjugates. Micelles prepared from PEG_{750}-DSPE or PEG_{2000}-DSPE also selectively accumulated in EL4 T lymphoma tumors in mice [76]. Some other recent data also clearly confirmed spontaneous EPR-mediated targeting of PEG-PE-based micelles to experimental tumors [74] in mice as well as into the damaged heart areas in rabbits with experimental myocardial infarction [111] (Figure 9.2). In the last case, after the injection of ^{111}In-labeled micelles, the accumulated radioactivity localized within the infarcted zones was revealed by the histochemical staining. The accumulation of micelles in the infarct was approximately tenfold higher than in normal heart tissue.

Thus, the transport efficacy and accumulation of microparticulates, including micelles, in tumors is, to a great extent, determined by their ability to penetrate the tumor vascular endothelium. Diffusion and accumulation parameters were shown to be strongly dependent on the cutoff size of the tumor blood vessel wall, and the cutoff size varies for different tumors [112,113]. As tumor vasculature permeability depends on the particular type of tumor [113], the use of micelles as drug carriers could be specifically reserved for tumors whose vasculature has the low cutoff size (below 200 nm). In these cases, small micelles should provide more efficient drug delivery into tumors than other nanoparticulate drug carriers. Thus, the micelle-incorporated model protein (soybean trypsin inhibitor) accumulated in subcutaneous Lewis lung carcinoma in mice to a higher extent than when the same protein was encapsulated in larger liposomes [110]. Also, adriamycin in polymeric micelles was shown to be much more efficient in the experimental treatment of murine solid tumor, colon adenocarcinoma, than the free drug [114].

Another targeting mechanism is based on the premise that many pathological processes are accompanied by a local temperature increase and/or acidosis [115,116]. Hence, the efficiency of the micellar carriers may be improved by making micelles capable of disintegration under the increased temperature or decreased pH values in pathological sites, i.e., by combining the EPR effect with stimuli responsiveness. For this purpose, micelles were made of thermo- or pH-sensitive components, such as poly(N-isopropylacrylamide) and its copolymers with poly(D,L-lactide) and other blocks, and such micelles possess the ability to disintegrate in target areas, releasing the micelle-incorporated drug [117–119]. pH-responsive polymeric micelles loaded with phtalocyanine seem to be promising carriers for the photodynamic cancer therapy [120], whereas doxorubicin-loaded polymeric micelles containing acid-cleavable linkages provided enhanced intracellular drug delivery into tumor cells and a higher antitumor efficiency [121]. Thermoresponsive polymeric micelles have been shown to demonstrate an increased drug release upon temperature changes [122].

As with other drug carriers, the efficiency of polymeric micelles may also be enhanced by attaching targeting ligands to the micelle surface. The attachment of various specific ligands to the water-exposed termini of hydrophilic blocks could be used to improve the targeting of micelles, micelle-incorporated drugs, and DNA [123]. Among those ligands, one can name various sugar moieties [124], transferrin [125], and folate residues [126] because many target cells, especially cancer cells, overexpress appropriate receptors (such as transferrin and folate receptors) on their surface. It has been shown that PEG-polylactide copolymer micelles modified with galactose or lactose specifically interact with lectins, thus targeting delivery of the micelles to hepatic sites [123,127]. Transferrin-bearing PEG-polyethyleneimine-based micelles target tumors overexpressing transferrin receptors [125]. Additionally, mixed micelle-like complexes of PEGylated DNA and PEI modified with transferrin [128,129] have also been designed for enhanced DNA delivery into cells overexpressing transferrin receptors. A similar targeting approach was successfully tested with folate-modified micelles [130]. Poly(L-histidine)-PEG and poly(L-lactic acid)-PEG block copolymer micelles carrying folate on their surface combined targetability and pH sensitivity, and effectively delivered adriamycin to tumor cells in vitro, demonstrating their potential for the treatment of solid tumors [131].

Because, among all specific ligands, antibodies provide the greatest opportunities in terms of diversity of targets and specificity of interaction, various attempts to covalently attach antibodies to a surfactant or to polymeric micelles have been made [22,74,123,125,132]. Thus, micelles modified with fatty-acid-conjugated Fab fragments of antibodies to antigens of brain glia cells (acid gliofibrillary antigen and alpha 2-glycoprotein) loaded with neuroleptic trifluoperazine increasingly accumulate in the rat brain upon intracarotid administration [22,132]. By adapting the coupling technique developed for attaching specific ligands to liposomes [133], PEG-PE-based immunomicelles were derivatized with monoclonal antibodies. The approach uses PEG-PE with the free PEG terminus activated with a p-nitrophenylcarbonyl (pNP) group. Diacyllipid fragments of such bifunctional PEG derivatives are firmly incorporated into the micelle core, whereas the water-exposed pNP group, stable at pH values below 6, efficiently interacts with amino groups of various ligands (including antibodies and their fragments) at pH values above 8.0 yielding a stable urethane (carbamate) bond (Figure 9.3a). Using fluorescently labeled proteins and SDS-PAGE, it was calculated that 10 to 20 antibody molecules could be attached to a single micelle [74,134]. Immunomicelles specifically recognize their target substrates as was confirmed by ELISA techniques with corresponding substrate monolayers. The analysis of micelle size and size distribution before and after attachment of various antibodies by the use of dynamic light scattering and freeze-fracture electron microscopy demonstrated that protein attachment did not affect the size of the micelles substantially [74].

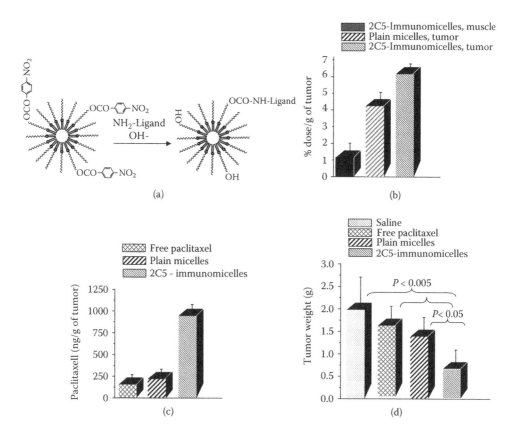

FIGURE 9.3 Immunomicelles: (a) the scheme of the attachment of amino-group-containing ligands to a PEG-based micelle containing *p*-nitrophenylcarbonyl groups on the distal termini of hydrophilic PEG blocks, (b) *in vivo* accumulation of paclitaxel-loaded mAb 2C5-immunomicelles in Lewis lung carcinoma (LLC) in mice 2 h post-administration; immunomicelles show the highest accumulation of all preparations, (c) *in vivo* delivery of paclitaxel by 2C5-immunomicelles to LLC tumor in mice; immunomicelles deliver the maximum quantity of drug to the tumor, (d) therapeutic effect of paclitaxel-loaded 2C5-immunomicelles in mice with LLC tumor; paclitaxel-loaded tumor-targeted PEG-PE micelles inhibit tumor growth by approximately 75% compared to 25% inhibition for the same dose of free drug and 35% inhibition with the drug in nontargeted micelles.

To specifically enhance the tumor accumulation of PEG-PE-based micelles, tumor-specific monoclonal antibodies were used [74,134]. Although anticancer antibodies are usually tumor-type-specific and unable to react with different tumors, we have shown that certain nonpathogenic monoclonal antinuclear autoantibodies with the nucleosome-restricted specificity (monoclonal antibody 2C5, mAb 2C5, among others) recognize the surface of numerous tumor, but not normal cells, via tumor cell surface-bound nucleosomes [135,136]. Fluorescently labeled mAb 2C5-immunomicelles effectively bind to the surface of various unrelated tumor cell lines, such as human BT20 and MCF-7 (breast adenocarcinomas) and murine LLC (Lewis lung carcinoma) and EL4 (T lymphoma) cells. Drug (paclitaxel)-loaded mAb 2C5-immunomicelles also demonstrated the same specific properties as "empty" immunomicelles and effectively bound to various tumors cells. Such specific recognition of cancer cells by drug-loaded mAb 2C5-immunomicelles results in dramatically improved cancer cell killing by such micelles compared to paclitaxel-loaded plain micelles or free drug, as shown *in vitro* with MCF-7 cells. *In vivo* experiments with LLC tumor-bearing mice revealed a dramatically enhanced tumor uptake of paclitaxel-loaded radiolabeled 2C5-immunomicelles as compared to nontargeted micelles (Figure 9.3b). Drug-loaded immunomicelles may also be better internalized by tumor cells in a similar manner to antibody-targeted liposomes [137] and thus deliver more drugs inside tumor cells than might be achieved with the simple EPR-effect-mediated tumor accumulation. By analyzing the absolute quantity of tumor-accumulated paclitaxel (HPLC) [138] delivered by different drug formulations, it was shown that mAb immunomicelles were capable of delivering to tumors substantially higher quantities of paclitaxel than was the case with paclitaxel-loaded nontargeted micelles or the free drug formulation (Figure 9.3c). As a result, a much higher therapeutic efficiency with paclitaxel-loaded mAb 2C5-micelles was observed *in vivo* in mice with LLC tumors (Figure 9.3d).

An interesting new approach is the intracellular delivery of micelles. As PEG-PE micelles have been found to carry a net negative charge [111], which might hinder their internalization by cells, the alteration of this negative charge by the addition of positively charged lipids to PEG-PE was suggested in order to improve the endocytic uptake of micelles by cancer cells, thus increasing the efficiency of this drug delivery system [109]. Moreover, after endocytosis, drug- or DNA-loaded particles are able to escape from the endosomes and enter the cytoplasm of most cells because of the interaction between cationic lipids and the endosomal membranes [139]. Therefore, it is possible that after enhanced endocytosis, paclitaxel-loaded PEG-PE: positively charged lipid mixed micelles could escape from endosomes and enter the cytoplasm of cancer cells, where paclitaxel could be slowly released from the micelles and kill cancer cells with a higher efficiency than the free drug or drugs in negatively charged PEG-PE micelles. The addition of positively charged lipids facilitated the intracellular uptake and cytoplasmic delivery of paclitaxel-containing micelles as evidenced by the fact that the anticancer effect of paclitaxel in mixed (positively-charged-lipid-containing) micelles was significantly greater than that of free paclitaxel and of paclitaxel in PEG-PE micelles in two cancer cell lines. In A2780 cancer cells, the IC50 values of free paclitaxel, paclitaxel in PEG-PE micelles, and paclitaxel in PEG-PE: positively charged lipid mixed micelles were 12.2, 3.9, and 0.7 μM, respectively. Similar results were also obtained with BT-20 cancer cells. The endosome-destabilizing effect and cytoplasmic delivery of drug-loaded mixed micelles were also confirmed by fluorescence microscopy. Similarly, PEG-PE-based micelles loaded with the anticancer vitamin K_3 and 1,8-diazabicyclo[5,4,0]undec-7-ene (DBU) were more cytotoxic than micelles with only vitamin K_3, because DBU facilitated endosomal destabilization and cytoplasmic delivery of vitamin K_3 [140].

9.5 POLYMERIC MICELLES AS CARRIERS OF IMAGING AGENTS

Medical diagnostic imaging modalities that can utilize micelle-based contrast agents include γ scintigraphy, magnetic resonance imaging (MRI), and computed tomography (CT). All these modalities require a certain quantity of reporter groups to be accumulated in the area under observation. To reach the required local concentration of a contrast agent, the use of micelles has been advocated; such micelles should be able to carry multiple reporter moieties for the efficient delivery of contrast agents selectively into the required areas [141,142]. See the generalized scheme of the contrast micelle in Figure 9.4a.

Chelated paramagnetic metal moieties (Gd, Mn, or Dy ions) are the major focus for the design of MR positive (T1) contrast agents. Often, chelated metal ions possess a hydrophilic character (for example, the complex of diethylenetriamine pentaacetic acid [DTPA] with Gd^{3+}). In order to be incorporated into micelles, such structures should be amphiphilic in nature. The synthesis of chelating agents, in which a hydrophilic chelating residue is covalently linked to a hydrophobic (lipid) chain that can be anchored into the micelle's hydrophobic core, whereas a more hydrophilic chelate is localized in the hydrophilic shell of the micelle, was described a long time ago [143]. Several chelating probes of this type have been developed for liposome membrane incorporation studies (DTPA-PE [144], DTPA-stearylamine [DTPA-SA] [145], and amphiphilic acylated paramagnetic complexes of Mn and Gd [146]). The amphiphilic chelating probes (paramagnetic Gd-DTPA-PE and radioactive ^{111}In-DTPA-SA) have been incorporated into PEG (5 kDa)-PE micelles and used *in vivo* for MRI and γ scintigraphy.

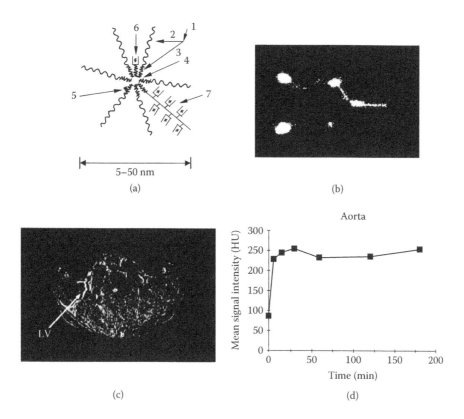

FIGURE 9.4 Polymeric micelles as carriers for imaging agents: (a) schematic representation of micelle loading with a contrast agent. The micelle is formed spontaneously in aqueous media from amphiphilic compound (1), the molecule of which consists of distinct hydrophilic (2) and hydrophobic (3) moieties. Hydrophobic moieties form the micelle core (4). Contrast agent (asterisk; or MR-active metal-loaded chelating group, or heavy elements such as iodine or bromine) can be directly coupled to the hydrophobic moiety within the micelle core (5) or incorporated into the micelle as an individual monomeric (6) or polymeric (7) amphiphilic unit; (b) *micelles in radioscintigraphy (γ-imaging)*. Rabbit lower-body radioscintigram 30 min after subcutaneous administration of 20 μCi ^{111}In-labeled (via DTPA-SA) PEG-PE micelles into the dorsum of both hind paws is shown; (c) *micelles in MRI*. Transverse MR image of axillary or subscapular lymph node areas in the rabbit 4 min after subcutaneous administration of PEG-PE micelles containing core-incorporated Gd-loaded amphiphilic chelate DTPA-PE (0.5-μmol Gd). Fast and clear visualization of the lymph vessel (LV) can be seen. Images were acquired using a 1.5 Tesla GE Signa MRI scanner operated at fat suppression mode and T1-weighted pulse sequence; (d) *micelles in CT*. CT signal intensity (Hounsfield units) from the rat blood pool (registered at the aorta area) at different times after intravenous administration of iodine-containing polymeric micelles (170 mg iodine/kg) is shown. Strong and prolonged blood opacification is observed.

In experiments on lymphatic imaging [147], amphiphilic chelating probes Gd(^{111}In)-DTPA-PE and ^{111}In-DTPA-SA were incorporated into PEG (5 kDa)-PE micelles (20 nm in diameter) and used in experimental percutaneous lymphography in rabbits utilizing scintigraphy and MRI. Figure 9.4b shows the localization of ^{111}In-labeled DTPA-SA/PEG (5kDa)-PE micelles in local lymphatics after subcutaneous administration of a 20 μCi dose into the dorsum of a rabbit's hind paw. The popliteal lymph node can be visualized already within seconds after injection. Figure 9.4c shows a T1-weighted transverse MR image of the axillary or subscapular lymph node area in a rabbit obtained after subcutaneous injection of small doses of Gd-DTPA-PE/PEG(5 kDa)-PE micelles. The collecting lymph vessel (LV) becomes visible only 4 min after administration of Gd-containing micelles.

To increase the loading of micelles with reporter metals and improve their contrast properties in different imaging modalities, novel amphiphilic polymers (polychelating amphiphilic polymers or PAPs), containing multiple chelating groups, which are suitable for incorporation into micelles, have been designed [148]. Polymer-attached chelating moieties provide high-affinity binding of the wide range of radioactive and nonradioactive heavy metal ions (Figure 9.4a). The polymeric backbone for the attachment of multiple chelating moieties has to contain a sufficient number of reactive groups. Poly-L-lysine (PLL) containing multiple free amino groups represents a frequent choice. To couple the chelator to a PLL, the reactive intermediate of the chelator is usually used, containing mixed anhydride, cyclic anhydride, N-hydroxysuccinimide ester, tetrafluorophenyl ester, isothiocyanate, etc. [149]. PLL-based polychelator with a PLL-N-terminus-attached lipid residue (PE) easily incorporates into the micelle core in the process of micelle preparation and sharply increases the number of chelated In or Gd atoms attached to a single lipid anchor. This enables the number of bound reporter metal atoms per single carrier particle, as well as the resulting signal, to be increased.

In case of MRI, the higher Gd content leads to better relaxivity and, consequently, to the greater MR signal intensity. Additionally, upon incorporation into the micelle core, metal atoms chelated into polymer-attached groups are directly exposed to the exterior water environment and have better access to the adjacent tissue water protons. This leads to the corresponding enhancement of the micelle contrast properties. As a result, amphiphilic polychelator-containing micelles have a higher relaxation influence on water protons compared to conventional preparations at the same phospholipid content. In addition to the enhanced relaxivity, the micelle corona formed by the PEG polymer can help in avoiding the contrast agent (both for gamma and MR imaging) uptake at the site of injection by resident phagocytic cells [150].

Computed tomography (CT) represents an imaging modality with high spatial and temporal resolution. However, because obtaining diagnostically significant imaging requires the contrast agent (iodine) concentration be on the order of millimoles per milliliter of tissue [151], large doses of low-molecular-weight CT contrast agent, such as iodine-containing organic molecules, are normally administered to patients. CT is especially attractive for the multipurpose diagnostic imaging of the blood pool. However, the selective blood enhancement upon the administration of traditional CT contrast agents is brief because of rapid extravasation and clearance of the contrast. In order to more specifically target contrast agents, attempts have been made to use contrast-agent-loaded microparticulate carriers for CT imaging [152,153]. Current particulate contrast agents possess a relatively large particle size (between 0.25 and 3.5 μm) and are actively cleared by phagocytosis. They often also contain small radiopaque molecules that are able to extravasate and dilute the signal. Long-circulating contrast-loaded micelles seem to be able to solve the aforementioned problems [154]. Synthesis and *in vivo* properties of the micelles made of a block copolymer comprising methoxy-poly(ethylene glycol) (MPEG) and iodine-substituted poly-L-lysine have been described [155,156]. These micelles are very stable, can be heavily loaded with iodine (up to 35% of iodine by weight), and have a size below 100 nm. When administered intravenously in rats and rabbits, these micelles provide a significant enhancement in the blood pool (aorta and heart) for at least 2 h following the injection (Figure 9.4d). Another important feature of these iodine-containing micelles is their ability to slowly dissociate into unimers and gradually be cleared from the body via the kidneys.

9.6 CONCLUDING REMARKS

Polymeric micelles demonstrate many attractive properties as pharmaceutical carriers. They are stable both *in vitro* and *in vivo*, can be loaded with a wide variety of poorly soluble pharmaceutical agents, effectively accumulate in pathological body areas with compromised vasculature (infarcts, tumors), and can be targeted by attaching various specific ligands to their surface. Both therapeutic and diagnostic micelles can be easily produced in substantial quantities. It appears that micellar carriers have a promising future.

REFERENCES

1. Shabner, B.A. and Collings J.M., Eds., *Cancer Chemotherapy: Principles and Practice*, Humana Press, Philadelphia, PA, 1990.
2. Yokogawa, K. et al., Relationships in the structure-tissue distribution of basic drugs in the rabbit, *Pharm. Res.,* 7, 691, 1990.
3. Hageluken, A. et al., Lipophilic beta-adrenoceptor antagonists and local anesthetics are effective direct activators of G-proteins, *Biochem. Pharmacol.,* 47, 1789, 1994.
4. Lipinski, C.A., Drug-like properties and the causes of poor solubility and poor permeability, *J. Pharmacol. Toxicol. Methods,* 44, 235, 2000.
5. Lipinski, C.A. et al., Experimental and computational approaches to estimate solubility and permeability in drug discovery and development settings, *Adv. Drug Delivery Rev.,* 46, 3, 2001.
6. Teicher, B.A., Ed., *Anticancer Drug Delivery Guide,* Humana Press, Philadelphia, PA, 1997.
7. Yalkowsky, S.H., Ed., *Techniques of Solubilization of Drugs*, Marcel Dekker, New York, 1981.
8. Thompson, D. and Chaubal, M.V., Cyclodextrins (CDS) — excipients by definition, drug delivery systems by function (part I: injectable applications), *Drug Delivery Technol.,* 2, 34, 2000.
9. Ray, R., *Handbook of Pharmaceutical Excipients,* APhA, Washington, D.C., 2003.
10. Ansel, H.C., Allen, L.V., and Popovich, N.G., *Pharmaceutical Dosage Forms and Drug Delivery Systems,* Kluwer, Philadelphia, PA, 1999.
11. Lasic, D.D. and Papahadjopoulos, D., Eds., *Medical Applications of Liposomes,* Elsevier, New York, 1998.
12. Constantinides, P.P. et al., Formulation development and antitumor activity of a filter-sterilizable emulsion of paclitaxel, *Pharm. Res.,* 17, 175, 2000.
13. Palmer, T.N. et al., The mechanism of liposome accumulation in infarction, *Biochim. Biophys. Acta,* 797, 363, 1984.
14. Gabizon, A.A., Liposome circulation time and tumor targeting: implications for cancer chemotherapy, *Adv. Drug Delivery Rev.,* 16, 285, 1995.
15. Maeda, H. et al., Tumor vascular permeability and the EPR effect in macromolecular therapeutics: a review, *J. Controlled Release,* 65, 271, 2000.
16. Mittal, K.L. and Lindman, B., Eds., *Surfactants in Solution,* Vol. 1–3, Plenum Press, New York, 1991.
17. Elworthy, P.H., Florence, A.T., and Macfarlane, C.B., Eds., *Solubilization by Surface Active Agents,* Chapman and Hall, London, 1968.
18. Attwood, D. and Florence, A.T., Eds., *Surfactant Systems,* Chapman and Hall, London, 1983.
19. Trubetskoy, V.S. and Torchilin, V.P., Use of polyoxyethylene-lipid conjugates as long-circulating carriers for delivery of therapeutic and diagnostic agents, *Adv. Drug Delivery Rev.,* 16, 311, 1995.
20. Kwon, G.S. and Kataoka, K., Block copolymer micelles as long-circulating drug vehicles, *Adv. Drug Delivery Rev.,* 16, 295, 1995.
21. Saletu, B. et al., Comparative bioavailability studies with a new mixed-micelles solution of diazepam utilizing radioreceptor assay, psychometry and EEG brain mapping, *Int. Clin. Psychopharmacol.,* 3, 287, 1988.
22. Kabanov, A.V. et al., The neuroleptic activity of haloperidol increases after its solubilization in surfactant micelles, *FEBS Lett.,* 258, 343, 1989.
23. Martinez-Coscolla, A. et al., Studies on the reliability of novel absorption-lipophilicity approach to interpret the effects of the synthetic surfactants on drug and xenobiotics absorption, *Drug. Res.,* 43, 699, 1993.
24. Masuda, Y. et al., The mode of enhanced enteral absorbtion of macrimolecules by lipid-surfactant mixed micelles, *J. Pharmacobio.-Dyn.,* 9, 793, 1986.
25. Lasic, D.D., Mixed micelles in drug delivery, *Nature* 355, 279–280, 1992.
26. Tengamnuay, P. and Mitra, A.K., Bile salt-fatty acid mixed micelles as nasal absorption promoters of peptides, *Pharm. Res.,* 7, 127, 1990.
27. Magnusson, G., Olsson, T., and Nyberg, J.-A., Toxicity of Pluronic F-68, *Toxicol. Lett.,* 30, 203, 1986.
28. Schmolka, I.R., A review of block polymer surfactants, *J. Am. Oil Chem. Soc.,* 54, 110, 1977.
29. Port, C.D., Garvin, P.J., and Ganote, C.E., The effect of Pluronic F-38 (poloxamer 108) administered intravenously in rats, *Toxicol. Appl. Pharmacol.,* 44, 401, 1978.
30. Yokoyama, M., Block copolymers as drug carriers, *CRC Crit. Rev. Ther. Drug Carrier Syst.,* 9, 213, 1992.

31. Zhang, L. and Eisenberg, A., Multiple morphologies of "crew-cut" aggregates of polystyrene-b-poly(acrylic acid) block copolymers, *Science,* 268, 1728, 1995.

32. Jones, M.-C. and Leroux, J.-C., Polymeric micelles — a new generation of colloidal drug carriers, *Eur. J. Pharm. Biopharm.,* 48, 101, 1999.

33. Martin, A., *Physical Pharmacy,* 4th ed., Williams and Wilkins, Baltimore, MD, 1993, p. 396.

34. La, S.B., Okano, T., and Kataoka, K., Preparation and characterization of the micelle-forming polymeric drug indomethacin-incorporated poly(ethylene oxide)-poly(beta-benzyl-L-aspartate) block copolymer micelles, *J. Pharm. Sci.,* 85, 85, 1996.

35. Kabanov, A.V., Batrakova, E.V., and Alakhov, V.Y., Pluronic block copolymers as novel polymer therapeutics for drug and gene delivery, *J. Controlled Release,* 82, 189, 2002.

36. Yokoyama, M. et al., Analysis of micelle formation of an adriamycin-conjugated poly(ethylene glycol)-poly(aspartic acid) block copolymer by gel permeation chromatography, *Pharm. Res.,* 10, 895, 1993.

37. Gao, Z. and Eisenberg, A., A model of micellization for block copolymers in solutions, *Macromolecules,* 26, 7353, 1993.

38. Cammas, S. et al., Thermoresponsive polymer nanoparticles with a core-shell micelle structure as site specific drug carriers, *J. Controlled Release,* 48, 157, 1997.

39. Kwon, G.S., Biodistribution of micelle-forming polymer-drug conjugates, *Pharm. Res.,* 10, 970, 1993.

40. Kwon, G. et al., Micelles based on AB block copolymers of poly(ethylene oxide) and poly(benzyl-aspartat), *Langmuir,* 9, 945, 1993.

41. Nagarajan, R. and Ganesh, K., Block copolymer self-assembly in selective solvents: theory of solubilization in spherical micelles, *Macromolecules,* 22, 4312, 1989.

42. Alexandridis, P., Holzwarth, J.F., and Hatton, T.A., Micellization of poly(ethylene oxide)-poly(propylene oxide)-poly(ethylene oxide) triblock copolymers in aqueous, *Macromolecules,* 27, 2414, 1994.

43. Alexandridis, P. et al., Surface activity of poly(ethylene oxide)-block-poly(propylene oxide)-block-poly(ethylene oxide) copolymers, *Langmuir,* 10, 2604, 1994.

44. Winnik, F.M. et al., Amphiphilic poly(N-isopropylacrylamide) prepared by using a lipophilic radical initiator: synthesis and solution properties in water, *Macromolecules,* 25, 1876, 1992.

45. Ringsdorf, H., Venzmer, J., and Winnik, F.M., Fluorescence studies of hydrophobically modified poly(N-isopropylacrylamides), *Macromolecules,* 24, 1678, 1991.

46. Nakamura, K., Endo, R., and Takeda, M., Study of molecular motion of block copolymers in solution by high-resolution proton magnetic resonance, *J. Polym. Sci. Polym. Phys. Ed.,* 15, 2095, 1977.

47. Allen, C., Maysinger, D., and Eisenberg, A., Nano-engineering block copolymer aggregates for drug delivery, *Coll. Surf. B: Biointerfaces,* 16, 1, 1999.

48. Torchilin, V.P. and Trubetskoy, V.S., Biodistribution of surface-modified liposomes and particles, in *Microparticulate Systems for the Delivery of Proteins and Vaccines,* Cohen, S. and Bernstein, H., Eds., Marcel Dekker, New York, 1996, chap. 8.

49. Gref, R., et al., The controlled intravenous delivery of drugs using PEG-coated sterically stabilized nanospheres, *Adv. Drug Delivery Rev.,* 16, 215, 1995.

50. Hagan, S.A. et al., Polylactide-poly(ethelene glycol) copolymers as drug delivery systems, 1. Characterization of water dispersible micelle-forming systems, *Langmuir,* 12, 2153, 1996.

51. Inoue, T. et al., An AB block copolymers of oligo(methyl methacrylate) and poly(acrylic acid) for micellar delivery of hydrophobic drugs, *J. Controlled Release,* 51, 221, 1998.

52. Müller, R.H., *Colloidal Carriers for Controlled Drug Delivery and Targeting,* Wissenschaftliche Verlagsgesellschaft, Stuttgart, Germany, and CRC Press, Boca Raton, FL, 1991.

53. Kuntz, R.M. and Saltzman, W.M., Polymeric controlled delivery for immunization, *Trends Biotechnol.,* 15, 364, 1997.

54. Marques, C.M., Bunchy micelles, *Langmuir,* 13, 1430, 1997.

55. Torchilin, V.P. and Trubetskoy, V.S., Which polymers can make nanoparticulate drug carriers long-circulating? *Adv. Drug Delivery Rev.,* 16, 141, 1995.

56. Kwon, G.S., Diblock copolymer nanoparticles for drug delivery, *CRC Crit. Rev. Ther. Drug Carrier Syst.,* 15, 481, 1998.

57. Schild, H.G. and Tirrel, D.A., Microheterogenous solutions of amphiphilic copolymers of N-isopropylacrylamide. An investigation via fluorescence methods, *Langmuir,* 7, 1319, 1991.

58. Torchilin, V.P. et al., Amphiphilic vinyl polymers effectively prolong liposome circulation time in vivo, *Biochim. Biophys. Acta,* 1195, 181, 1994.

59. Torchilin, V.P. et al., New synthetic amphiphilic polymers for steric protection of liposomes in vivo, *J. Pharm. Sci.,* 84, 1049, 1995.

60. Miller, D.W. et al., Interactions of pluronic block copolymers with brain microvessel endothelial cells: evidence of two potential pathways for drug absorption, *Bioconjugate Chem.,* 8, 649, 1997.

61. Yokoyama, M. et al., Characterization and anticancer activity of the micelle-forming polymeric anticancer drug adriamycin-conjugated poly(ethylene glycol)-poly(aspartic acid) block copolymer, *Cancer Res.,* 50, 1693, 1990.

62. Harada, A. and Kataoka, K., Novel polyion complex micelles entrapping enzyme molecules in the core. Preparation of narrowly-distributed micelles from lysozyme and poly(ethylene glycol)-poly(aspartic acid) block copolymer in aqueous medium, *Macromolecules,* 31, 288, 1998.

63. Kwon, G.S. et al., Block copolymer micelles for drug delivery: loading and release of doxorubicin, *J. Controlled Release,* 48, 195, 1997.

64. Jeong, Y.I. et al., Clonazepam release from core-shell type nanoparticles in vitro, *J. Controlled Release,* 51, 169, 1998.

65. Kim, S.Y. et al., Methoxy poly(ethylene glycol) and ε-caprolactone amphiphilic block copolymeric micelle containing indomethacin, II. Micelle formation and drug release behaviors, *J. Controlled Release,* 51, 13, 1998.

66. Allen, C. et al., Polycaprolactone-b-poly(ethylene oxide) block copolymer micelles as a novel drug delivery vehicle for neurotrophic agents FK506 and L-685,818, *Bioconjugate Chem.,* 9, 564, 1998.

67. Ramaswamy, M. et al., Human plasma distribution of free paclitaxel and paclitaxel associated with diblock copolymers, *J. Pharm. Sci.,* 86, 460, 1997.

68. Hagan, S.A. et al., Polylactide-poly(ethylene glycol) copolymers as drug delivery systems, 1. Characterization of water dispersible micelle-forming systems, *Langmuir,* 12, 2153, 1996.

69. Kabanov, A.V. and Kabanov, V.A., Interpolyelectrolyte and block ionomer complexes for gene delivery: physico-chemical aspects, *Adv. Drug Delivery Rev.,* 30, 49, 1998.

70. Trubetskoy, V.S. et al., Block copolymer of polyethylene glycol and polylysine as a carrier of organic iodine: design of a long circulating particulate contrast medium for x-ray computed tomography, *J. Drug Target.,* 4, 381, 1997.

71. Yu, K., Zhang, L., and Eisenberg, A., Novel morphologies of "crew-cut" aggregates of amphiphilic diblock copolymers in dilute solutions, *Langmuir,* 12, 5980, 1996.

72. Klibanov, A.L. et al., Amphipathic polyethyleneglycols effectively prolong the circulation time of liposomes, *FEBS Lett.,* 268, 235, 1990.

73. Trubetskoy, V.S. and Torchilin, V.P., Polyethylene glycol based micelles as carriers of therapeutic and diagnostic agents, *S.T.P. Pharm. Sci.,* 6, 79, 1996.

74. Torchilin, V.P. et al., Immunomicelles: Targeted pharmaceutical carriers for poorly soluble drugs, *Proc. Natl. Acad. Sci. U.S.A.,* 100, 6039, 2003.

75. Rosen, M.J., Ed., *Surfactants and Interfacial Phenomena,* Wiley-Interscience, New York, 1989.

76. Lukyanov, A.N. et al., Polyethylene glycol-diacyllipid micelles demonstrate increased accumulation in subcutaneous tumors in mice. *Pharm. Res.,* 19, 1424, 2002.

77. Weissig, V., Lizano, C., and Torchilin, V.P., Micellar delivery system for dequalinium — a lipophilic cationic drug with anticarcinoma activity, *J. Liposome Res.,* 8, 391, 1998.

78. Gabizon, A.A., Liposome circulation time and tumor targeting: implications for cancer therapy, *Adv. Drug Delivery Rev.,* 16, 285, 1995.

79. Maruyama, K. et al., Phosphatidyl polyglycerols prolong liposome circulation in vivo, *Int. J. Pharm.,* 111, 103, 1994.

80. Woodle, M.C., Engbers, C.M., and Zalipsky, S., New amphipathic polymer-lipid conjugates forming long-circulating reticuloendothelial system-evading liposomes, *Bioconjuagate Chem.,* 4, 493, 1994.

81. Torchilin, V.P. et al., Amphiphilic poly-N-vinylpyrrolidones: synthesis, properties and liposome surface modification, *Biomaterials,* 22, 3035, 2001.

82. Torchilin, V.P., Structure and design of polymeric surfactant-based drug delivery systems, *J. Controlled Release,* 73, 137, 2001.

83. Xing, L. and Mattice, W.L., Large internal structures of micelles of triblock copolymers with small insoluble molecules in their cores, *Langmuir,* 14, 4074, 1998.

84. Teng, Y. et al., Release kinetics studies of aromatic molecules into water from block polymer micelles, *Macromolecules,* 31, 3578, 1998.

85. Donbrow, M., Ed., *Microcapsules and Nanoparticles in Medicine and Pharmacy,* CRC Press, Boca Raton, FL, 1992.

86. Alakhov, V.Y. and Kabanov, V.A., Block copolymeric biotransport carriers as versatile vehicles for drug delivery, *Exp. Opin. Invest. Drugs,* 7, 1453, 1998.

87. Zhang, X. et al., An investigation of the antitumor activity and biodistribution of polymeric micellar paclitaxel, *Cancer Chemother. Pharmacol.,* 40, 81, 1997.

88. Gao, Z. et al., PEG-PE/ Phosphatidylcholine mixed Immunomicelles specifically deliver encapsulated taxol to tumor cells of different origin and promote their efficient killing, *J. Drug Target.,* 11, 87, 2003.

89. Alkan-Onyuksel, H. et al., A mixed micellar formulation suitable for the parenteral administration of taxol, *Pharm. Res.,* 11, 206, 1994.

90. Lin, S.Y. and Kawashima, Y., The influence of three poly(oxyethylene)poly(oxypropylene) surface-active block copolymers on the solubility behavior of indomethacin, *Pharm. Acta Helv.,* 60, 339, 1985.

91. Lin, S.Y. and Kawashima, Y., Pluronic surfactants affecting diazepam solubility, compatibility, and adsorption from i.v. admixture solutions, *J. Parenter. Sci. Technol.,* 41, 83, 1987.

92. Yokoyama, M., Okano, T., and Kataoka, K., Improved synthesis of adriamycin-conjugated poly(ethylene oxide)-poly(aspartic acid) block copolymer and formation of unimodal micellar structure with controlled amount of physically entrapped adriamycin, *J. Controlled Release,* 32, 269, 2004.

93. Yokoyama, M. et al., Characterization of physical entrapment and chemical conjugation of adriamycin in polymeric micelles and their design for in vivo delivery to a solid tumor, *J. Controlled Release,* 50, 79, 1998.

94. Batrakova, E.V. et al., Anthracycline antibiotics non-covalently incorporated into the block copolymer micelles: in vivo evaluation of anti-cancer activity, *Br. J. Cancer,* 74, 1545, 1996.

95. Kabanov, A.V. et al., Water-soluble block polycations as carriers for oligonucleotide delivery, *Bioconjugate Chem.,* 6, 639, 1996.

96. Matsumura, Y. et al., Reduction of the side effects of an antitumor agent, KRN5500, by incorporation of the drug into polymeric micelles, *Jpn. J. Cancer Res.,* 90, 122, 1999.

97. Kwon, G.S. et al., Enhanced tumor accumulation and prolonged circulation times of micelles-forming poly(ethylene oxide-aspartate) block copolymers-adriamycin conjugates, *J. Controlled Release,* 29, 17, 1997.

98. Kataoka, K. et al., Block-copolymer micelles as vehicles for drug delivery, *J. Controlled Release,* 24, 119, 1993.

99. Kwon, G.S. and Okano, T., Polymeric micelles as new drug carriers, *Adv. Drug Delivery Rev.,* 21, 107, 1996.

100. Kwon, G.S. and Okano, T., Soluble self-assembled block copolymers for drug delivery, *Pharm. Res.,* 16, 597, 1999.

101. Allen, C. et al., Polycaprolactone-b-poly(ethylene oxide) copolymer micelles as a delivery vehicle for dihydrotestosterone, *J. Controlled Release,* 63, 275, 2000.

102. Gao, Z. et al., Diacyl-polymer micelles as nanocarriers for poorly soluble anticancer drugs, *Nano Lett.,* 2, 979, 2002.

103. Wang J. et al., Preparation and in vitro synergistic anticancer effect of Vitamin K# and 1,8-diazabicyclo[5,4,0]undec-7-ene in poly(ethylene glycol)-diacyllipid micelles, *Int. J. Pharm.,* 272, 129, 2004.

104. Samadi-Boboli, M. et al., Low density lipoprotein for cytotoxic drug targeting: improved activity of elliptinium derivative against B16 melanoma in mice, *Br. J. Cancer,* 68, 319, 1993.

105. Katayose, S. and Kataoka, K., Remarkable increase in nuclease resistance of plasmid DNA through supramolecular assembly with poly(ethylene glycol)-poly(L-lysine) block copolymer, *J. Pharm. Sci.,* 87, 160, 1998.

106. Seymour, L.W., Kataoka, K., and Kabanov, A.V., Cationic block copolymers as self-assembling vectors for gene delivery, in *Self-Assembling Complexes for Gene Delivery. From Laboratory to Clinical Trial,* Kabanov, A.V., Seymour, L.W., and Felgner, P., Eds., John Wiley & Sons, Chichester, 1998, p. 219.

107. Katayose, S. and Kataoka, K., Water-soluble polyion complex associates of DNA and poly(ethylene glycol)-poly(L-lysine) block copolymer, *Bioconjugate Chem.,* 8, 702, 1997.

108. Yokoyama, M. et al., Incorporation of water-insoluble anticancer drug into polymeric micelles and control of their particle size, *J. Controlled Release,* 55, 219, 1998.

109. Wang, J., Mongayt, D., and Torchilin, V.P., Polymeric micelles for delivery of poorly soluble drugs: preparation and anticancer activity in vitro of paclitaxel incorporated into mixed micelles based on poly(ethylene glycol)-lipid conjugate and positively charged lipids, *J. Drug Target,* 2004, in press.

110. Weissig, V., Whiteman, K.R., and Torchilin, V.P., Accumulation of liposomal- and micellar-bound protein in solid tumor, *Pharm. Res.,* 15, 1552, 1998.

111. Lukyanov, A.N., Hartner, W.C., and Torchilin, V.P., Increased accumulation of PEG-PE micelles in the area of experimental myocardial infarction in rabbits, *J. Controlled Release,* 94, 187, 2004.

112. Yuan, F. et al., Microvascular permeability and interstitial penetration of sterically-stabilized (stealth) liposomes in human tumor xenograft, *Cancer Res.,* 54, 3352, 1994.

113. Yuan, F. et al., Vascular permeability in a human tumor xenograft: molecular size dependence and cutoff size, *Cancer Res.,* 55, 3752, 1995.

114. Yokoyama, M. et al., Selective delivery of adriamycin to a solid tumor using a polymeric micelle carrier system, *J. Drug Target,* 7, 171, 1999.

115. Helmlinger, G. et al., Interstitial pH and pO2 gradients in solid tumors in vivo: high-resolution measurements reveal a lack of correlation, *Nat. Med.,* 3, 177, 1997.

116. Tannock, I.F. and Rotin, R., Acid pH in tumors and its potential for therapeutic exploitation, *Cancer Res.,* 49, 4373, 1998.

117. Cammas, S. et al., Thermorespensive polymer nanoparticles with a core-shell micelle structure as site specific drug carriers, *J. Controlled Release,* 48, 157, 1997.

118. Chung, J.E. et al., Effect of molecular architecture of hydrophobically modified poly(N-isopropy-lacrylamide) on the formation of thermoresponsive core-shell micellar drug carriers. *J. Controlled Release,* 53, 119, 1998.

119. Meyer, O., Papahadjopoulos, D., and Leroux, J.C., Copolymers of N-isopropylacrylamide can trigger pH sensitivity to stable liposomes, *FEBS Lett.,* 41, 61, 1998.

120. Le Garrec, D. et al., Optimizing pH-responsive polymeric micelles for drug delivery in a cancer photodynamic therapy model, *J. Drug Target,* 10, 429, 2002.

121. Yoo, H.S., Lee, E.A., and Park, T.G., Doxorubicin-conjugated biodegradable polymeric micelles having acid-cleavable linkages, *J. Controlled Release,* 82, 17, 2002.

122. Chung, J.E. et al., Thermo-responsive drug delivery from polymeric micelles constructed using block copolymers of poly(N-isopropylacrylamide) and poly(butylmethacrylate), *J. Controlled Release,* 62, 115, 1999.

123. Torchilin, V.P., Structure and design of polymeric surfactant-based drug delivery systems, *J. Controlled Release,* 73, 137, 2001.

124. Nagasaki, Y. et al., Sugar-installed block copolymer micelles: their preparation and specific interaction with lectin molecules, *Biomacromolecules,* 2, 1067, 2001.

125. Vinogradov, S. et al., Polyion complex micelles with protein-modified corona for receptor-mediated delivery of oligonucleotides into cells, *Bioconjugate Chem.,* 10, 851, 1999.

126. Leamon, C.P., Weigl, D., and Hendren, R.W., Folate copolymer-mediated transfection of cultured cells, *Bioconjugate Chem.,* 10, 947, 1999.

127. Jule, E., Nagasaki, Y., and Kataoka, K., Lactose-installed poly(ethylene glycol)-poly(D,L-lactide) block copolymer micelles exhibit fast-rate binding and high affinity toward a protein bed simulating a cell surface. A surface plasmon resonance study, *Bioconjugate Chem.,* 14, 177, 2003.

128. Ogris, M. et al., PEGylated DNA/transferrin-PEI complexes: reduced interaction with blood components, extended circulation in blood and potential for systemic gene delivery, *Gene Ther.,* 6, 595, 1999.

129. Dash, P.R. et al., Decreased binding to proteins and cells of polymeric gene delivery vectors surface modified with a multivalent hydrophilic polymer and retargeting through attachment of transferring, *J. Biol. Chem.* 275, 3793, 2000.

130. Leamon, C.P. and Low, P.S., Folate-mediated targeting: from diagnostics to drug and gene delivery, *Drug Discovery Today,* 6, 44, 2001.

131. Lee, E.S., Na, K., and Bae, Y.H., Polymeric micelle for tumor pH and folate-mediated targeting, *J. Controlled Release,* 91, 103, 2003.

132. Chekhonin, V.P. et al., Fatty acid acylated Fab-fragments of antibodies to neurospecific proteins as carriers for neuroleptic targeted delivery in brain, *FEBS Lett.,* 287, 14, 1991.

133. Torchilin, V.P. et al., p-Nitrophenylcarbonyl-PEG-PE-liposomes: fast and simple attachment of specific ligands, including monoclonal antibodies, to distal ends of PEG chains via p-nitrophenylcarbonyl groups, *Biochim. Biophys. Acta,* 1511, 397, 2001.

134. Gao, Z. et al., PEG-PE/phosphatidylcholine mixed immunomicelles specifically deliver encapsulated taxol to tumor cells of different origin and promote their efficient killing, *J. Drug Target,* 11, 87, 2003.

135. Iakoubov, L.Z. and Torchilin, V.P., A novel class of antitumor antibodies: nucleosome-restricted antinuclear autoantibodies (ANA) from healthy aged nonautoimmune mice, *Oncol. Res.,* 9, 439, 1997.

136. Torchilin, V.P., Iakoubov, L.Z., and Estrov, Z., Therapeutic potential of antinuclear autoantibodies in cancer, *Cancer Ther.,* 1, 179, 2003.

137. Park, J.W. et al., Tumor targeting using anti-HER2 immunoliposomes, *J. Controlled Release,* 74, 95, 2001.

138. Sharma, A., Conway, W.D., and Straubinger, R.M., Reversed-phase high-performance liquid chromatographic determination of taxol in mouse plasma, *J. Chromatogr. B: Biomed. Appl.,* 655, 315, 1994.

139. Hafez, I.M., Maurer, N., and Cullis, P.R., On the mechanism whereby cationic lipids promote intracellular delivery of polynucleic acids, *Gene Ther.,* 8, 1188, 2001.

140. Wang, J. et al., Preparation and in vitro synergistic anticancer effect of Vitamin K# and 1,8-diazabicyclo[5,4,0]undec-7-ene in poly(ethylene glycol)-diacyllipid micelles, *Int. J. Pharm.,* 272, 129, 2004.

141. Wolf, G.L., Targeted delivery of imaging agents: an overview, in *Handbook of Targeted Delivery of Imaging Agents,* Torchilin, V.P., Ed., CRC Press, Boca Raton, FL, 1995, p. 3.

142. Torchilin, V.P., Pharmacokinetic considerations in the development of labeled liposomes and micelles for diagnostic imaging, *Quat. J. Nucl. Med.,* 41, 141, 1997.

143. Jasanada, F. and Nepveu, F., Synthesis of amphiphilic chelating agents: bis(hexadecylamide) and bis(octadecylamide) of diethylenetriaminepentaacetic acid, *Tetrahed. Lett.,* 33, 5745, 1992.

144. Grant, C.W.M., Karlik, S., and Florio, E., A liposomal MRI contrast agent: phosphatidyl ethanolamine, *Magn. Res. Med.,* 11, 236, 1989.

145. Kabalka, G. et al., Gadolinium-labeled liposomes containing paramagnetic amphiphatic agents: targeted MRI contrast agent for the liver, *Magn. Res. Med.,* 8, 89, 1989.

146. Unger, E. et al., Manganese-based liposomes: comparative approaches, *Invest. Radiol.,* 28, 933, 1993.

147. Trubetskoy, V.S. et al., Stable polymeric micelles: lymphangiographic contrast media for gamma scintigraphy and magnetic resonance imaging, *Acad. Radiol.,* 3, 232, 1996.

148. Trubetskoy, V.S. and Torchilin, V.P., New approaches in the chemical design of Gd-containing liposomes for use in magnetic resonance imaging of lymph nodes, *J. Liposome Res.,* 4, 961, 1994.

149. Slinkin, M.A., Klibanov, A.L., and Torchilin, V.P., Terminal-modified polylysine-based chelating polymers: highly efficient coupling to antibody with minimal loss in immunoreactivity, *Bioconjugate Chem.,* 2, 342, 1991.

150. Torchilin, V.P., Polymeric micelles in diagnostic imaging, *Coll. Surf. B: Biointerfaces,* 16, 305, 1999.

151. Wolf, G.L., Delivery of diagnostic agents: achievements and challenges, *Adv. Drug Delivery Rev.,* 37, 1, 1999.

152. Gazelle, G.S. et al., Nanoparticulate computed tomography contrast agents for blood pool and liver-spleen imaging, *Acad. Radiol.,* 1, 273, 1994.

153. Leander, P., A new liposomal contrast medium for CT of the liver: an imaging study in a rabbit tumor model, *Acta Radiol.,* 37, 63, 1996.

154. Trubetskoy, V.S. and Torchilin, V.P., Use of polyoxyethylene-lipid conjugates as long-circulating carriers for delivery of therapeutic and diagnostic agents, *Adv. Drug Delivery Rev.,* 16, 311, 1995.

155. Trubetskoy, V.S. et al., Block copolymer of polyethylene glycol and polylysine as a carrier of organic iodine: design of a long circulating particulate contrast medium for X-ray computed tomography, *J. Drug Target,* 4, 381, 1997.

156. Torchilin, V.P., Frank-Kamenetsky, M.D., and Wolf, G.L., CT visualization of blood pool in rats by using long-circulating, iodine-containing micelles, *Acad. Radiol.,* 6, 61, 1999.

10 Polymeric Vesicles

Ijeoma Florence Uchegbu, Shona Anderson,
and Anthony Brownlie

CONTENTS

10.1 INTRODUCTION

This chapter will examine what is known about polymeric vesicles (Figure 10.1) and highlight future drug delivery applications. Closed bilayer systems arise when amphiphilic molecules self-assemble in aqueous media in an effort to reduce the high-energy interaction between the hydrophobic portion of the amphiphile and the aqueous disperse phase and to maximize the low-energy interaction between the hydrophilic head group and the disperse phase (Figure 10.1). Vesicular self-assemblies reside in the nanometer to micrometer size domain. Excellent reviews exist on the self-assembly of amphiphiles [4], and hence this topic will not be dealt with in great detail here.

Liposomes were the first synthetic self-assembling vesicular systems to be described [7], and they are the result of phospholipids. Phospholipids are the building blocks of our cell membranes. Liposomes were discovered in 1965 [7] and licensed for clinical use in the mid-1990s. Liposome-encapsulated drugs, e.g., liposome-encapsulated doxorubicin, known as Doxil® or Caelyx® [15], have since been used by cancer patients in many parts of the world. The commercial liposome-encapsulated

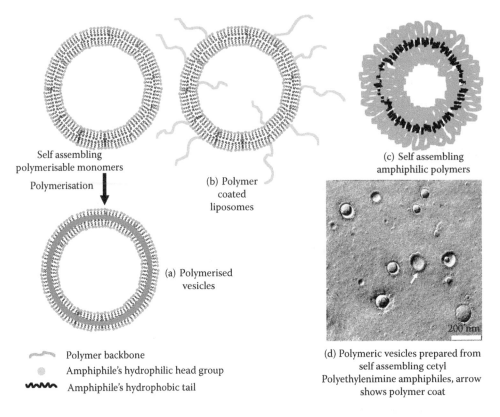

Self assembling
polymerisable monomers

Polymerisation

(b) Polymer
coated
liposomes

(c) Self assembling
amphiphilic polymers

(a) Polymerised
vesicles

⌇⌇ Polymer backbone
• Amphiphile's hydrophilic head group
〰〰 Amphiphile's hydrophobic tail

(d) Polymeric vesicles prepared from
self assembling cetyl
Polyethylenimine amphiphiles, arrow
shows polymer coat

FIGURE 10.1 Polymeric vesicles may arise from (a) the self-assembly of polymerizable monomers that are subsequently polymerized, (b) the cooperative self-assembly of lipids and polymers, or the self-assembly of amphiphilic polymers, both block (c) and random copolymers (d).

doxorubicin formulation is the only polymeric vesicle formulation licensed for clinical use [15]. This formulation consists of poly(oxyethylene)-coated liposomes.

Polymeric vesicles were first investigated as a means of stabilizing the metastable vesicles formed from low-molecular-weight amphiphiles, with the polymer providing a kinetic trap for the self-assembled system [11,20]. A wealth of polymer architectures are now known to assemble into vesicles: block copolymers [21,22], random graft copolymers [19], polymerized self-assembling monomers [20], and polymers-bearing lipid pendant groups [12,20,23] (Figure 10.2). Additionally, polymeric vesicles, although not normally termed as such, arise from the self-assembly of amphiphilic polymers and lipids [24] or amphiphilic polymers and surfactants [25] (Figure 10.1).

As may be inferred from the list in the preceding paragraph that there are two main ways in which polymeric vesicles may be formed, either from the self-assembly of polymers or from the polymerization of monomers subsequent to self-assembly (Figure 10.1). Vesicular self-assembly is not a spontaneous process and normally requires an input of energy, for example, in the form of probe sonication [19]. It is known that vesicle formation from low-molecular-weight amphiphiles in aqueous media is controlled by two opposing forces, namely, the steric or ionic repulsion between hydrophilic head groups, which maximizes the interfacial area per molecule, and the attractive forces between hydrophobic groups, which serves to reduce the interfacial area per molecule [4]. Attaining a minimal interfacial energy is thus served by the formation of a closed spherical bilayer. In general terms, the less hydrophobic amphiphiles form micelles, whereas amphiphiles of intermediate hydrophobicity form vesicles [4]. The self-assembly of

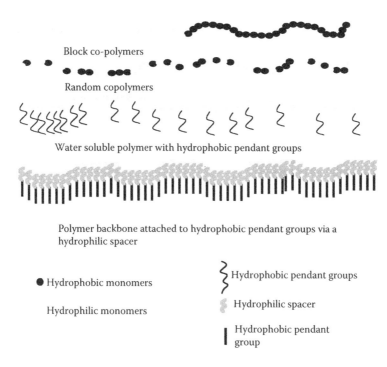

Block co-polymers

Random copolymers

Water soluble polymer with hydrophobic pendant groups

Polymer backbone attached to hydrophobic pendant groups via a
hydrophilic spacer

● Hydrophobic monomers

Hydrophilic monomers

Hydrophobic pendant groups

Hydrophilic spacer

Hydrophobic pendant
group

FIGURE 10.2 Schematic representation of self-assembling vesicle-forming polymers.

polymers into vesicles is governed by similar constraints, and as such the hydrophobic–lipophilic balance of polymers determines whether a polymer will self-assemble into vesicles in a manner similar to that found in liposomes and niosomes [22]. There is a clear relationship between the hydrophobic content of polymers and self-assembly. Low levels of hydrophobicity (less than 50% of the polymer molecular weight consisting of hydrophobic moieties) favors the formation of micelles [26], intermediate levels of hydrophobicity (50 to 80%) favors the formation of bilayer vesicles [18, 26–28], and higher levels of hydrophobicity (above 60 to 80%) favors the formation of dense nanoparticles [18]. This is true for both block copolymers and polymers bearing hydrophobic pendant groups. For the self-assembly of block copolymers it has been established that generally the surfactant parameter $(\frac{v}{al})$ should approach unity for vesicular self-assemblies to prevail [22], where v is the volume of the hydrophobic block; l, the length of the hydrophobic block; and a, the area of the hydrophilic block.

There are some polymer-specific factors that impact on vesicle-forming ability. For example, the degree of polymerization is critical to the vesicle-forming ability, and generally very high degrees of polymerization prevent vesicle formation [10,19]. Furthermore, the flexibility of the hydrophobic block in block copolymers determines which self-assemblies will be formed, with the more flexible hydrophobic portions of the polymer being able to form vesicles and the more rigid polymers being unable to self-assemble into three-dimensional structures [22]. Polymeric vesicles appear to be largely unilamellar [3,12], and unilamellarity is favored when the molecular weight of the amphiphile increases [18].

Polymeric vesicles often possess superior mechanical stability [22], are often less susceptible to degradation by organic solvents and soluble surfactants [22], and are frequently less permeable to low-molecular-weight solutes when compared to monomeric vesicles [20,29]. The widespread exploitation of these fascinating nanocarriers for the development of responsive and biomimetic nanomedicines with superior stability characteristics is awaited.

10.2   SELF-ASSEMBLING POLYMERS

One of the routes to the formation of a polymeric vesicle is the self-assembly of amphiphilic polymers. Amphiphilic polymers, whether in the form of block copolymers, random copolymers, or hydrophobically substituted water-soluble polymers (Figure 10.2), may either assemble into vesicles alone or self-assemble into vesicles in the presence of amphiphilic lipids or surfactants. These classes of polymeric vesicles will be dealt with in this section.

10.2.1   POLYMERS AND LIPOSOMES OR NIOSOMES

10.2.1.1   Amphiphilic Polymers

It can be said that the formulation of liposomes with poly(ethylene oxide) amphiphiles such as distearolyphosphatidylethanolamine–poly(ethylene glycol) (polymer 1; Figure 10.3), [24] was the crucial step that allowed liposomes to become clinically relevant drug delivery systems. The resulting liposome possesses, as shown schematically in Figure 10.1, a hydrophilic polymer surface, which prevents recognition and clearance of the particles from the blood by the liver and spleen macrophages, [24, 30] thus increasing the liposomes' circulation time and allowing tumor targeting [31]. This is further discussed in Section 10.4. Niosomes (nonionic surfactant vesicles), when formulated with a water-soluble poly(oxyethylene) cholesteryl ether (polymer 2; Figure 10.3), also circulate for prolonged periods in the blood, accumulate in tumor tissue, and improve tumoricidal activity [32]. As well as stabilizing vesicles in the blood, poly(oxyethylene) amphiphiles also stabilize vesicles against aggregation, thus promoting vesicle colloidal stability [33].

Poly(oxyethylene) amphiphiles have a large hydrophilic head group (Figure 10.3) and are thus more hydrophilic than the vesicle-forming amphiphiles, hence the level of the former must be kept low to avoid solubilisation of the membrane and the formation of mixed micelles [34,35]. It has been observed that only 10 mol% poly(ethylene oxide)–lipid amphiphiles may be incorporated into liposomes [36] or niosomes [33,35] without a loss of vesicle integrity. In actual fact, unusual

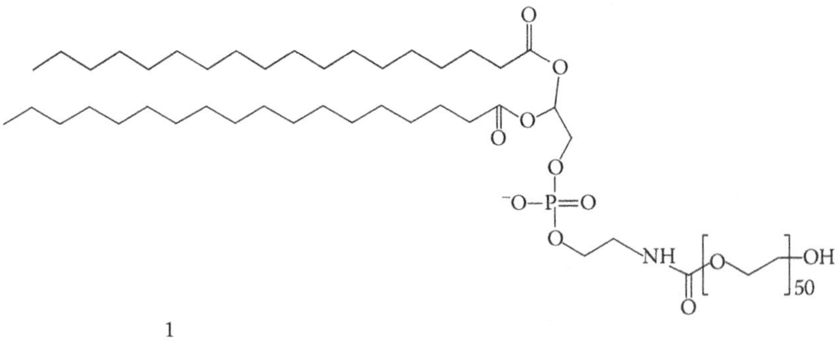

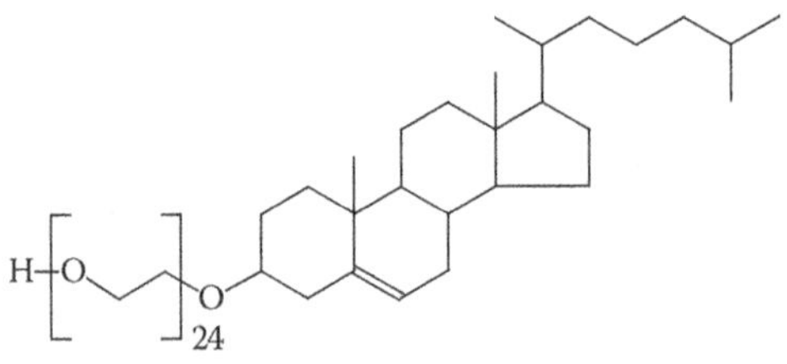

FIGURE 10.3 Poly(oxyethylene) amphiphiles used to give a poly(oxyethylene) coating to vesicles. These polymers prolong the vesicles' blood circulation, allowing them to accumulate in tumors.

morphologies [35] result from the incorporation of sufficient quantities of polymer 2 (Figure 10.3) in niosomes. When polymer 2 is added to diglycerol hexadecyl ether niosomes, micelles are formed, but before the formation of micelles giant vesicles (discomes) of 25 to 100 μm in size are formed [35]. Discomes contain polymer 2 at a level of 20 to 40 mol% [35] and have been studied as ocular drug delivery agents [37].

When vesicles are destabilized by amphiphilic polymers, the nature of the hydrophobic group appears to be important in the destabilization process. The interaction of hydrophobically modified poly(sodium acrylates) with oppositely charged vesicles leads to a disruption of the bilayer if there is a mismatch in the hydrophobic pendant groups of the polymer and that of the bilayer [38], and as such poly(sodium acrylates)-bearing *n*-dodecyl chains do not disrupt vesicles formed from sodium di-*n*-dodecylphosphate, whereas poly(sodium acrylates)-bearing *n*-nonyl or *n*-octadecyl chains do disrupt the said membranes. Generally destabilization appears to proceed by an adsorption of the amphiphilic polymer onto the surface of the vesicles, followed by a penetration of the hydrophobic portion of the amphiphile into the bilayer [39] and, ultimately, the formation of mixed micelles with bilayer components [40]. Depending on the nature and relative levels of the polymer and vesicle, vesicle disruption can be slow, extending over hours or days [40,41], or fast and complete within minutes [35].

At subdegradation levels, the poly(oxyethylene)–amphiphile membrane is stabilized by an asymmetric distribution of the hydrophilic polymer between the inner and outer bilayer leaflets [36], with the polymer preferring to localize on the outer leaflet [36]. Preferred residence in the outer leaflet is favored because the greater repulsion between the longer hydrophilic corona molecules on the outer leaflet stabilizes the vesicle curvature [42]. The asymmetric distribution of the amphiphilic polymer is the driving force for vesicle formation [36]. Steric stabilization of vesicles may also be achieved with amphiphilic ABA block copolymers such as poly(oxyethylene)-*block*-poly(oxypropylene)-*block*-poly(oxyethylene) [43,44].

10.2.1.2 Water-Soluble Polymers

Liposome bilayers are also destabilized by water-soluble non-amphiphilic polymers. Such studies on vesicle polymer interactions provide an insight into the *in vivo* interactions between liposomes and biomacromolecules, and as such it is interesting to observe that egg phosphatidylcholine liposomes are destabilized by water-soluble polymers such as poly-α,β-[*N*-(2-hydroxyethyl)-L-aspartamide [45]. Destabilization is mediated by the hydrogen bonding between the liposome bilayer components and the polymer. This hydrogen bonding alters the lipid packing in the bilayer, with resultant leakage of the liposome contents. The degradation of liposomes in the blood is known to be mediated via the interaction with blood proteins [46]. It is possible that some similarities exist between the mechanism of protein destabilization of liposomes *in vivo* and the *in vitro* destabilization of liposomes by synthetic hydrophilic polymers.

Some water-soluble polymers also promote the fusion of vesicles. When plain poly(oxyethylene) is mixed with cationic dioctadecyldimethylammonium bromide vesicles, fusion due to intervesicular polymer depletion is observed; this depletion is mediated by the polymer avoiding the entropically unfavorable intervesicular spaces [47], which causes vesicles to make contact with one another and undergo fusion so that they share a bilayer. Fusion is necessary to avoid the electrostatic repulsion energy penalty associated with the two vesicles making contact.

Contrary to the destabilizing properties outlined earlier for water-soluble polymer and vesicle interactions, oppositely charged water-soluble polyelectrolytes may also promote vesicle formation from non-vesicle-forming water-soluble amphiphiles [48]. Examples of this vesicle-promoting ability include the fact that vesicles emerge when lecithin–sodium dodecyl sulfate mixtures [48] or sodium dodecyl sulfate–decanol mixtures [49] are added to poly(diallyldimethylammonium chloride). The cationic polyelectrolyte partially neutralizes the sodium dodecyl sulfate anionic charge by adsorption onto the bilayer surface, thus shifting the balance of electrostatic repulsion

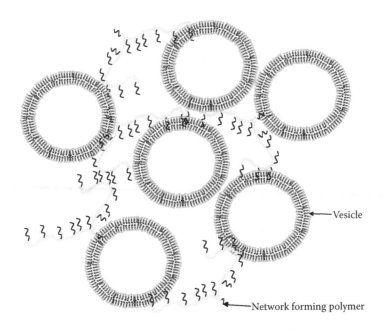

FIGURE 10.4 Polymer–vesicle gel networks. Polymers and vesicles have opposite charges.

vs. hydrophobic attractive forces to the point where vesicle formation is favored [48]. In a similar manner, vesicles are formed when dodecyl trimethylammonium bromide is incubated with partially hydrolyzed polyacrylamide (containing free carboxylate groups) [50].

10.2.1.3 Polymer–Vesicle Gels

Amphiphilic polymers interact with preformed surfactant vesicles to form interesting gel systems, as depicted schematically in Figure 10.4. Catanionic vesicles, composed of anionic and cationic surfactants with a net anionic charge, on interaction with hydrophobically modified cationic polyelectrolytes form gels due to vesicle cross-linking by the polymer [51]. Cross-linking is facilitated by the electrostatic interaction between the polymer and the vesicles and also by the insertion of hydrophobic grafts into the vesicle bilayer. It is conceivable that these gel matrices may be exploited for the controlled delivery of drugs. Additionally, polyelectrolytes devoid of hydrophobic units also interact with anionic vesicles to form gels [51]. Eventually, at higher concentrations, these latter polyelectrolytes lead to vesicle disruption.

10.2.2 BLOCK COPOLYMERS

Block copolymer vesicles, termed *polymersomes*, are fairly new discoveries, first reported in the 1990s [52]. Polymersomes have been prepared from a variety of block copolymers, some examples of which are given in Figure 10.5a. Other vesicle-forming block copolymers include: poly(ethylene oxide)-*block*-poly(ethylethylene) [3], poly(ethylene oxide)-*block*-poly(caprolactone) [27], poly(ethylene oxide)-*block*-poly([3-(trimethyoxy-silyl)propyl methacrylate] [53,54], poly(ethylene oxide)-*block*-polybutadiene [55–57], poly(ethylene oxide)-*block*-poly(propylene sulfide) [58], and poly(ethylene oxide)-*block*-polystyrene [52]. Vesicle sizes are varied and range from tens of nanometres [59] to tens of microns [60]. Polymersome membranes are thicker than conventional vesicle membranes (Figure 10.5b) [3]. Polymersome membranes possess 8- to 21-nm hydrophobic cores, and these are 2 to 5 times thicker than the 4-nm hydrophobic cores displayed by conventional low-molecular-weight amphiphile membranes [3,4,27,28,59]. The thickness of the membrane is

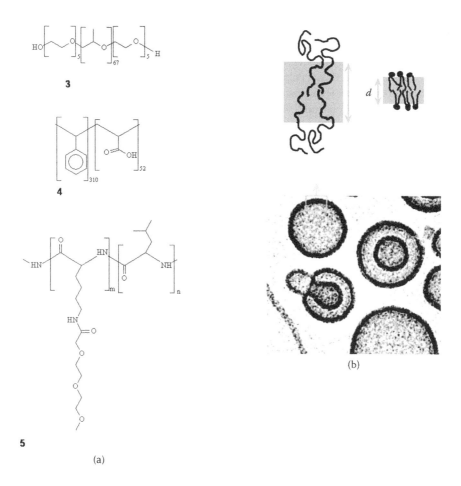

(a)

(b)

FIGURE 10.5 (a) Examples of some vesicle-forming block copolymers: polymer 3 (see Schillen, K., Bryskhe, K., and Mel'nikova, Y.S., Vesicles formed from poly(oxyethylene)-poly(oxypropylene)-poly(oxyethylene) triblock copolymer in dilute aqueous solution, *Macromolecules,* 32, 6885–6888, 1999), polymer 4 (see Burke, S.E. and Eisenberg, A., Kinetic and mechanistic details of the vesicle-to-rod transition in aggregates of PS310-b-PAA(52) in dioxane-water mixtures, *Polymer,* 42, 9111–9120, 2001), and polymer 5 (see Bellomo, E.G., Wyrsta, M.D., Pakstis, L., Pochan, D.J., and Deming, T.J., Stimuli-responsive polypeptide vesicles by conformation-specific assembly, *Nat. Mater.,* 3, 244–248, 2004); (b) polymersome membranes are thicker (8 nm thick) than lipid membranes as shown by Discher and coworkers shows schematic representation of thickness of polymerosome membrane (top left) and lipid membrane (top right), transmission electron micrograph of polymerosomes are also shown (bottom). (see Discher, B., Won, Y.Y., Ege, J.C.M., Bates, F.S., Discher, D., and Hammer, D.A., Polymersomes: tough vesicles made from diblock copolymers, *Science,* 284, 1143–1146, 1999). This affects the permeability as well as stability of these vesicle membranes. Reproduced with permission from D.E. Discher, University of Pennsylvania, Philadelphia.

determined by the degree of polymerization in the hydrophobic block [28]. These extra-thick membranes confer exceptional stability to organic solvents and water soluble surfactants [22] and also result in vesicles with superior mechanical stability [3,22,61,62]. Polymersomes are thus less likely to rupture on perturbation [3], and this diminished likelihood increases with polymer molecular weight [28]. Polymersomes have an asymmetric distribution of the polymers in the inner and outer leaflets of the bilayer [42]. The polymers with a large hydrophilic chain length are preferentially localized to the exterior leaflet, and vice versa, for the reasons stated earlier [42].

Polymersomes have been prepared in aqueous media, organic media, and organic aqueous mixtures, depending on the particular block copolymer used [52,59], and the morphology of the self-assembly may be drastically changed by altering the polarity of the disperse phase [6,63]. For example, vesicle-to-rod transitions are facilitated with polystyrene-*block*-poly(acrylic acid) vesicles by increasing the level of dioxane in an aqueous vesicle dispersion [6]. The transition is mediated by a decrease in the interfacial tension between the hydrophobic portion of the aggregating polymer and the disperse phase as the level of dioxane increases. Also, in a reverse of the aforementioned transition; a rod-to-vesicle transition may be facilitated by an increase in the water content in the dioxane–water system [64].

Vesicle stability is a desirable characteristic for vesicle-containing medicines, and as such a great deal of scientific effort has been expended on producing ever more stable systems. As the drive for nanomedicines (medicines incorporating functional nanoparticles) grows, stability issues will need to be adequately addressed to ensure the widespread adoption of such systems. In actual fact, the early workers in the polymeric vesicle field were primarily driven by this need to produce stable drug carriers. Extremely stable systems are possible on polymerization of block copolymers subsequent to self-assembly. Poly(ethylene oxide)-*block*-poly[3-(trimethoxysilyl)propyl methacrylate] copolymer vesicles in water–methanol–triethylamine mixtures produced polymerized polymersomes that are stable for up to 1 yr [53]. Triethylamine hydrolyzes the trimethoxysilyl groups and then catalyzes their polycondensation to yield an extremely stable hydrophobic polysilsesquioxane core [53,54]. Additionally, poly(ethylene oxide)-*block*-poly(butadiene) vesicles on crosslinking produce vesicles that are organic-solvent resistant [56].

10.2.3 POLYMERS BEARING HYDROPHOBIC PENDANT GROUPS

The first report on the use of preformed polymers to prepare polymeric bilayer vesicles was presented in 1981 by Kunitake and others [1]. In this study, bilayer vesicles were prepared from polymer 6 shown in Figure 10.6a. Polymer 6 comprises a hydrophilic polyacrylamide backbone and dialkyl hydrophobic pendant groups separated from the polymer backbone by hydrophilic oligooxyethylene spacers (shown schematically in Figure 10.2). The hydrophilic spacer group between the dialkyl moieties was shown by Ringsdorf and others to be essential for vesicle formation for these polyacrylamide-type polymers [20]. The hydrophilic spacer allows the decoupling of the polymer motion from the ordering of the bilayer [29].

The introduction of essentially water-soluble carbohydrate (e.g., polymer 7 [12,13]; Figure 10.6a), polyamine (e.g., polymers 8–10 [18]; Figure 10.6a), and polyamino acid (e.g., polymer 11 [19]; Figure 10.6a) polymer backbones bearing hydrophobic pendant groups is a fairly recent development. The bilayer arrangement is as depicted in Figure 10.6b, and the thick polymer coat is clearly visible on micrographs (Figure 10.1). For drug delivery applications, it is important to appreciate that the conversion of the poly(L-lysine) into vesicles reduces its cytotoxicity [65], thus potentially allowing this molecule to be exploited as a pharmaceutical excipient.

Poly(ethylenimine) (polymer 10; Figure 10.6a [18]) and poly(L-lysine) (polymer 11; Figure 10.6a [19,66]) based amphiphiles have been studied in some detail, and the formation of vesicles from these amphiphiles is dependant on the level of lipid pendant groups. Hydrophobically modified poly(ethylenimines), for example, form dense nanoparticles, bilayer vesicles, or micellar self-assemblies, depending on their hydrophobic content [18]. Hence, poly(ethylenimine) amphiphiles with a hydrophobic content of 58% and above favor dense nanoparticle self-assemblies, whereas a hydrophobic content of 43 to 58% favors bilayer vesicle assemblies and a hydrophobic content of less than 43% favors the formation of micellar assemblies [18].

A remarkably similar trend has been reported for the poly(oxyethylene)-*block*-poly(lactic acid) system in that a poly(lactic acid) fraction equal to or more than 80% favors dense nanoparticles, whereas a poly(lactic acid) fraction of 58 to 80% favors bilayer vesicle assemblies and a poly(lactic acid) fraction of less than 50% favors the production of micellar self-assemblies [27].

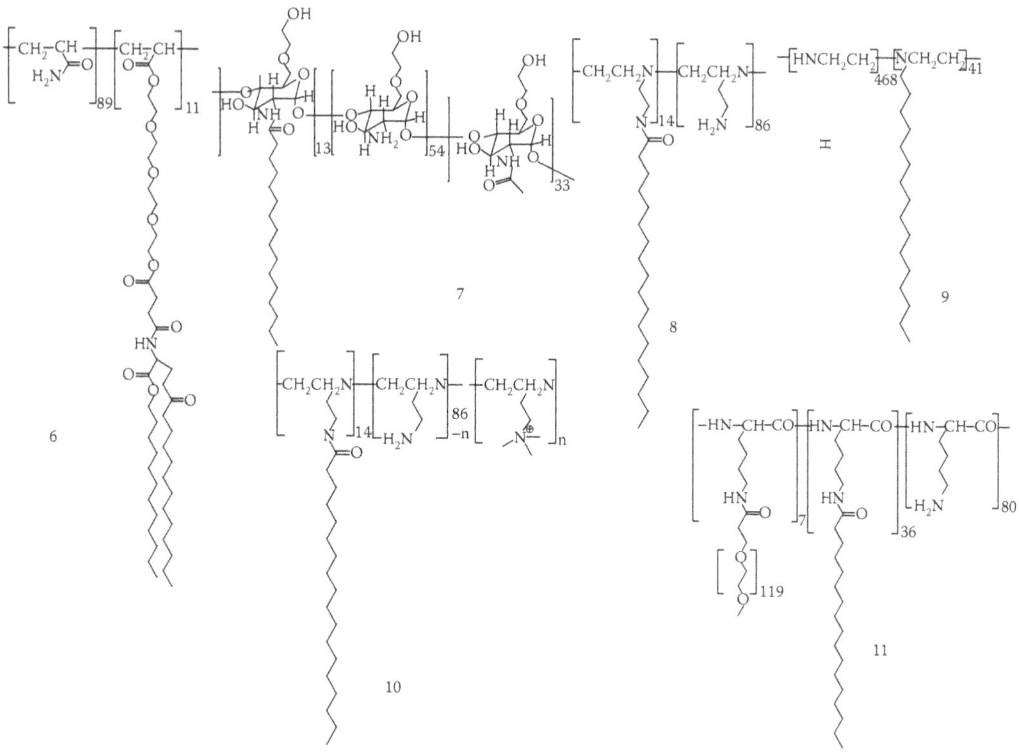

(a)

FIGURE 10.6 (a) Representative vesicle-forming polymers from the polyacrylamide, polymer 6 (see Kunitake, T., Nakashima, K., Takarabe, M., Nagai, A., Tsuge, A., and Yanagi, H., Vesicles of polymeric bilayer and monolayer membranes, *J. Am. Chem. Soc.*, 103, 5945–5947, 1981), chitosan, polymer 7 (see Uchegbu, I.F., Schatzlein, A.G., Tetley, L., Gray, A.I., Sludden, J., Siddique, S., and Mosha, E., Polymeric chitosan-based vesicles for drug delivery, *J. Pharm. Pharmacol.*, 50, 453–458, 1998 and Wang, W., McConaghy, A.M., Tetley, L., and Uchegbu, I.F., Controls on polymer molecular weight may be used to control the size of palmitoyl glycol chitosan polymeric vesicles, *Langmuir*, 17, 631–636, 2001), polyamine, polymers 8–10 (see Brownlie, A., Uchegbu, I.F., and Schatzlein, A.G., PEI based vesicle-polymer hybrid gene delivery system with improved biocompatibility, *Int. J. Pharm.*, 274, 41–52, 2004 and Wang, W., Qu, X., Gray, A.I., Tetley, L., and Uchegbu, I.F., Self-assembly of cetyl linear polyethylenimine to give micelles, vesicles and nanoparticles is controlled by the hydrophobicity of the polymer, *Macromolecules*, 37, 9114–9122, 2004), and polyamino acid, polymer 11 (see Wang, W., Tetley, L., and Uchegbu, I.F., The level of hydrophobic substitution and the molecular weight of amphiphilic poly-L-lysine-based polymers strongly affects their assembly into polymeric bilayer vesicles, *J. Coll. Interf. Sci.*, 237, 200–207, 2001), classes of polymers bearing hydrophobic pendant groups; (b) the polyethylenimine polymers (polymers 8 and 10) are arranged in the bilayer as shown. Micrograph shows a negative stained transmission electron image of polymer 8, cholesterol (2: 199^{-1}) vesicles.

The sizes of the vesicle and dense nanoparticle assemblies formed from amphiphilic poly(ethylenimines) (e.g., polymer 9, Figure 10.6a) are also dependant on polymer levels of hydrophobic modification (mol% cetylation), and the relationships shown in Equation 10.1 and Equation 10.2 have been developed [18].

$$d_v = 1.95Ct + 139 \tag{10.1}$$

$$d_n = 2.31Ct + 5.6 \tag{10.2}$$

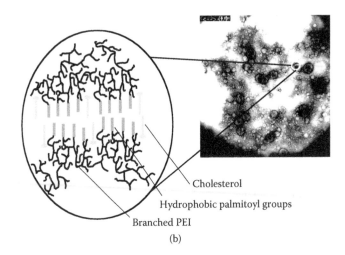

Cholesterol

Hydrophobic palmitoyl groups

Branched PEI

(b)

FIGURE 10.6 (Continued).

where d_v is the z-averaged mean vesicle hydrodynamic diameter; Ct, the mol% cetylation; and d_n, the z-averaged mean nanoparticle hydrodynamic diameter.

The molecular weight of the polymer is also an important factor to consider when choosing vesicle-forming polymers. The importance of this parameter has been demonstrated with the poly(L-lysine) vesicle system [19] (e.g., polymer 9; Figure 10.6a). With these amphiphiles a vesicle formation index (F) was computed:

$$F = \frac{H}{L\,DP} \tag{10.3}$$

where H is the mol% unreacted L-lysine units; L, the mol% L-lysine units substituted with palmitic acid; and DP, the degree of polymerization of the polymer. An F value in excess of 0.168 was found to be necessary for vesicle formation [19].

Additionally, not only does the molecular weight of the polymer impact on vesicle formation but it also is a direct controller of vesicle mean size, and for the palmitoyl glycol chitosan system [13], the relationship shown in Equation 10.4 has been developed

$$\sqrt{MW} = 0.782d_v + 107 \tag{10.4}$$

where MW is the polymer molecular weight and d_v, the vesicle z-averaged mean hydrodynamic diameter.

10.3 POLYMERIZATION AFTER SELF-ASSEMBLY

Polymerization after self-assembly may take the form of the polymerization of amphiphilic monomers after self-assembly (Figure 10.1) or of a hydrophobic [9,16] (Figure 10.7) or hydrophilic [67] non-amphiphilic monomer after monomer equilibration with vesicle membranes, and in all cases extremely interesting potential drug carriers result. The main advantage of this technology is the production of systems that are extremely stable and thus resist degradation from detergents [68,69] and organic solvents [8,69,70]. However, as polymerization involves fairly reactive species, this technology is best applied prior to drug loading, and thus has some limitations.

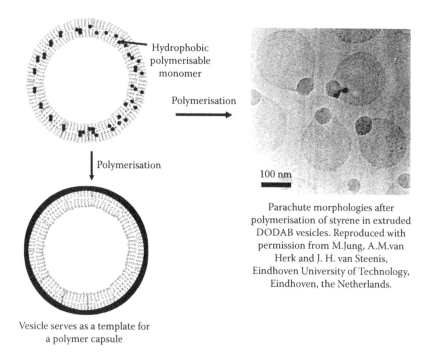

Parachute morphologies after polymerisation of styrene in extruded DODAB vesicles. Reproduced with permission from M.Jung, A.M.van Herk and J. H. van Steenis, Eindhoven University of Technology, Eindhoven, the Netherlands.

FIGURE 10.7 The polymerization of hydrophobic monomers yields either phase-separated parachute morphologies (see Jung, M., den Ouden, I., Montoya-Goni, A., Hubert, D.H.W., Frederik, P.M., van Herk, A.M., and German, A.L., Polymerization in polymerizable vesicle bilayer membranes, *Langmuir*, 16, 4185–4195, 2000 and Jung, M., Hubert, D.H.W., Bomans, P.H.H., Frederik, P.M., Meuldijk, J., van Herk, A.M., Fischer, H., and German, A.L., New vesicle-polymer hybrids: the parachute architecture, *Langmuir*, 13, 6877–6880, 1997) or polymer nanocapsules (see McKelvey, C.A., Kaler, E.W., Zasadzinski, J.A., Coldren, B., and Jung, H.T., Templating hollow polymeric spheres from catanionic equilibrium vesicles: synthesis and characterization, *Langmuir*, 16, 8285–8290, 2000).

10.3.1 POLYMERIZATION OF NON-AMPHIPHILIC MONOMERS IN PREFORMED VESICLES

The polymerization of a hydrophobic monomer in a bilayer membrane was first reported in 1986 for the dioctadecyldimethylammonium bromide–styrene/divinyl benzene system [71]. Evidence now exists, confirming that there are two possible outcomes of using this technique (Figure 10.7). The polymerization of a hydrophobic monomer within a vesicle bilayer yields either a phase-separated latex particle [9] or, alternatively, a polymer shell [16] that may optionally be isolated from the vesicle template (Figure 10.7).

The phase-separated morphologies, christened *"parachute" morphologies*, arise when dioctadecyldimethylammonium bromide vesicles are incubated with polymerizable monomers, such as styrene, and subsequently polymerized [9,72–76]. Latex beads are visible on representative micrographs (Figure 10.7). Whether these two component structures will find particular use in drug delivery remains an unanswered question.

To obtain polymer shells, in which the vesicle serves as a template, amphiphiles with styrene moieties attached to the hydrophobic tail (polymer 12; Figure 10.8) have been used to prepare vesicles, followed by an incubation of these styrene-functionalized vesicles with styrene monomers and, finally, polymerization [5]. Polymerization appears to occur throughout the length of the bilayer without the phase separation of the growing polymer [5]. A copolymerization between the styrene monomer and styrene-functionalized amphiphile is thought to be the reason why phase separation is not observed [5]. Others have successfully utilized the vesicle as a polymer shell template by

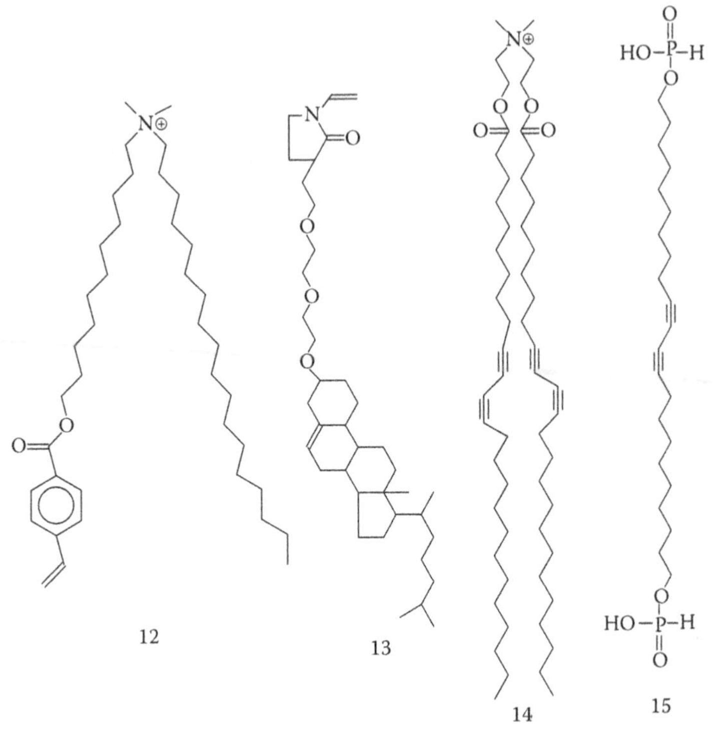

FIGURE 10.8 Polymerizable vesicle-forming monomers used to make polymerized vesicles by Jung et al. (polymer 12; see Jung, M., den Ouden, I., Montoya-Goni, A., Hubert, D.H.W., Frederik, P.M., van Herk, A.M., and German, A.L., Polymerization in polymerizable vesicle bilayer membranes, *Langmuir,* 16, 4185–4195, 2000), Cho et al. (polymer 13; see Cho, I., Dong, S., and Jeong, S.W., Vesicle formation by nonionic polymerizable cholesterol-based amphiphiles, *Polymer,* 36, 1513–1515, 1995), Hub et al. (polymer 14; see Hub, H.H., Hupfer, B., Koch, H., and Ringsdorf, H., Polymerizable phospholipid analogues — new stable biomembrane cell models, *Angew. Chem. Int. Ed. Engl.,* 19, 938–940, 1980) and Bader et al. (polymer 15; see Bader, H. and Ringsdorf, H., Liposomes from alpha, omega-dipolar amphiphiles with a polymerizable diyne moiety in the hydrophobic chain, *J. Polym. Sci. Polym. Chem. Ed.,* 20, 1623–1628, 1982).

using vesicles prepared from fluorinated phospholipids with polymerizable hydrocarbon poly(iso-decylacrylate) monomers [77]. The polymer is distributed homogenously throughout the hydrophobic core of the vesicle bilayer. This is explained by the fact that the fluorinated section of the bilayer is segregated from the hydrocarbon section of the bilayer; it is the latter in which the monomer resides. The confinement of the monomer to the hydrocarbon region prevents its phase separation into a latex particle and the polymer is forced to grow with limited dimensionality [77].

The use of catanionic surfactant (comprising both cationic and anionic surfactants) vesicles in the polymerizable hydrophobic monomer–vesicle system also results in the production of extremely stable polymer shells [16]. When styrene or divinylbenzene are incorporated into cetyltrimethylammonium tosylate–dodecylbenzene sulfonate vesicles at up to 12% by weight and the system polymerized, polymer shells result, which may be isolated as a dry powder by dialyzing out the catanionic surfactants [16]. The shells may then be stabilized in aqueous media using either water-soluble surfactants or the introduction of surface sulfonate groups [16]. The polymer shell has a thickness of 6 nm and a diameter of about 100 nm [78].

Polymer shells utilizing a vesicle template are also achieved by the incubation of cationic (diocatdecyldimethylammonium bromide) vesicles with tetramethyl orthosilicate; the latter of which is hydrolyzed and condensed to give silica [79]. Silica deposits as a 10-nm layer on the surface of the vesicles.

Finally, hydrophilic monomers, as well as hydrophobic monomers, associated with vesicles may be polymerized to yield polymer shells [67]. In the example presented by Ringsdorf and others, the polymerization of choline methacrylate counterions surrounding dihexadecylphosphate vesicles yields a polymer coat on the exterior or optionally (by removing the external ions prior to polymerization) on the interior of the vesicles [67]. The resulting tough polymer coat is highly impermeable to entrapped solutes.

10.3.2 SELF-ASSEMBLING POLYMERIZABLE MONOMERS

Polymerized vesicles may also be prepared by utilizing self-assembling polymerizable amphiphiles, followed by the polymerization of the resulting vesicular self-assembly (Figure 10.1). Examples of some polymerizable vesicle-forming monomers are shown in Figure 10.8, and others include N,N-dimethyl-N-[11-(p-vinylbenzoyloxyl)undecyl]octadecylammonium bromide, [5] 1,2-di(2,4-octadecadienoyl)-sn-glycerol-3-phosphocholine [68], 2-[N-methyl-N-[O-tocopheryloligo(oxyethylene)oxycarbonyl]methylamino]ethyl methacrylate [80], 1-ethenyl-3-(8-cholest-5-en-3β-yloxy)-3,6-dioxaoctyl-0-2-pyrrolidone [8], 1-carboxy-10,12-docosadiynyl-22-(22,4-dicarboxy)benzoate [81], and [[(cholesteryloxycarbonyl]methyl][2-(methacryloyloxy)ethyl]dimethylammonium chloride [69]. This method of producing polymerized vesicles is the oldest form of this technology [11,82].

Polymerised vesicles prepared using polymerized self-assembling monomers are essentially polymer shells, and it is unclear how much of the bilayer assembly actually survives the polymerization step. The advantage, however, is that they are extremely stable, resisting degradation by detergents [68,69,83] or organic solvents [8,69,70,84]. Polymerized vesicles are also less leaky [70], thermostable [80], and, because the vesicle-forming components are kinetically trapped by the polymerization process, have improved colloidal stability [8]. A major advantage of these nanosystems is that they may be isolated as dry powders that are readily dispersible in water to give 50- to 100-nm particles [69], thus potentially allowing the formulation of solid vesicle dosage forms.

As well as from unsaturated hydrocarbon monomers [20,85] (e.g., Figure 10.8), polymerized vesicles may be prepared from thiol [86] and isocyano [84] monomers. The former are polymerized by oxidation with hydrogen peroxide and depolymerized using dithiothreitol [86], wheras the latter are polymerized in the presence of a nickel catalyst [84]. However, the polymerized thiol vesicles do not have the diminished permeability advantages usually associated with polymeric vesicles [86].

When producing vesicles for the carriage of a hydrophilic load, care must be taken when polymerizing monomers that are not localized within the bilayer because the resulting polymer could take up valuable space within the vesicles. Liposomes have been formed entrapping a polymer network comprising N-isopropylacrylamide and tetraethylene glycol dimethacrylate by loading liposomes, bearing 1,2-disteary-l-3-octaethylene glycol ether methacrylate in their bilayers with N-isopropylacrylamide and tetraethylene glycol dimethacrylate, and followed by photopolymerisation with the initiator 2,2-diethoxyacetophenone [83]. High loads of N-isopropylacrylamide cause the network to fill the whole of the interior liposome space, whereas low levels cause the network to merely line the interior space of the liposome [87].

10.4 DRUG DELIVERY APPLICATIONS

Polymeric vesicles exist in three main varieties as illustrated in Figure 10.1. Although polymeric vesicles in which a hydrophilic polymer, poly(oxyethylene), functionalizes the surface to give reticuloendothelial-system-avoiding ability have been used in licensed medicines as detailed earlier; polymeric vesicles in which the polymeric backbone not only coats but actually comprises an integral part of the vesicle bilayer are yet to be exploited to enhance the properties of medicines. This latter group of polymeric vesicles is a suitable candidate for the development of robust, controllable, and responsive nanomedicines. This section, while summarizing the drug delivery application of poly(oxyethylene) coated liposomes, will also offer an insight into the drug delivery potential of some of the other polymeric vesicle types.

10.4.1 Drug Targeting

Poly(oxyethylene) amphiphiles such as polymer 1 [24] and polymer 2 [32] (Figure 10.3), on incorporation into liposomes [24] and niosomes [32], respectively, result in intravenously injected liposomes and niosomes enjoying a prolonged residence time in the blood. This prolonged circulation is clearly mediated by an avoidance of clearance by the liver and spleen [88] and is primarily achieved by reduced protein binding to the vesicles in the blood [89]; the latter makes vesicles unrecognizable to the macrophages of the liver and spleen. The prolonged blood residence time may also involve a decrease in liposome aggregation in plasma [90]. Decreased intravascular aggregation would prevent liposomes from being trapped in various capillary beds. Ultimately, the long circulation of such liposomes [88] and niosomes [32] leads to tumor targeting because of the leaky nature of the poorly developed tumor vascular endothelium [91]. An increased accumulation of drug within tumor tissue is associated with superior tumoricidal activity in animals [32, 88] and in man [92]. Polymer-coated doxorubicin liposomes are now licensed for clinical use and marketed as Caelyx in Europe and Doxil in the U.S. [15].

Only 10 mol% poly(ethylene oxide)–lipid amphiphiles may be incorporated into liposomes [36] or niosomes [33,35] without a loss of vesicle integrity, which is because of the preferred tendency of the hydrophilic poly(oxyethylene) amphiphile to form micelles. Polymersomes composed of poly(ethylene oxide)-*block*-poly(butadiene) or poly(ethylene oxide)-*block*-poly(ethylethylene) in which the entire vesicle surface is covered with the poly(ethylene oxide) coat have been studied as long-circulating nanocarriers for drug delivery [93]. The circulation time of poly(ethylene oxide) polymersomes is directly dependant on the length of the poly(ethylene oxide) block, and polymersome half-lives of up to 28 h have been recorded in rats with a poly(ethylene oxide) having a degree of polymerisation of 50 [93]. This half-life compares favorably with a half-life of 14 h recorded for poly(oxyethylene)-coated liposomes [89]. It is assumed that the 100% surface coverage of the polymeric vesicles is responsible for the reduced clearance of these polymersomes from the blood [62]. The long half-life of these polymersomes makes them excellent candidates for the development of antitumor medicines.

Furthermore, drug release may be further controlled in the polymersomes by controlling the hydrolysis rate of the hydrophobic blocks [27]. This has been demonstrated with poly(L-lactic acid)-*block*-poly(ethylene glycol) and poly(caprolactone)-*block*-poly(ethylene glycol) vesicles [27]. Hydrolysis of the hydrophobic block causes the polymer to move from a vesicular to a micellar assembly as the overall level of hydrophobic content diminishes, and this in turn leads to drug release [27]. Hydrolysis rates, and implicitly release rates, may be controlled by varying the relative level of the hydrophobic blocks.

The concepts outlined earlier may be used to achieve passive targeting, in which vesicles are homed in to the particular anatomical site. Strategies aimed at actively targeting vesicles to particular parts of the anatomy or particular areas of pathology by exploiting ligand–receptor interactions have utilized such poly(ethylene glycol) liposomes (PEGylated liposomes) bearing targeting ligands [94,95]. An important consideration when preparing these formulations is to ensure that the targeting ligand is attached to the distal end of the poly(oxyethylene) chains and not directly on the bilayer [94]. The adherence of such ligands to their targets is hindered if the targeting ligand is attached to the lipid surface of poly(oxyethylene)-coated vesicles instead of to the ends of the poly(oxyethylene) chains. Evidence exists to indicate that ligand–receptor binding is even hindered by neighboring poly(oxyethylene) chains when the ligands are indeed attached to the distal ends of the polymer chains [55]. It is for this reason that a sufficient coating density of ligands relative to the overall level of poly(oxyethylene) chains should be used.

TABLE 10.1
Biological Activity of Poly(ethylenimine)[a] and Poly(L-lysine)[b] Vesicles

Polymer	A431 Cells		A549 Cells	
	IC50 (μg ml^{-1})	Gene Transfer Relative to Parent Polymer	IC50 (μg ml^{-1})	Gene Transfer Relative to Parent Polymer
Poly(ethylenimine)	1.9	1	5.2	1
Polymer 8 (Figure 10.6a)	16.9	0.2	12.6	0.08
Polymer 8, cholesterol vesicles 2: 1 (g g^{-1})	15.9	0.2	11	0.08
Poly(L-lysine)	7	1	7	1
Polymer 11, cholesterol (Figure 10.6a)	74	7.8	63	2.3

[a] From Brownlie, A., Uchegbu, I.F., and Schatzlein, A.G., PEI-based vesicle-polymer hybrid gene delivery system with improved biocompatibility, *Int. J. Pharm.*, 274, 41–52, 2004.

[b] From Brown, M.D., Schatzlein, A., Brownlie, A., Jack, V., Wang, W., Tetley, L., Gray, A.I., and Uchegbu, I.F., Preliminary characterization of novel amino acid based polymeric vesicles as gene and drug delivery agents, *Bioconjugate Chem.*, 11, 880–891, 2000.

10.4.2 CATIONIC POLYMERIC VESICLES IN DRUG AND GENE DELIVERY

Poly(L-lysine) based vesicles, prepared from polymer 11 (Figure 10.6), have been used for gene delivery [65,96] because these vesicles are less toxic than unmodified poly(L-lysine) and produced higher levels of gene transfer (Table 10.1) [65]. The production of polymeric vesicles and the resultant reduction in cytotoxicity enables poly(L-lysine) derivatives to be used as an *in vivo* gene carriers because the unmodified polymer is too toxic for use as an *in vivo* gene-transfer system. When the targeting ligand galactose was bound to the distal ends of the poly(oxyethylene) chains, gene expression was increased in HepG2 cells *in vitro* [96]. However, *in vivo* targeting to the liver hepatocytes was not achieved with these systems [96].

A similar procedure with the poly(ethylenimine) vesicles prepared using polymer 8 (Figure 10.6) also resulted in a reduction in the cytotoxicity of the polymer (Table 10.1) [17], although in this case the poly(ethylenimine) vesicles were not as efficient gene-transfer agents as the free polymer.

Carbohydrate polymeric vesicles may also be used as drug-targeting agents. Vesicles prepared from glycol chitosan improve the intracellular delivery of hydrophilic macromolecules [97] and anticancer drugs [98]; the latter is achieved with the help of a transferrin ligand attached to the surface of the vesicle. These carbohydrate vesicles improve the *in vivo* tolerability of the cytotoxic agent doxorubicin; however, they are not active against subcutaneously implanted A431 tumors.

10.4.3 RESPONSIVE RELEASE

The ultimate goal of all drug delivery efforts is the simple fabrication of responsive systems that are capable of delivering precise quantities of their payload in response to physiological or, more commonly, pathological stimuli. Preprogrammable and intelligently responsive pills, implants, and injectables are so far merely the unobtainable ideal. However, polymeric systems have been fabricated with responsive capability, and it is possible that in the future these may be fine-tuned to produce truly intelligent and dynamic drug delivery systems.

The various environmental stimuli that may be used to trigger the release of encapsulated drug are outlined in the following subsections, and examples of existing developments in the area are given. However, in addition to the areas covered here, it may be possible in the future for pathology-specific molecules to interact with polymeric vesicles and trigger release.

10.4.3.1 pH

Hydrophobically modified pH-sensitive poly(*N*-isopropylacrylamide) polymers, i.e., random copolymers of poly(*N*-isopropylacrylamide)-*co*-poly(met acrylic acid)-*co*-poly(octadecylacrylate) when incorporated into liposomes and niosomes form pH-sensitive vesicles that are able to preferentially release their payload at acid pH [99]. Such polymers improve the cytotoxicity of cytosine arabinofuranoside, a drug that is usually degraded in the intracellular lysosomal compartment, presumably by enabling its release in the acidic early endosomes [99].

The pH-responsive perturbation of stearoylphosphatidylcholine, cholesterol liposomes [100], and myristoylphosphatidylcholine liposomes [101] by poly(2-ethacrylic acid) may also be used to fabricate acid-sensitive drug delivery systems. Poly(2-ethacrylic acid) at low pH becomes more hydrophobic and hence destabilizes the membranes of liposomes in a pH-dependant manner [100]. Cholesterol appears to inhibit the uptake of the protonated polymer by the bilayers, whereas the presence of a poly(oxyethylene) surface does not prevent the protonated polymer from interacting with the membrane and causing contents release [100]. The destabilisation of liposomes by poly(2-ethacrylic acid) may also be photoinduced by employing 3,3-dicarboxydiphenyliodonium salts as a photosensitive proton source; acidification of the polymer on irradiation leads to a destabilisation of the membrane [101]. Attaching poly(2-ethacrylic acid) to preformed vesicles also results in the formation of acid-sensitive vesicles, which release most of their contents on mild acidification [102]. Hence, coating vesicles with poly(2-ethacrylic acid) may be a feasible method of facilitating the intracellular (endosomal) release of drugs, thus localizing drug activity to the interior of the cell.

Diblock polypeptides in which the hydrophilic block consists of ethylene glycol derivatised amino acids (L-lysine) and the hydrophobic block consists of poly(L-leucine) (polymer 5; Figure 10.5a) form pH-responsive vesicles that disaggregate at low pHs, provided the level of L-leucine and the polymer chain length is maintained within defined limits of about 12 to 25 mol% and the polymer has a degree of polymerization of less than 200 [10]. Once again these L-lysine systems may be applied to facilitate endosome-specific release.

10.4.3.2 Temperature

Temperature-responsive liposomes have also been developed from mixtures of dimyristoylphosphatidylcholine and hydrophobically modified poly-*N*-isopropylacrylamide, a polymer with a lower critical solution temperature of about 32°C [103]. The polymer is anchored in the membrane by its hydrophobic groups, and on heating the liposome suspension to above the lowest critical solution temperature (LCST), the hydrodynamic radius of the polymer hydrophilic head group decreases, forcing the polymer hydrophobic groups to rearrange within the bilayer, such rearrangement giving rise to a perturbation of the liposome bilayer and the eventual release of liposome contents. This temperature-responsive system may be used to localize drugs to particular regions of pathology by employing localized hyperthermia.

10.4.3.3 Enzyme

Vesicles that release their contents in the presence of an enzyme may be formed by loading polymeric vesicles with an enzyme-activated prodrug (Figure 10.9). The particulate nature of the drug delivery system should allow the drug to accumulate in tumors, for example, where the particulates may be activated by an externally applied enzyme in a similar manner to the antibody-directed enzyme prodrug therapeutic strategy. The antibody-directed enzyme prodrug therapeutic strategy enables an enzyme to be homed in to tumors by using antibodies followed by the application of an enzyme-activated prodrug [104]. Alternatively, a membrane-bound enzyme may be used to control and ultimately prolong the activity of either an entrapped hydrophilic (entrapped in the vesicle aqueous core) or hydrophobic (entrapped in the vesicle membrane) drug as illustrated in Figure 10.9. It is possible that the enzyme may be chosen such that it is

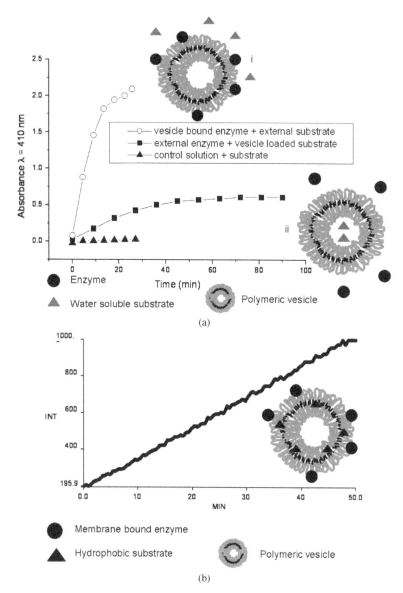

(a)

(b)

FIGURE 10.9 (a) Enzyme-activated polymeric vesicles. Vesicles bearing membrane-bound enzyme (i) were formed by probe sonicating polymer 7 (Figure 10.6a), cholesterol, N-biotinylated dipalmitoyl phosphatidyl ethanolamine (8:4:1 g g[1]) in sodium phosphate monobasic (0·1m, 2ml) isolation of the vesicles by ultracentrifugation (150,000 g), redispersion in a similar volume of sodium phosphate monobasic (0·1m), and incubation of the vesicles with β-galactosidase streptavidin (3 U). The membrane-bound enzyme (0.2 ml) was then incubated with o-nitrophenyl-β-D-galactoside (2.1 mM, 2-ml substrate) and the absorbance monitored (λ = 410 nm). The control solution contained similar levels of substrate but no enzyme. Vesicles encapsulating o-nitrophenyl-β-D-galactoside (ii) were prepared by probe sonicating polymer 7 and cholesterol (8: 4 g g[1]) in the presence of o-nitrophenyl-β-D-galactoside solution (34 mM, 2 ml), isolation of the vesicles by ultracentrifugation, and redispersion in sodium phosphate monobasic (0·1m) buffer. These latter vesicles (0.4 ml) were then incubated with β-D-galactosidase (2 U ml[−1], 0·1 ml) and the absorbance once again monitored; (b) enzyme-activated polymeric vesicles. Vesicles-bearing membrane-bound enzyme and containing the hydrophobic substrate fluorescein di-β-D-galactospyranoside were formed by probe sonicating polymer 7 (Figure 10.6a), cholesterol, N-biotinylated dipalmitoyl phosphatidyl ethanolamine, fluorescein di-β-D-galactospyranoside (8: 4: 1: 0.0005 g g[1]) in sodium phosphate monobasic (0·1m) and incubation of the resulting vesicles with b-galactosidase streptavidin (0.3 U). The fluorescence of the enzyme-hydrolyzed substrate was monitored (excitation wavelength = 490 nm, emission wavelength = 514 nm). 1·0 unit of enzyme (1·O U) is the amount of enzyme causing transformation of 1·0 µm of substrate per minute at 25°C under optimal conditions of measurement.

activated in the presence of pathology-specific molecules, thus achieving pathology-responsive and localized drug activity.

10.4.3.4 Magnetic Field

Magnetically-responsive polymerized liposomes composed of 1,2-di(2,4-octadecadienoyl)-*sn*-glycerol-3-phosphorylcholine, loaded with ferric oxide, and subsequently polymerized may be localized by an external magnetic field to the small intestine and specifically the Peyer's patches [68]. These polymerized vesicles are stable to the degradative influence of solubilizing surfactants such as triton-X 100 [68], and hence should not suffer excessive bile-salt-mediated degradation during gut transit. These magnetically-responsive polymeric vesicles may be used to improve the absorption of drugs via the oral route, and the authors of this report found higher levels of a radioactive marker in the liver of magnetically treated mice when compared to control animals that had not been subjected to magnetic treatment [68].

10.4.3.5 Oxygen

Block copolymer vesicles that are destabilized by oxidative mechanisms have been constructed from poly(oxyethylene)-*block*-poly(propylene sulfide)-*block*-poly(oxyethylene) ABA block copolymers [58]. These polymeric vesicles are destabilized on oxidation of the central sulfide block to give sulfoxides and ultimately sulfones [58]. On oxidation, the vesicles are transformed to worm-like micelles and finally spherical micelles, eventually releasing their contents.

10.5 CONCLUSIONS

In summary, polymeric vesicles may be fabricated from a variety of macromolecular amphiphile architectures, which include: block copolymers, random graft copolymers, and polymers bearing hydrophobic low-molecular-weight pendant or terminal groups. These tough particles, which reside in the nanometre and micrometer size domains, may be used for drug targeting, the preparation of responsive release systems, and other drug delivery applications.

REFERENCES

1. Kunitake, T., Nakashima, K., Takarabe, M., Nagai, A., Tsuge, A., and Yanagi, H., Vesicles of polymeric bilayer and monolayer membranes, *J. Am. Chem. Soc.,* 103, 5945–5947, 1981.
2. Schillen, K., Bryskhe, K., and Mel'nikova, Y.S., Vesicles formed form poly(oxyethylene)-poly(oxypropylene)-poly(oxyethylene) triblock copolymer in dilute aqueous solution, *Macromolecules,* 32, 6885–6888, 1999.
3. Discher, B., Won, Y.Y., Ege, J.C.M., Bates, F.S., Discher, D., and Hammer, D.A., Polymersomes: tough vesicles made from diblock copolymers, *Science,* 284, 1143–1146, 1999.
4. Israelachvili, J., *Intermolecular and Surface Forces.* 2nd ed., London, Academic Press, 1991.
5. Jung, M., den Ouden, I., Montoya-Goni, A., Hubert, D.H.W., Frederik, P.M., van Herk, A.M., and German, A.L., Polymerization in polymerizable vesicle bilayer membranes, *Langmuir,* 16, 4185–4195, 2000.
6. Burke, S.E. and Eisenberg, A., Kinetic and mechanistic details of the vesicle-to-rod transition in aggregates of PS310-b-PAA(52) in dioxane-water mixtures, *Polymer,* 42, 9111–9120, 2001.
7. Bangham, A.D., Standish, M.M., and Watkins, J.C., Diffusion of univalent ions across the lamellae of swollen phospholipids, *J. Mol. Biol.,* 13, 238–252, 1965.
8. Cho, I., Dong, S., and Jeong, S.W., Vesicle formation by nonionic polymerizable cholesterol-based amphiphiles, *Polymer,* 36, 1513–1515, 1995.
9. Jung, M., Hubert, D.H.W., Bomans, P.H.H., Frederik, P.M., Meuldijk, J., van Herk, A.M., Fischer, H., and German, A.L., New vesicle-polymer hybrids: the parachute architecture, *Langmuir,* 13, 6877–6880, 1997.

10. Bellomo, E.G., Wyrsta, M.D., Pakstis, L., Pochan, D.J., and Deming, T.J., Stimuli-responsive polypeptide vesicles by conformation-specific assembly, *Nat. Mater.,* 3, 244–248, 2004.

11. Hub, H.H., Hupfer, B., Koch, H., and Ringsdorf, H., Polymerizable phospholipid analogues — new stable biomembrane cell models, *Angew. Chem. Int. Ed. Engl.,* 19, 938–940, 1980.

12. Uchegbu, I.F., Schatzlein, A.G., Tetley, L., Gray, A.I., Sludden, J., Siddique, S., and Mosha, E., Polymeric chitosan-based vesicles for drug delivery, *J. Pharm. Pharmacol.,* 50, 453–458, 1998.

13. Wang, W., McConaghy, A.M., Tetley, L., and Uchegbu, I.F., Controls on polymer molecular weight may be used to control the size of palmitoyl glycol chitosan polymeric vesicles, *Langmuir,* 17, 631–636, 2001.

14. Bader, H. and Ringsdorf, H., Liposomes from alpha, omega-dipolar amphiphiles with a polymerizable diyne moiety in the hydrophobic chain, *J. Polym. Sci. Polym. Chem. Ed.,* 20, 1623–1628, 1982.

15. Gabizon, A.A., Pegylated liposomal doxorubicin: metamorphosis of an old drug into a new form of chemotherapy, *Cancer Invest.,* 19, 424–436, 2001.

16. McKelvey, C.A., Kaler, E.W., Zasadzinski, J.A., Coldren, B., and Jung, H.T., Templating hollow polymeric spheres from catanionic equilibrium vesicles: synthesis and characterization, *Langmuir,* 16, 8285–8290, 2000.

17. Brownlie, A., Uchegbu, I.F., and Schatzlein, A.G., PEI based vesicle-polymer hybrid gene delivery system with improved biocompatibility, *Int. J. Pharm.,* 274, 41–52, 2004.

18. Wang, W., Qu, X., Gray, A.I., Tetley, L., and Uchegbu, I.F., Self assembly of cetyl linear polyethylenimine to give micelles, vesicles and nanoparticles is controlled by the hydrophobicity of the polymer, *Macromolecules,* 37, 9114–9122, 2004.

19. Wang, W., Tetley, L., and Uchegbu, I.F., The level of hydrophobic substitution and the molecular weight of amphiphilic poly-L-lysine-based polymers strongly affects their assembly into polymeric bilayer vesicles, *J. Coll. Interf. Sci.,* 237, 200–207, 2001.

20. Ringsdorf, H., Schlarb, B., and Venzmer, J., Molecular architecture and function of polymeric oriented systems: models for the study of organisation, surface recognition, and dynamics of biomembranes, *Angew. Chem., Int. Ed. Engl.,* 27, 113–158, 1988.

21. Discher, D.E. and Eisenberg, A., Polymer vesicles, *Science,* 297, 967–973, 2002.

22. Antonietti, M. and Forster, S., Vesicles and liposomes: a self-assembly principle beyond lipids, *Adv. Mater.,* 15, 1323–1333, 2003.

23. Wakita, M. and Hashimoto, M., Bilayer vesicle formation of N-octadecylchitosan, *Kobun. Ronbun.,* 52, 589–593, 1995.

24. Blume, G. and Cevc, G., Liposomes for the sustained drug release in vivo, *Biochim. Biophys. Acta,* 1029, 91–97, 1990.

25. Uchegbu, I.F. and Florence, A.T., Nonionic surfactant vesicles (niosomes) — physical and pharmaceutical chemistry, *Adv. Coll. Interf. Sci.,* 58, 1–55, 1995.

26. Kukula, H., Schlaad, H., Antonietti, M., and Forster, S., The formation of polymer vesicles or peptosomes by polybutadiene-block-poly(L-glutamate)s in dilute aqueous solution, *J. Am. Chem. Soc.,* 124, 1658–1663, 2002.

27. Ahmed, F. and Discher, D.E., Self-porating polymersomes of PEG-PLA and PEG-PCL: hydrolysis-triggered controlled release vesicles, *J. Controlled Release,* 96, 37–53, 2004.

28. Bermudez, H., Brannan, A.K., Hammer, D.A., Bates, F.S., and Discher, D.E., Molecular weight dependence of polymerosome membrane structure, elasticity, and stability, *Macromolecules,* 35, 8203–8208, 2002.

29. Elbert, R., Lashewsky, A., and Ringsdorf, H., Hydrophilic spacer groups in polymerizable lipids: formation of biomembrane models from bulk polymerised lipids, *J. Am. Chem. Soc.,* 107, 4134–4141, 1985.

30. Allen, T.M., Hansen, C., Martin, F., Redemann, C., and Yau-Young, A., Liposomes containing synthetic lipid derivatives of poly(ethylene glycol) show prolonged circulation half-lives in vivo, *Biochim. Biophys. Acta,* 1066, 29–36, 1991.

31. Huang, S.K., Lee, K.-D., Hong, K., Friend, D.S., and Papahadjopoulos, D., Microscopic localisation of sterically stabilized liposomes in colon carcinoma bearing mice, *Cancer Res.,* 52, 5135–5142, 1992.

32. Uchegbu, I.F., Double, J.A., Turton, J.A., and Florence, A.T., Distribution, metabolism and tumoricidal activity of doxorubicin administered in sorbitan monostearate (Span 60) niosomes in the mouse, *Pharm. Res.,* 12, 1019–1024, 1995.

33. Beugin-Deroo, S., Ollivon, M., and Lesieur, S., Bilayer stability and impermeability of nonionic surfactant vesicles sterically stabilized by PEG-cholesterol conjugates, *J. Coll. Interf. Sci.,* 202, 324–333, 1998.

34. Bedu-Addo, F.K., Tang, P., Xu, Y., and Huang, L., Effects of polyethylene glycol chain length and phospholipid acyl chain composition on the interaction of polyethyleneglycol-phospholipid conjugates with phospholipid: implications in liposomal drug delivery, *Pharm. Res.,* 13, 710–717, 1996.

35. Uchegbu, I.F., Bouwstra, J.A., and Florence, A.T., Large disk-shaped structures (discomes) in nonionic surfactant vesicle to micelle transitions, *J. Phys. Chem.,* 96, 10548–10553, 1992.

36. Rovira-Bru, M., Thompson, D.H., and Szleifer, I., Size and structure of spontaneously forming liposomes in lipid/PEG-lipid mixtures, *Biophys. J.,* 83, 2419–2439, 2002.

37. Vyas, S.P., Mysore, N., Jaitely, V., and Venkatesan, N., Discoidal niosome based controlled ocular delivery of timolol maleate, *Pharmazie,* 53, 466–469, 1998.

38. Kevelam, J., Engberts, J., Blandamer, M.J., Briggs, B., and Cullis, P.M., Anchoring of hydrophobically modified poly(sodium acrylate)s into DDP vesicle bilayers: hydrophobic match and mismatch, *Coll. Polym. Sci.,* 276, 190–194, 1998.

39. Kang, S.Y., Park, M.K., and Jung, H.T., Self-association between nano-sized bilayer and amphiphilic polymer, *J. Ind. Eng. Chem.,* 9, 45–50, 2003.

40. Ladaviere, C., Toustou, M., Gulik-Krzywicki, T., and Tribet, C., Slow reorganization of small phosphatidylcholine vesicles upon adsorption of amphiphilic polymers, *J. Coll. Interf. Sci.,* 241, 178–187, 2001.

41. Ladaviere, C., Tribet, C., and Cribier, S., Lateral organization of lipid membranes induced by amphiphilic polymer inclusions, *Langmuir,* 18, 7320–7327, 2002.

42. Luo, L. and Eisenberg, A., Thermodynamic stabilization mechanism of block copolymer vesicles, *J. Am. Chem. Soc.,* 123, 1012–1013, 2001.

43. Kostarelos, K., Tadros, T.F., and Luckham, P.F., Physical conjugation of (tri-) block copolymers to liposomes toward the construction of sterically stabilized vesicle systems, *Langmuir,* 15, 369–376, 1999.

44. Kostarelos, K., Luckham, P.F., and Tadros, T.F., Steric stabilization of phospholipid vesicles by block copolymers — Vesicle flocculation and osmotic swelling caused by monovalent and divalent cations, *J. Chem. Soc. Farad. Trans.,* 94, 2159–2168, 1998.

45. Zhang, L., Peng, T., Cheng, S.X., and Zhuo, R.X., Destabilization of liposomes by uncharged hydrophilic and amphiphilic polymers, *J. Phys. Chem. B,* 108, 7763–7770, 2004.

46. Scherphof, G., Roerdink, F., Waite, M., and Parks, J., Disintegration of phosphatidylcholine liposomes in plasma as a result of interaction with high density lipoproteins, *Biochim. Biophys. Acta,* 542, 296–307, 1978.

47. Caria, A., Regev, O., and Khan, A., Surfactant-polymer interactions: phase diagram and fusion of vesicle in the didodecyldimethylammonium bromide-poly(ethylene oxide)-water system, *J. Coll. Interf. Sci.,* 200, 19–30, 1998.

48. Robertson, D., Hellweg, T., Tiersch, B., and Koetz, J., Polymer-induced structural changes in lecithin/sodium dodecyl sulfate-based multilamellar vesicles, *J. Coll. Interf. Sci.,* 270, 187–194, 2004.

49. Kotz, J., Tiersch, B., and Bogen, I., Polyelectrolyte-induced vesicle formation in lamellar liquid-crystalline model systems, *Coll. Polymer Sci.,* 278, 164–168, 2000.

50. Huang, J.B., Zhu, Y., Zhu, B.Y., Li, R.K., and Fu, H.I., Spontaneous vesicle formation in aqueous mixtures of cationic surfactants and partially hydrolyzed polyacrylamide, *J. Coll. Interf. Sci.,* 236, 201–207, 2001.

51. Antunes, F.E., Marques, E.F., Gomes, R., Thuresson, K., Lindman, B., and Miguel, M.G., Network formation of catanionic vesicles and oppositely charged polyelectrolytes: effect of polymer charge density and hydrophobic modification, *Langmuir,* 20, 4647–4656, 2004.

52. Yu, K.H. and Eisenberg, A., Bilayer morphologies of self-assembled crew-cut aggregates of amphiphilic PS-b-PEO copolymers in solution, *Macromolecules,* 31, 3509–3518, 1998.

53. Du, J.Z. and Chen, Y.M., Preparation of organic/inorganic hybrid hollow particles based on gelation of polymer vesicles, *Macromolecules,* 37, 5710–5716, 2004.

54. Du, J.Z., Chen, Y.C., Zhang, Y., Han, C.C., Fishcer, K., and Schmidt, M., Organic/inorganic hybrid vesicles based on a reactive block copolymer, *J. Am. Chem. Soc.,* 125, 14710–14711, 2003.

55. Lin, J.J., Silas, J.A., Bermudez, H., Milam, V.T., Bates, F.S., and Hammer, D.A., The effect of polymer chain length and surface density on the adhesiveness of functionalized polymersomes, *Langmuir*, 20, 5493–5500, 2004.

56. Ahmed, F., Hategan, A., Discher, D.E., and Discher, B.M., Block copolymer assemblies with cross-link stabilization: From single-component monolayers to bilayer blends with PEO-PLA, *Langmuir*, 19, 6505–6511, 2003.

57. Bermudez, H., Aranda-Espinoza, H., Hammer, D.A., and Discher, D.E., Pore stability and dynamics in polymer membranes, *Europhys. Lett.*, 64, 550–556, 2003.

58. Napoli, A., Valentini, M., Tirelli, N., Muller, M., and Hubbell, J.A., Oxidation-responsive polymeric vesicles, *Nat. Mater.*, 3, 183–189, 2004.

59. Discher, B.M., Hammer, D.A., Bates, F.S., and Discher, D.E., Polymer vesicles in various media, *Curr. Opin. Coll. Interf. Sci.*, 5, 125–131, 2000.

60. Haluska, C.K., Gozdz, W.T., Dobereiner, H.G., Forster, S., and Gompper, G., Giant hexagonal super-structures in diblock-copolymer membranes, *Phys. Rev. Lett.*, 89, Art. No. 238302, 2002.

61. Dimova, R., Seifert, U., Pouligny, B., Forster, S., and Dobereiner, H.G., Hyperviscous diblock copolymer vesicles, *Eur. Phys. J. E*, 7, 241–250, 2002.

62. Lee, J.C.M., Bermudez, H., Discher, B.M., Sheehan, M.A., Won, Y.Y., Bates, F.S., and Discher, D.E., Preparation, stability, and in vitro performance of vesicles made with diblock copolymers, *Biotechnol. Bioeng.*, 73, 135–145, 2001.

63. Shen, H.W. and Eisenberg, A., Morphological phase diagram for a ternary system of block copolymer PS310-b-PAA(52)/dioxane/H_2O, *J. Phys. Chem.*, 103, 9473–9487, 1999.

64. Chen, L., Shen, H.W., and Eisenberg, A., Kinetics and mechanism of the rod-to-vesicle transition of block copolymer aggregates in dilute solution, *J. Phys. Chem. B*, 103, 9488–9497, 1999.

65. Brown, M.D., Schatzlein, A., Brownlie, A., Jack, V., Wang, W., Tetley, L., Gray, A.I., and Uchegbu, I.F., Preliminary characterization of novel amino acid based polymeric vesicles as gene and drug delivery agents, *Bioconjugate Chem.*, 11, 880–891, 2000.

66. Uchegbu, I.F., Tetley, L., and Wang, W., Nanoparticles and polymeric vesicles from new poly-L-lysine based amphiphiles, in *Biomaterials for Drug Delivery and Tissue Engineering*, Mallapragada, S. Tracy, M., Narasimhan, B., Mathiowitz, B., Korsmeyer, R., Eds. Materials Research Society, Pennsylvania, 2001, pp. NN6.8.1–NN6.8.6.

67. Ringsdorf, H., Schlarb, B., Tyminski, P.N., and O'Brien, D.F., Permeability characteristics of liposomes in a net-membranes of dihexadecyl phosphate with polymerizable gegenions, *Macromolecules*, 21, 671–677, 1988.

68. Chen, H.M. and Langer, R., Magnetically-responsive polymerized liposomes as potential oral delivery vehicles, *Pharm. Res.*, 14, 537–540, 1997.

69. Cho, I. and Chung, K.C., Cholesterol-containing polymeric vesicles — syntheses, characterization, and separation as a solid powder, *Macromolecules*, 21, 565–571, 1988.

70. Cho, I. and Kim, Y.D., Synthesis and properties of tocopherol-containing polymeric vesicle systems, *Macromol. Symp.*, 118, 631–640, 1997.

71. Murtagh, J. and Thomas, J.K., Mobility and reactivity in colloid aggregates with motion restricted by polymerization, *Faraday Discuss. Chem. Soc.*, 81, 127–136, 1986.

72. Hubert, D.H.W., Jung, M., and German, A.L., Vesicle templating, *Adv. Mater.*, 12, 1291–1294, 2000.

73. Jung, M., Hubert, D.H.W., Bomans, P.H.H., Frederik, P., van Herk, A.M., and German, A.L., A topology map for novel vesicle-polymer hybrid architectures, *Adv. Mater.*, 12, 210–213, 2000.

74. Jung, M., Hubert, D.H.W., van Herk, A.M., and German, A.L., The parachute morphology as equilibrium morphology of vesicle-polymer hybrids? *Macromol. Symp.*, 151, 393–398, 2000.

75. Jung, M., Hubert, D.H.W., van Veldhoven, E., Frederik, P., van Herk, A.M., and German, A.L., Vesicle-polymer hybrid architectures: A full account of the parachute architecture, *Langmuir*, 16, 3165–3174, 2000.

76. Jung, M., van Casteren, I., Monteiro, M.J., van Herk, A.M., and German, A.L., Pulsed-laser polymerization in compartmentalized liquids. 1. Polymerization in vesicles, *Macromolecules*, 33, 3620–3629, 2000.

77. Krafft, M.P., Schieldknecht, L., Marie, P., Giulieri, F., Schmutz, M., Poulain, N., and Nakache, E., Fluorinated vesicles allow intrabilayer polymerization of a hydrophobic monomer, yielding polymerized microcapsules, *Langmuir*, 17, 2872–2877, 2001.

78. McKelvey, C.A. and Kaler, E.W., Characterization of nanostructured hollow polymer spheres with small-angle neutron scattering (SANS), *J. Coll. Interf. Sci.,* 245, 68–74, 2002.

79. Hubert, D.H.W., Jung, M., Frederik, P.M., Bomans, P.H.H., Meuldijk, J., and German, A.L., Vesicle-directed growth of silica, *Adv. Mater.,* 12, 1286–1290, 2000.

80. Cho, I. and Kim, Y.D., Formation of stable polymeric vesicles by tocopherol-containing amphiphiles, *Macromol. Rapid Commun.,* 19, 27–30, 1998.

81. Bader, H. and Ringsdorf, H., Membrane-spanning symmetric and asymmetric diene amphiphiles, *Faraday Discuss. Chem. Soc.,* 81, 329–337, 1986.

82. Eaton, P.E., Jobe, P.G., and Kayson, N., Polymerised vesicles, *J. Am. Chem. Soc.,* 102, 6638–6640, 1980.

83. Stauch, O., Uhlmann, T., Frohlich, M., Thomann, R., El-Badry, M., Kim, Y.K., and Schubert, R., Mimicking a cytoskeleton by coupling poly(N-isopropylacrylamide) to the inner leaflet of liposomal membranes: effects of photopolymerization on vesicle shape and polymer architecture, *Biomacromolecules,* 3, 324–332, 2002.

84. Roks, M.F.M., Visser, H.G.J., Zwikker, J.W., Verkley, A.J., and Nolte, R.J.M., Polymerized vesicles derived from an isocyano amphiphile: electron microscope evidence of the polymerized state, *J. Am. Chem. Soc.,* 105, 4507–4510, 1983.

85. Fendler, J.H. and Tundo, P., Polymerised surfactant aggregates: characterization and utilization, *Acc. Chem. Res.,* 17, 3–8, 1984.

86. Samuel, N.K.P., Singh, M., Yamaguchi, K., and Regen, S.L., Polymerised-depolymerised vesicles: reversible thiol-disulphide-based phosphatidylcholine membranes, *J. Am. Chem. Soc.,* 107, 42–47, 1985.

87. Stauch, O., Schubert, R., Savin, G., and Burchard, W., Structure of artificial cytoskeleton containing liposomes in aqueous solution studied by static and dynamic light scattering, *Biomacromolecules,* 3, 565–578, 2002.

88. Unezaki, S., Maruyama, K., Ishida, O., Suginaka, A., Hosoda, J., and Iwatsuru, M., Enhanced tumor targeting and improved antitumor activity of doxorubicin by long-circulating liposomes containing amphipathic poly(ethylene glycol), *Int. J. Pharm.,* 126, 41–48, 1995.

89. Blume, G. and Cevc, G., Molecular mechanism of the lipid vesicle longevity in vivo, *Biochim. Biophys. Acta,* 1146, 157–168, 1993.

90. Yoshioka, H., Surface modification of haemoglobin-containing liposomes with poly(ethylene glycol) prevents liposome aggregation in blood plasma, *Biomaterials,* 12, 861–864, 1991.

91. Yuan, F., Dellian, M., Fukumura, D., Leunig, M., Berk, D.A., Torchilin, V.P., and Jain, R.K., Vascular permeability in a human tumor xenograft: molecular size dependence and cutoff size, *Cancer Res.,* 55, 3752–3756, 1995.

92. Gabizon, A., Isacson, R., Libson, E., Kaufman, B., Uziely, B., Catane, R., Bendor, C.G., Rabello, E., Cass, Y., Peretz, T., Sulkes, A., Chisin, R., and Barenholz, Y., Clinical-studies of liposome-encapsulated doxorubicin, *Acta Oncol.,* 33, 779–786, 1994.

93. Photos, P.J., Bacakova, L., Discher, B., Bates, F.S., and Discher, D.E., Polymer vesicles in vivo: correlations with PEG molecular weight, *J. Controlled Release,* 90, 323–334, 2003.

94. Blume, G., Cevc, G., Crommelin, M., Bakkerwoudenberg, I., Kluft, C., and Storm, G., Specific targeting with poly(ethylene glycol)-modified liposomes — coupling of homing devices to the ends of the polymeric chains combines effective target binding with long circulation times, *Biochim. Biophys. Acta,* 1149, 180–184, 1993.

95. Allen, T.M., Long-circulating (sterically stabilized) liposomes for targeted drug delivery, *Trend. Pharmacol. Sci.,* 15, 215–220, 1994.

96. Brown, M.D., Gray, A.I., Tetley, L., Santovena, A., Rene, J., Schatzlein, A.G., and Uchegbu, I.F., In vitro and in vivo gene transfer with polyamino acid vesicles, *J. Controlled Release,* 93, 193–211, 2003.

97. Dufes, C., Schatzlein, A.G., Tetley, L., Gray, A.I., Watson, D.G., Olivier, J.C., Couet, W., and Uchegbu, I.F., Niosomes and polymeric chitosan based vesicles bearing transferrin and glucose ligands for drug targeting, Pharm. Res., 17, 1250–1258, 2000.

98. Dufes, C., Muller, J.-M., Couet, W., Olivier, J.C., Uchegbu, I.F., and Schatzlein, A., Anticancer drug delivery with transferrin targeted polymeric chitosan vesicles, *Pharm. Res.,* 21, 101–107, 2004.

99. Roux, E., Francis, M., Winnik, F.M., and Leroux, J.C., Polymer based pH-sensitive carriers as a means to improve the cytoplasmic delivery of drugs, *Int. J. Pharm.,* 242, 25–36, 2002.

100. Needham, D., Mills, J., and Eichenbaum, G., Interactions between poly(2-ethylacrylic acid) and lipid bilayer membranes: effects of cholesterol and grafted poly(ethylene glycol), *Faraday Discuss,* 103–110, 1998.

101. You, H. and Tirrell, D.A., Photoinduced polyelectrolyte-driven release of contents of phosphatidyl-choline bilayer vesicles, *J. Am. Chem. Soc.,* 113, 4022–4023, 1991.

102. Maeda, M., Kumano, A., and Tirrell, D.A., H+-induced release of contents of phosphatidylcholine vesicles bearing surface bound polyelectrolyte chains, *J. Am. Chem. Soc.,* 110, 7455–7459, 1988.

103. Ringsdorf, H., Venzmer, J., and Winnik, F.M., Interaction of hydrophobically-modified poly-N-isopropylacrylamides with model membranes — or playing a molecular accordion, *Angew. Chem. Int. Ed. Engl.,* 30, 315–318, 1991.

104. Bagshawe, K.D., Sharma, S.K., Springer, C.J., Antoniw, P., Boden, J.A., Rogers, G.T., Burke, P.J., Melton, R.G., and Sherwood, R.F., Antibody directed enzyme prodrug therapy (ADEPT): clinical report, *Dis. Mark.,* 9, 233–238, 1991.

11 Polymer–Drug Conjugates

Vaikunth Cuchelkar and Jindřich Kopeček

CONTENTS

11.1 INTRODUCTION

Polymers have been extensively studied as drug delivery vehicles, especially for anticancer drugs. Such polymer–drug conjugates, broadly referred to as *macromolecular therapeutics*, afford therapeutic, pharmacokinetic, and pharmaceutical advantages in comparison to conventional low-molecular-weight therapeutics. A better understanding of the principles of polymeric drug delivery complemented with an increasing awareness of the systemic action of current therapeutics has spurred interest in developing polymeric delivery systems to increase drug efficacy and decrease unwanted drug effects. This chapter will discuss some basic principles and examples of polymeric delivery systems; it is hoped that this overview will stimulate the reader to further research this exciting field.

Conjugation of drugs to polymers was first attempted in 1955 when Jatzkewitz attached mescaline to poly(N-vinylpyrrolidone) using a dipeptide (glycyl-L-leucine) spacer [1] to develop a depot formulation for the hallucinogenic alkaloid. Ushakov's group synthesized numerous water-soluble polymer–drug conjugates in the 1960s and the 1970s [2,3]. In the 1970s, de Duve et al., discovered that macromolecules localize in the lysosome following their incubation with cells [4]. This information was used to formulate a rational design of polymeric–drug conjugates that are stable in the blood stream during circulation but could release the free drug specifically in the cells by the use of lysosomally degradable linkers. The first clear concept for the use of polymer–drug conjugates was presented by Ringsdorf in 1975 [5]. Since then numerous polymer–drug conjugates have been synthesized and evaluated for their efficacy.

In the 1980s, Matsumura and Maeda discovered that polymeric carriers localize preferentially in the tumor tissue [6]; this has made complexes of polymers and anticancer agents especially attractive. Enhancements involving the use of tissue-targeting moieties and peptide transduction domains have been developed more recently to further increase the efficacy of these conjugates. It must be mentioned that polymeric delivery systems may be used in conjunction with other classes of drugs. However, the advantage of developing such conjugates is limited, for example, to increasing the circulating half-life; whereas in the case of anticancer agents, conjugation with polymers increases their specificity for tumor tissue, reduces their systemic toxicity, and increases their circulating half-life.

11.2 POLYMERS WITH INTRINSIC ACTIVITY

Certain polymers of natural origin demonstrate intrinsic biological activity; synthetic polymers have also been developed mimicking these natural polymers. The result is the emergence of polymeric drugs (polymers that demonstrate biological activity) as a rapidly developing class of therapeutics with significant clinical applications (Table 11.1). These polymeric drugs are not the focus of this chapter; details can be found elsewhere [7–21].

TABLE 11.1
Polymers with Intrinsic Activity

Polymer	Activity	References
Dextrin-2-sulfate	Antiviral (including HIV) effect; antiangiogenic effect	7–9
COPAXONE ® (a random copolymer of L-alanine, L-lysine, L-glutamic acid and L-tyrosine)	Minimizes autoimmune response to myelin basic protein (MBP); slows the progression and the frequency of relapse in multiple sclerosis (MS)	10–13
Poly(allylamines)	Sequesters phosphorus in the serum and reduce serum phophorus levels, which are elevated in end stage renal disease	14–17
DEAE-dextran (Diethylaminoethyl-dextran)	Activity *in vivo* against NJA leukemia, JBI ascites, plasmocytoma in mice, and Yoshida ascites in rats	18–20
Poly(Arg-Gly-Asp)	Inhibits formation of lung metastasis and migration of B16-BL6 melanoma in mice	21

11.3 BIOLOGICAL RATIONALE

Current low-molecular-weight anticancer agents are hydrophobic agents that enter the cell by diffusion and subsequently distribute to all the subcellular compartments. In contrast, soluble polymers are limited in the mode of entry to endocytosis [4]. Endocytosis in the case of soluble macromolecules can occur by three different mechanisms: (1) fluid-phase endocytosis (also known as bulk-fluid endocytosis), (2) adsorptive endocytosis, and (3) receptor-mediated endocytosis (Figure 11.1). The essential features of the three processes are enumerated in Table 11.2.

Receptor-mediated endocytosis involves the interaction of macromolecules with specific cells bearing the relevant recognition moieties. Hence, this mechanism enhances distribution to specific body compartments, consequently affecting the biodistribution.

11.3.1 Manipulation of Subcellular Fate of Polymer–Drug Conjugates by Use of Appropriate Spacers Linking the Drug and Polymer

Following internalization, macromolecules are localized in the lysosomal compartment. However, the lysosomal membrane is not permeable to macromolecules [29], and the polymer–drug conjugates cannot cross into the surrounding cytoplasm. Incorporation of linkers degradable in the lysosomal environment can allow for release of free drug and subsequent drug redistribution in the cell. Linkers that could be used include pH-sensitive linkers, disulfide bonds, and lysosomal enzyme-sensitive linkers.

Acid-labile linkers that are rapidly hydrolyzed at the acidic pH in the lysosomal and prelysosomal compartments, such as hydrazone linkages [30] and *cis*-aconityl spacers [31], demonstrate decreased intravascular stability as the pH in the blood is only two units higher than that in the lysosomes. Disulfide bonds [32] linking the drug to the polymer are relatively nonspecifically degraded in the bloodstream and at the level of the cell membrane. Nonspecific release of the free drug results in the development of side effects.

The lysosome contains enzymes of several different classes (e.g., nucleases, proteases, lipases, and phosphatases). Drugs can be attached to polymer backbones by enzymatically degradable spacers [33], for example, oligopeptide sequences. These linkers are stable in circulation and can be specifically cleaved in the lysosome releasing the free drug. Such polymer-drug conjugates combine the advantages of higher efficacy (as free drug is more efficacious than the polymer-bound drug) and intravascular stability with relative specificity for tumor tissue because of the enhanced permeability and retention effect afforded by polymer–drug conjugates (as described in Section 11.4). Detailed studies with various oligopeptide spacers have been performed to determine optimal linker sequences [34]. The linker glycylphenylalanylleucylglycyl (GFLG), which is susceptible to lysosomal cathepsin B (a cysteine protease) [35], is stable in the bloodstream [36] and is commonly used for the synthesis of polymer–drug conjugates.

11.4 ADVANTAGES OF POLYMER–DRUG CONJUGATES

Polymer–drug conjugates afford several advantages over the free drug (Figure 11.2):

1. Enhanced permeability and retention effect: Current anticancer agents are mainly low-molecular-weight chemicals that redistribute to all the tissues of the body following intravenous administration. The subsequent cytotoxic action manifested all over the body results in the majority of toxic side effects produced by chemotherapeutic regimens. Polymeric delivery systems modify the biodistribution of drugs and localize them to the tumor due to anatomical and physiological differences between normal and tumor tissue (Figure 11.3). Tumor morphology is characterized by the presence of a very permeable microvasculature. Secretion of various biologically active molecules [37–39] increases the vascular permeability in tumor tissue (Table 11.3). In addition, the lymphatics draining

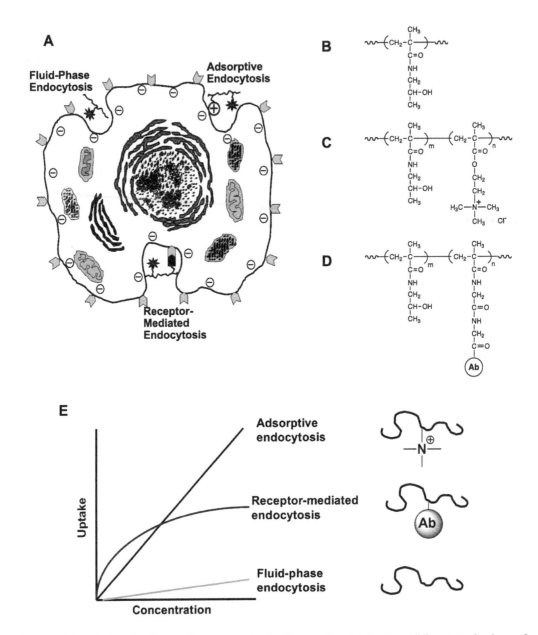

FIGURE 11.1 Modes of cell entry for macromolecular therapeutics: (a) the three different mechanisms of endocytosis possible in the case of tumor cells. Structures of polymers that can be internalized by these mechanisms — fluid-phase endocytosis, adsorptive endocytosis, and receptor-mediated endocytosis are shown; (b) poly(HPMA) is internalized by fluid-phase endocytosis, because it does not interact with cell membrane structures and is completely dissolved in the interstitial fluid; (c) a copolymer of HPMA and methacryloyloxyethyltrimethylammonium chloride will be internalized by adsorptive endocytosis. The copolymer is positively charged at physiological pH and adsorbs to the cell membrane (which is negatively charged because of the action of the Na^+–K^+ ATPase pump); (d) an HPMA copolymer that bears a pendant antibody which will bind a receptor on the cell surface (for example, OV-TL16, which binds the OA3 antigen overexpressed on the surface of ovarian carcinoma cells) will be internalized by receptor-mediated endocytosis; (e) the relative amounts of polymers endocytosed via the three methods. Fluid-phase endocytosis results in a slow rate of internalization. Both adsorptive and receptor-mediated endocytosis proceed at a faster rate; however, receptor-mediated endocytosis shows saturation at higher concentrations of the macromolecule (as there are a limited number of receptors or antigens on the cell surface).

TABLE 11.2
Mechanisms of Endocytosis

	Fluid-Phase Endocytosis	Adsorptive Endocytosis	Receptor-Mediated Endocytosis
Interactions with the Cell Surface	No interaction between the macromolecule and the cell surface	Macromolecules are adsorbed nonspecifically to the cell surface	Macromolecules are bound specifically to the cell surface
Occurrence	Macromolecules are dissolved in liquid surrounding the cells	Macromolecules adsorb to the cell surface because of hydrophobic interactions [22] or charge interactions [23] (positively charged molecules with a negatively charged membrane)	Macromolecules attach to the cell surface because of binding of moieties specific to cell surface molecules [24] (receptors or antigens) and initiate endocytotic processes
Rate of Internalization	Dependent on concentration in extracellular fluid, therefore, generally regarded as a slower method of internalization	Following adsorption, the increased local concentration translates into an increased rate of internalization as compared to fluid phase endocytosis	Binding initiates endocytosis, resulting in an increased rate of internalization as compared to fluid phase endocytosis
Example	Polymer consisting of HPMA [25] (Figure 11.1b)	HPMA-based polymer-bearing pendant positively charged moieties [23] (Figure 11.1c)	HPMA-based polymer-bearing moieties specific for cell surface receptors which internalize following complex formation [26–28] (Figure 11.1d)

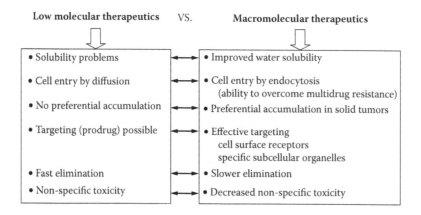

FIGURE 11.2 Comparison of low-molecular-weight therapeutics with macromolecular therapeutics.

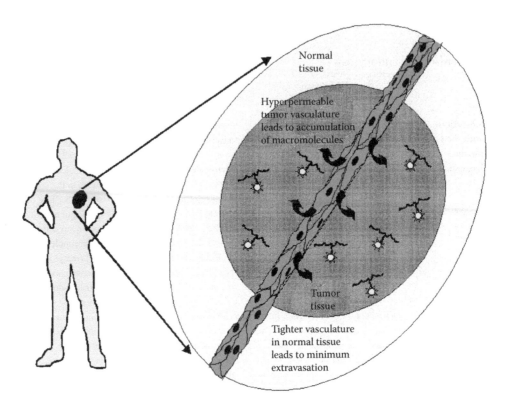

FIGURE 11.3 Enhanced permeability and retention effect. Tumor morphology is characterized by an enhanced permeability (due to various bioactive molecules) resulting in the permeation and trapping of macromolecular therapeutics in tumor tissue. This, when combined with decreased lymphatic drainage, contributes to high local concentrations of the polymer–drug conjugate in the tumor interstitium.

the tumor tissue are usually blocked, resulting in poor tissue drainage. The combination of deficient lymphatic drainage with increased vascular permeability and lack of lymphatic capillaries results in a pooling of high-molecular-weight agents in the tumor tissue [6,37] — a phenomenon called the *enhanced permeability and retention* (EPR) effect. Other factors that influence the EPR effect include the presence of an increased vascular density with defective smooth muscle cells [45,46] lacking autoregulatory mechanisms [39]. The EPR effect results in preferential localization of macromolecular therapeutics in tumor tissue and, consequently, decreased drug accumulation in other tissues. This translates into an increase in the specificity of the therapeutic agent and diminished side effects.

2. Renal elimination is size (and therefore molecular weight) dependent. Polymers and macromolecular therapeutics are excreted slower from the body and have a longer

TABLE 11.3
Biologically Active Molecules Involved in the EPR Effect

Factor	References
Vascular endothelial growth factor (VEGF) (vascular permeability factor)	38
Nitric oxide (NO)	40–42
Peroxynitrite (ONOO⁻)	41,42
Prostaglandins	39
TNF-α, IFN-γ, and bradykinin	43,44

circulating half-life. An increase in the molecular weight (and hence the hydrodynamic volume) of the macromolecular therapeutic reduces its rate of excretion, thereby prolonging its duration of action [47–49].

3. Polymers can sterically shield high-molecular-weight compounds such as antibodies from the antigen-presenting cells (APCs), which initiate the immune response and reduce the immunogenicity of immunogenic drugs [50].

4. Hydrophilic polymer backbones can increase the solubility of hydrophobic drugs and make them convenient for intravenous administration.

5. Polymers afford the facile attachment of targeting moieties [51].

6. Low-molecular-weight anticancer drugs that enter the cell by diffusion are exposed to cell membrane efflux pumps for example, the P-glycoprotein efflux pump [52]. Macromolecular therapeutics internalize via endocytotic mechanisms and localize in membrane-bound organelles. The exclusion of the drugs from the cytoplasm renders the efflux pumps ineffective. Polymeric drug conjugates thus bypass some of the common mechanisms of multidrug resistance [53]. In addition, higher amounts of energy are required to extrude macromolecular drug conjugates from the cell as compared to low-molecular-weight agents.

7. Following exposure to low-molecular-weight drugs, the concentration gradient that gets established decreases from the cell membrane to the nucleus (which is often the most susceptible subcellular compartment). As lysosomes are located in the perinuclear region, a higher nuclear concentration exists following release of the drug from the polymer [27,28], thereby translating into an enhanced therapeutic effect.

11.5 POLYMERIC DRUG CARRIERS

Fundamental requirements of polymeric drug carriers are listed in Table 11.4. Both natural and synthetic polymers can be used as carriers for drugs. Biodegradable polymeric drug carriers have been traditionally designed from natural polymers, such as polysaccharides and poly(amino acids), in the hope that natural catabolic processes will act to break down the macromolecules to smaller fragments that can be easily eliminated [54]. However, substitution of drugs along the polymeric carrier may prevent formation of enzyme–substrate complexes and result in the inability of a normally biodegradable macromolecule to be degraded into easily eliminated fragments [54,55]. In addition, degradation of drug-modified macromolecules, such as poly(amino acids) [56] or polysaccharides [57], may yield fragments that cannot penetrate the lysosomal membrane. Consequently, polymer–drug conjugates using naturally occurring polymers are usually considered nonbiodegradable [58].

Synthetic macromolecules may be preferred as drug carriers because they can be tailor-made to have properties matching the requirements of the biological situation. Synthetic chemistry can be used to obtain polymers having specific three-dimensional structures with defined compositions

---

TABLE 11.4
Requirements for Polymeric Drug Carriers

(1) Well characterized.

(2) Hydrophilic for intravenous drug delivery.

(3) Biocompatible (nontoxic and nonimmunogenic). Metabolic products generated from the parent polymers must also be biocompatible.

(4) Functionality to allow conjugation of the drug in sufficient amounts.

(5) Allow for drug linkage, which is stable in circulation.

(6) Result in a construct that allows convenient administration.

(7) Eliminated from the body once they have performed their function or metabolized to smaller fragments that are below the renal threshold and are subsequently eliminated.

and specific orientations of functional groups for precise drug conjugation [59]. Polymer–drug conjugates using synthetic polymers as backbones are usually nondegradable. Synthetic polymers have a molecular weight distribution (as compared to natural polymers that have fixed molecular weights), and hence complete elimination via renal processes requires synthetic polymers to have their entire molecular weight distribution under the renal threshold. Newer methods of synthesis broadly termed as *controlled/living radical polymerization* (LRP) methods (for example, *reversible addition fragmentation transfer* [RAFT] [60,61] and *atom transfer radical polymerization* (ATRP) [62,63]) can enable the synthesis of macromolecules with a better control of molecular weight and polydispersity.

11.6 FACTORS AFFECTING THE BIODISTRIBUTION OF POLYMER–DRUG CONJUGATES

Several factors affect the biodistribution of polymer conjugates, the major ones being hydrodynamic volume, polymer conformation and flexibility, effective charge on the polymer, and hydrophobicity. The *hydrodynamic volume* (of a polymer) is defined as the volume of a hydrodynamically equivalent sphere [64] and is intimately related to the molecular weight of the polymer. Macromolecules with a size below the renal threshold may be completely eliminated from the body by glomerular filtration, resulting in low circulating half-lives. The higher the molecular weight of the polymer, the higher is the retention time in the body [47–49]; increased circulation time allows for macromolecular accumulation in the tumor interstitium by the EPR effect and generates an enhanced therapeutic effect.

The shape and flexibility of the polymer–drug conjugate influence its penetration into the interstitial tissue and its reabsorption from the renal tubular epithelium, thereby affecting the relative biodistribution [54]. Negatively charged molecules can activate coagulation and stimulate cytokine release from cells of the immune system [59]. On the other hand, positively charged molecules can cause hemolysis and activate the complement cascade [59]. Activation of the complement cascade may subsequently initiate the coagulation and immune pathways. Positively charged conjugates also undergo adsorptive endocytosis (as mentioned in Section 11.3), thereby increasing uptake. Adsorptive endocytosis can also be achieved by increasing the hydrophobicity of polymer–drug conjugates.

High-molecular-weight polymer–drug conjugates can be designed by incorporating biodegradable linkers (susceptible to tumor enzymes) cross-linking polymer chains. Such conjugates demonstrate long circulating times [65,66] and are degraded to easily eliminated low-molecular-weight chains in the tumor interstitium. This approach combines the advantages of increased half-lives and high tumor accumulation with the possibility for easy elimination [66].

11.7 DRUG ATTACHMENT MODIFIES THE PROPERTIES OF POLYMERS

The behavior of macromolecules usually changes after the addition of a drug to the polymer backbone. At high substituent concentrations, hydrophobic moieties (for example, drug molecules) attached to a hydrophilic polymer may aggregate to form micelles with the hydrophilic polymer chains on the outside. Formation of micelles may affect the biodistribution and the efficacy of the polymeric conjugate. For example, such aggregates may not be able to move freely between body compartments. In addition, the increase in hydrodynamic volume may result in an increased intravascular half-life. Drug release from the macromolecular aggregates is also impaired.

Drugs may act as haptens [51] and activate the antigen-presenting cells (APCs), resulting in an immune response following substitution on the polymeric carriers (which may be nonimmunogenic in their native form). Incorporation of targeting moieties, especially antibodies, influences the biodistribution of the polymer–drug conjugate. Attachment of antibodies dramatically increases the molecular weight. Such conjugates achieve relatively higher concentrations in certain body compartments because of biorecognition. Furthermore, antibodies may induce an immune response and result in the uptake of such conjugates by the reticuloendothelial system (RES).

It is thus obvious that the properties and biodistribution of polymer–drug conjugates may be entirely different from that of native polymers. This necessitates the verification of biocompatibility and determination of biodistribution with the actual therapeutic agent. The influence of attachment of drugs and targeting moieties need to be taken into consideration when designing polymer–drug conjugates.

11.8 ENHANCING THE EFFICACY OF POLYMER–DRUG CONJUGATES

Passive localization of polymer–drug conjugates in tumor tissue by the EPR effect is nonselective and hence nonspecific. Furthermore, as internalization occurs through the natural endocytotic process, the rate of internalization (and therefore the intracellular concentration) is dependent on the rate of endocytosis and the interstitial drug concentration. These factors impose limitations on maximum intracellular drug concentrations. Hence, strategies need to be evolved to obtain optimal therapeutic effects while limiting potential side effects. Such modifications include the enhancement of intracellular drug concentrations by the incorporation of specific cellular targeting moieties, the use of protein transduction domains to enhance internalization, subcellular targeting to increase the efficacy of polymer–drug conjugates, and polymer-directed enzyme prodrug therapy (PDEPT), which increases the efficacy and specificity afforded by polymer–drug conjugates.

11.8.1 Tumor Targeting by Active-Targeting Mechanisms

Use of targeting moieties (complementary to molecules on the surface of the cell) (Table 11.5) can increase the specificity of polymeric conjugates for tumor tissue. Incorporation of targeting moieties results in cell surface binding with a concurrent increase in the local concentration. This enhances the amount of the polymeric conjugate being internalized. In certain cases, specific targeting moieties can induce receptor-mediated endocytosis, further increasing the rate of uptake and enhancing the intracellular concentration (as compared to fluid-phase or adsorptive endocytosis).

A design for an HPMA (N-(2-hydroxypropyl)methacrylamide) copolymer-based targetable polymeric delivery system is shown in Figure 11.4. HPMA copolymers are biocompatible, nonimmunogenic, and increase the solubility for hydrophobic drugs; they are commonly used as carriers for hydrophobic anticancer drugs. The features of an ideal targeting antigen are enlisted in Table 11.6.

The rate of uptake of polymer–drug conjugates can be increased by the incorporation of two or more types of targeting moieties (specific to different types of cellular recognition moieties). Such polyvalent interactions are collectively stronger than monovalent interactions [84]. In addition, use of different types of targeting moieties serves to enhance the specificity.

TABLE 11.5
Cellular Recognition Moieties That Can Be Used in Targetable Polymeric Delivery Systems

Target	Type of Moiety	Example	References
Cell-specific antigens	Antibodies (for example, OV-TL16 antibody)	OA-3 antigen overexpressed on ovarian carcinoma cells (in the case of OV-TL16 antibody)	27,67
Vitamin receptors	Vitamins or analogs	Folate-binding receptor	68,69
		Transferrin receptor	70,71
Cell-efflux pumps	Antibodies	P-glycoprotein pumps	72
Hormone receptors	Hormones or analogs	Insulin receptor	73,74
Growth-factor receptors	Proteins	VEGF receptor	75
		FGF-2 receptor	76
		EGF receptor	77–81
Cell-surface receptors	Modified sugars	asialoglycoprotein receptors in hepatoma cells	82,83

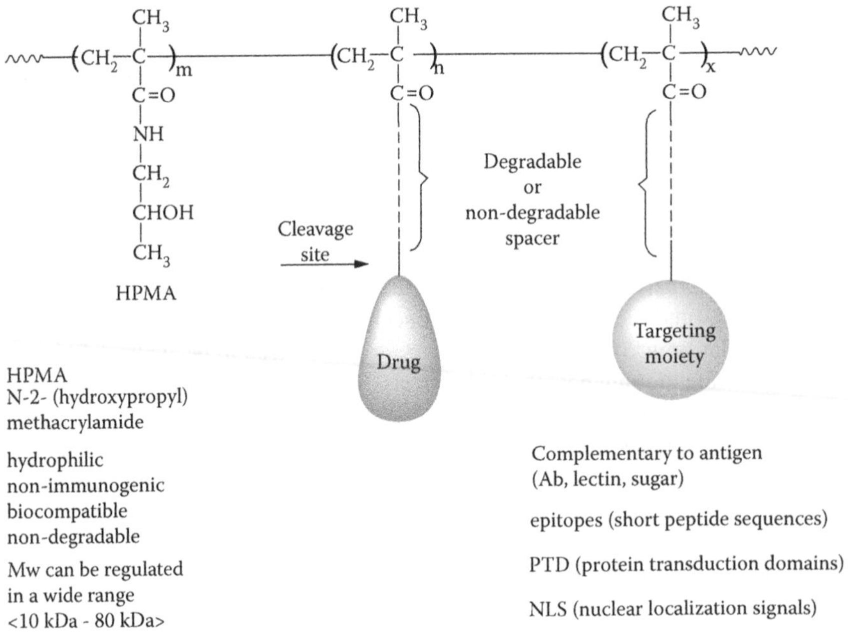

FIGURE 11.4 Design of a targetable drug delivery system using an HPMA backbone. The drug is linked to the polymeric backbone by a spacer that may or may not be biodegradable (to allow for the release of free drug). The choice of spacer is dictated by the requirements in each individual situation. The cellular targeting moiety is usually attached at a different point on the polymer backbone. HPMA as a polymer is hydrophilic, biocompatible, nonimmunogenic, and allows for regulation of molecular weight.

11.8.2 Subcellular Targeting

Drugs exert their action at specific subcellular sites depending on their mechanism of action. Directing drugs to these subcellular compartments can increase their local concentration and enhance the therapeutic effect almost exponentially; for example, photosensitizers demonstrate higher efficacy when they are directed to the nucleus or the mitochondria. Targeting these compartments requires smaller amounts of drug to achieve the same therapeutic effect. Subcellular targeting can be achieved by attaching specific localization sequences to the polymeric drug conjugate (Table 11.7).

11.8.3 Use of Protein Transduction Domains

Protein transduction domains (PTDs) (also referred to as cell-penetrating peptides) are known to translocate across the cell membrane into the cytoplasm in an energy-independent manner. Some examples

---

TABLE 11.6
Features of an Ideal Targeting Antigen

(1) Uniquely present on tumor cells resulting in a preferential attachment of the macromolecular conjugate, with reduced effects on noncancerous cells; this is referred to as the "binding site barrier."

(2) Present universally and stably on all tumor cells; for example, receptors necessary for cell proliferation or other vital functions.

(3) Induces receptor-mediated endocytosis of the conjugate; this results in a higher intracellular concentration.

TABLE 11.7
Specific Subcellular-Targeting Sequences

Organelle Targeted	Signal Sequence	References
Nucleus–monopartite	PPKKKRKV	85,86
	VSRKRPR	87
	GKKRSKV	88
	KSRKRKL	89
Nucleus–bipartite	KRPAATKKAGQAKKKKLDK	90
	RKKRKTEEESPLKDKAKKSK	91
	KKYENVVIKRSPRKRGRPRK	92
Peroxisomes	SKL–(C terminal)	93
	(N terminal)–MHRLQVVLGHL	94
Golgi apparatus	KTKKL–(C terminal)	95
Endoplasmic	KKSL–(C terminal)	96
reticulum	KPRRE–(C terminal)	97
Mitochondria	MLSLRQSIRFFK	98
	MSSESGKPIAKPIRKPGYTNPALKALG	99
Lysosome	KFERQ	100,101

of PTDs include the drosophila homeotic transcription factor antp, transcription factor VP22 from Herpes simplex virus type-1, and HIV-1 transactivating factor Tat protein.

Shorter sequences of the Tat protein, for example, the Tat peptide, (Y_{47}GRKKRRQRRR$_{57}$) have been shown to be effective in mediating transport across the cell membrane. PTDs have been successfully employed as vectors for cytoplasmic and nuclear macromolecular transport. The exact import mechanism remains to be determined in a large number of PTDs. Some examples in which PTDs have been used to transport molecules across biological barriers are mentioned in Table 11.8.

11.8.4 PDEPT

PDEPT is a new paradigm in polymeric delivery of drugs to anticancer tissue developed by Satchi-Fainaro and Duncan [111,112]. This strategy is a modification of ADEPT (antibody-directed enzyme prodrug therapy) [113], which uses a tumor-selective antibody conjugated to an enzyme. In ADEPT, antibody–enzyme conjugates are administered to the patient (usually intravenously) and allowed to localize at the tumor site. The antibody ensures the selective localization of the enzyme at the

TABLE 11.8
Protein Transduction Domains Used for Transporting Cargo Across the Cytoplasmic Membrane

Protein Transduction Domain	Cargo	References
Tat peptide (Y_{47}GRKKRRQRRR$_{57}$)	β-galactosidase	102
	Liposomes (200 nm)	103–105
	Chelates of technetium-99m and rhenium	106
	2-O-methyl phosphorothioate antisense oligonucleotides	107
	Poly[N-(2-hydroxypropyl)methacrylamide]	108
antp	2-O-methyl phosphorothioate antisense oligonucleotides	107
VP22	Green fluorescent protein	109
	Plasmid	110

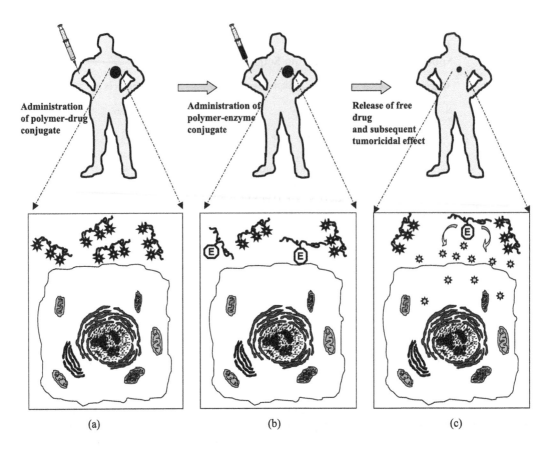

FIGURE 11.5 Strategy of PDEPT: (a) PDEPT involves the administration of a polymer–drug conjugate containing an enzymatically degradable spacer, (b) after allowing for the accumulation of the therapeutic in the tumor, a polymer–enzyme conjugate is administered, (c) the enzyme chosen specifically cleaves the linker connecting the drug to the polymer. Free drug then acts to reduce tumor bulk.

tumor site. Following the clearance of the conjugate from the blood, a prodrug of a cytotoxic agent is then administered to the patient. The enzyme converts the prodrug into its active form and kills the tumor cells selectively with reduced systemic side effects. An essential feature of this approach involves the selection of the prodrug that can be selectively activated by the enzyme.

PDEPT involves the administration of a polymer–drug conjugate containing an enzymatically degradable spacer. After allowing for the accumulation of the therapeutic in the tumor, a polymer–enzyme conjugate is administered (Figure 11.5). The enzyme chosen specifically cleaves the linker connecting the drug to the polymer, releasing the free drug. For example, an HPMA copolymer linked to Doxorubicin, using a GFLG spacer, can be followed by the administration of a HPMA copolymer-bound cathepsin B [111]. The polymer-bound cathepsin B will degrade the GFLG spacer, releasing free Doxorubicin in the vicinity of the tumor cells.

The polymer–enzyme conjugates used in PDEPT are less immunogenic [114] as compared to the antibody–enzyme conjugates [115] used in ADEPT. The administration of a polymeric drug followed by the administration of the activating enzyme as a polymeric conjugate in PDEPT may prevent premature release of the drug [111], thereby increasing the specificity and reducing systemic side effects.

11.9 SYNTHETIC PROCEDURES

Generally, macromolecule–drug conjugates can be synthesized using two methods — polymer-analogous reactions or copolymerization of polymeric precursors.

11.9.1 POLYMER-ANALOGOUS REACTIONS

This involves the attachment of a drug to a preformed polymeric carrier. A prerequisite of this approach is the matching of the reactive groups on the polymer backbone and the drug. Polymer backbones can be synthesized with reactive end groups on side chains that are complementary to functional groups on the drug molecule. The polymer can then be reacted with the drug and result in the formation of a polymer–drug conjugate. The free drug can be removed by dialysis or size exclusion chromatography (SEC). For example, a polymer-bearing reactive *p*-nitrophenol ester end group at side-chain termini can be synthesized, followed by a reaction with the drug bearing a reactive amino group, to synthesize polymer–drug conjugates. It may be essential to modify the reactive groups (either on the drug or polymer side chains) to enable the reaction to proceed in certain cases.

As an example, we will consider the synthesis of doxorubicin (DOX) bound to an HPMA copolymer backbone via a biodegradable GFLG (glycylphenylalanylleucylglycyl) spacer. The conjugate (P-GFLG-DOX, where P is the HPMA copolymer backbone) can be prepared using polymer-analogous techniques in a two-step method–the first step involves the synthesis of a copolymer of HPMA and MA-GFLG-ONp (*N*-methacryloylglycylphenylalanylleucylglycine *p*-nitrophenyl ester) to form a polymer precursor [116]. Details of the synthesis of HPMA and MA-GFLG-ONp can be found elsewhere [116]. Doxorubicin is reacted with the polymer precursor in the next step to synthesize the desired polymeric delivery system [116] (Figure 11.6).

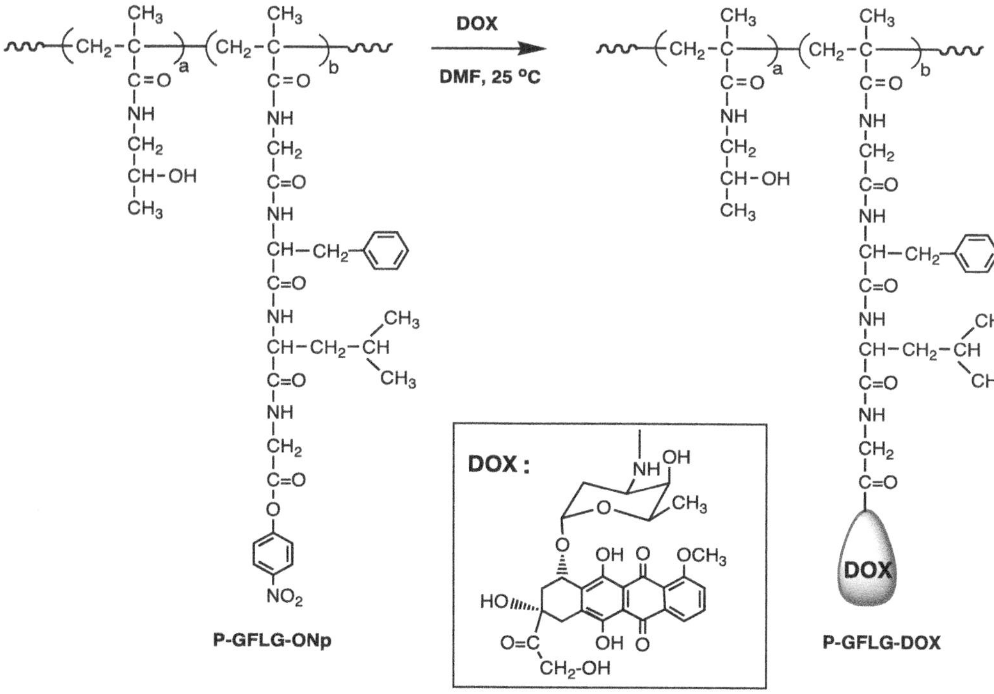

FIGURE 11.6 Polymer-analogous reaction for the synthesis of Doxorubicin bound to HPMA copolymer via a biodegradable GFLG spacer. P-GFLG-ONp (Poly[HPMA-*co*-(MA-GFLG-ONp)]), a copolymer of HPMA (*N*-(2-hydroxypropyl)methacrylamide) and MA-GFLG-ONp (*N*-methacryloylglycylphenylalanylleucylglycine *p*-nitrophenyl ester), is reacted with Doxorubicin to form P-GFLG-DOX. The chemical reaction involved is the aminolysis of reactive *p*-nitrophenyl ester groups by amino groups of Doxorubicin.

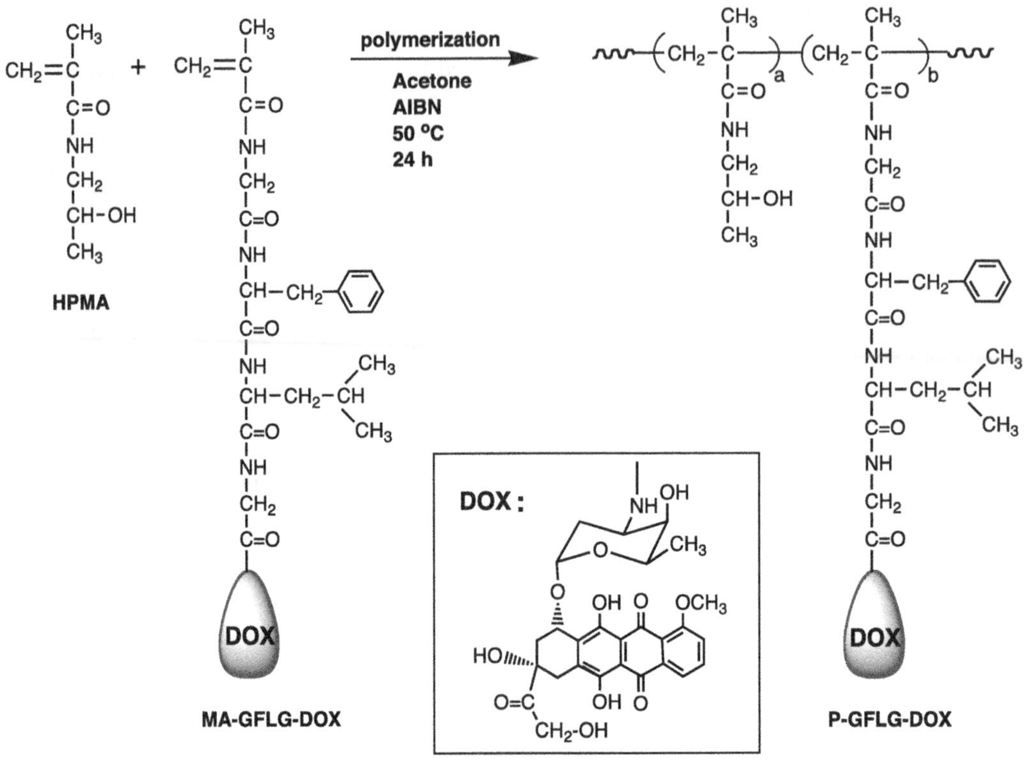

FIGURE 11.7 Copolymerization of HPMA and MA-GFLG-DOX to synthesize HPMA copolymer-based delivery system for Doxorubicin. The reaction is performed by the copolymerization of HPMA (*N*-(2-hydroxypropyl)methacrylamide) and MA-GFLG-Doxorubicin to form P-GFLG-DOX (Poly[HPMA-*co*-(MA-GFLG-DOX)]). The reaction is performed using 2,2-azobisisobutyronitrile (AIBN) as initiator and acetone as solvent at 50°C.

11.9.2 COPOLYMERIZATION OF POLYMERIZABLE DRUG DERIVATIVES WITH MONOMERS

An essential feature in this approach involves the synthesis of a polymerizable drug derivative by reacting the drug with a polymerizable molecule (monomer). This derivative can be purified and then polymerized with suitable monomers to form the polymer–drug conjugate. An advantage of this approach is the avoidance of some side reactions that occur during polymer-analogous reactions.

The polymeric drug conjugate (P-GFLG-DOX) can be synthesized by the copolymerization of HPMA with MA-GFLG-DOX (Figure 11.7). MA-GFLG-DOX is synthesized by reacting MA-GFLG-ONp with Doxorubicin as described in Reference 116.

Notice that both the synthetic methods (polymer-analogous reactions and copolymerization of polymeric precursors) can yield similar polymer–drug conjugates as in the case of P-GFLG-DOX. The method of synthesis selected depends on the individual requirements in each case.

11.9.3 ATTACHMENT OF TARGETING MOIETIES

Incorporation of targeting moieties in the structure of the polymer–drug conjugate can also be done using strategies similar to polymer-analogous or copolymerization reactions. Polymer–drug conjugates

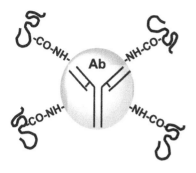

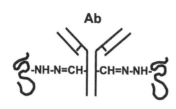

Type 1
Random attachment
by **amide** linkage

Type 2
Site-specific attachment
by **hydrazone linkage**
(via sugar chains near
the hinge region)

Type 3
Site-specific attachment
by **thioether linkage**
(via sulfhydryl group
generated in Fab')

FIGURE 11.8 Synthesis of antibody-targeted polymeric drug conjugates. Three different schemes are shown for the attachment of antibodies (or their fragments) to polymer backbones: (1) aminolysis of reactive esters on side-chain termini of polymers with surface amino groups on antibodies, (2) hydrazone linkages between reactive hydrazide residues on polymers with aldehyde groups on oxidized antibodies, and (3) thioether linkages between sulfhydryl groups on Fab fragments with maleimido groups on side-chain termini of polymers. (From Omelyanenko, V. et al., HPMA copolymer-anticancer drug-OV-TL16 antibody conjugates. 1. Influence of the method of synthesis on the binding affinity to OVCAR-3 ovarian carcinoma cells in vitro, *J. Drug Target.*, 3(5), 357, 1996.)

can be synthesized with pendant reactive groups on side-chain termini. Reactive groups are selected such that they can specifically bind the targeting moiety. For example, antibodies can be attached to polymer backbones using three different methods (Figure 11.8). Antibodies have accessible surface amino groups (predominantly ε-amino groups of lysine residues), and hence binding to polymer backbones can be performed via amide bonds formed by aminolysis of active ester groups on polymer side chains [67]. Another technique involves binding the antibody via hydrazone linkages formed by the reaction of aldehyde groups (generated by the oxidation of the saccharide moieties located near the hinge region) on the oxidized antibody with hydrazide reactive groups on side chains of the polymers [67]. Antibody binding may also be performed via thioether bonds formed by reacting sulfhydryl groups of Fab' fragments (of antibodies) with maleimide groups on side-chain termini of polymers [67]. A disadvantage of the aminolysis method lies in the possibility of attachment of multiple copolymer chains to the antibody molecule; this may restrict the flexibility of antibodies and affect biorecognition. The other techniques (via hydrazone or thioether bonds) may cause minor modifications to antibody structure and afford better control over biological activity.

Another strategy to synthesize antibody-targeted conjugates is to synthesize a polymerizable derivative of an antibody or its Fab' fragment [117,118]. These derivatives can be synthesized by the reaction of the antibody or its Fab' fragment with a polymerizable monomer, using chemistries similar to those mentioned in the previous section. Incorporation of these derivatives in polymerization reactions can yield targeted constructs. Care must be taken to perform these polymerization reactions under mild conditions to avoid denaturation of antibodies.

11.10 EXAMPLES OF SOME *N*-(2-HYDROXYPROPYL)METHACRYLAMIDE COPOLYMER–DRUG CONJUGATES

We will consider two polymeric drug conjugates based on poly(*N*-(2-hydroxypropyl)methacrylamide) in order to illustrate some of the features and enhancements that could be incorporated in the design of a polymeric delivery system. Experiments proving the efficacy of polymer–drug conjugates for the delivery of anticancer agents have been performed *in vivo*; some of these

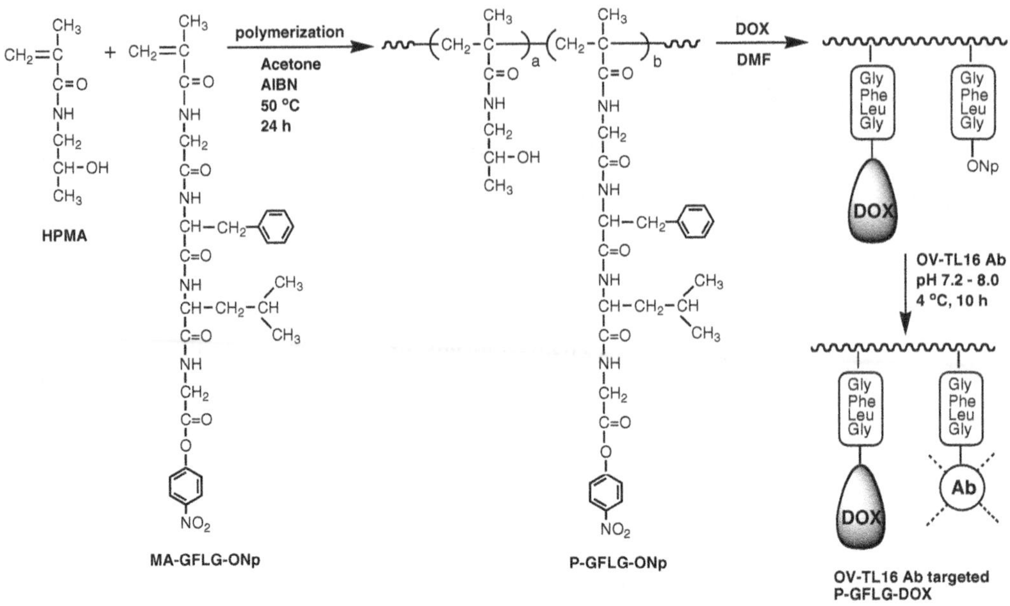

FIGURE 11.9 Synthetic scheme for the OV-TL16-targeted HPMA copolymer-based polymeric delivery system for Doxorubicin. The first step involves the polymerization of HPMA (*N*-(2-hydroxypropyl)methacrylamide) and MA-GFLG-ONp (*N*-methacryloylglycylphenylalanylleucylglycine *p*-nitrophenyl ester) to form the polymer precursor, P-GFLG-ONp. The polymer precursor is then serially aminolyzed with Doxorubicin and OV-TL16 antibody to synthesize the desired targeted delivery system. The OV-TL16 antibody enables recognition of the macromolecular therapeutic by OA-3 antigen on ovarian carcinoma cells, followed by receptor-mediated endocytosis. This enables favorable biodistribution and enhanced intracellular concentration to achieve a better therapeutic effect.

experiments will also be considered here. It is hoped that these illustrations will serve as a primer for understanding specific polymer–drug conjugates that the reader is interested in.

11.10.1 OV-TL16-Targeted HPMA Copolymer-Based Delivery System for Doxorubicin

The OV-TL 16 antibody is produced from hybridoma cells and is specific for OA-3 antigens that are associated with ovarian carcinoma cells. Targeted polymer–drug conjugates were synthesized by the aminolysis of HPMA copolymer-bearing pendant ONp groups (connected to the polymer backbone by lysosomally degradable GFLG spacers [67]) with Doxorubicin. The intermediate was then isolated, characterized, dissolved in buffer, and aminolyzed with the OV-TL16 antibody (Figure 11.9) [67]. The GFLG spacer allows for the release of Doxorubicin from the conjugate in the lysosome and consequent diffusion into the other subcellular compartments. Release of free Doxorubicin allows its intercalation with DNA, which is an important mechanism for its cytotoxic effect [119–122]. About 30% of the total amount of cell-associated conjugate was internalized within 90 min [67]. This internalization was inhibited by the presence of free OV-TL16 antibody in the cell culture medium, indicating the role of receptor-mediated endocytosis.

Confocal microscopy performed after incubating the cells for 24 h with the drug demonstrated localization of Doxorubicin in the nucleus. The IC_{50} values, which are measures of cytotoxicity (efficacy), in an ovarian carcinoma cell line (NIH: OVCAR-3) are listed in Table 11.9. Values are

TABLE 11.9
IC_{50} Values in OVCAR-3 Ovarian Carcinoma Cells

Compound	IC_{50} Value (μM)
Free DOX	2 ± 1
P-GFLG-DOX	150 ± 10
P-GFLG-DOX - OV-TL16	4.4 ± 1

Source: Adapted from Omelyanenko, V. et al., HPMA copolymer-anticancer drug-OV-TL16 antibody conjugates. II. Processing in epithelial ovarian carcinoma cells in vitro, *Int. J. Cancer,* 75(4), 600–608, 1998.

expressed as mean ± standard deviation — this is a standard way of denoting cytotoxicity of conjugates. The lower the IC_{50} value, the higher is the cytotoxicity.

The nontargeted HPMA copolymer with Doxorubicin, attached via a biodegradable GFLG spacer (P-GFLG-DOX), demonstrates a higher IC_{50} value as compared to the free Doxorubicin; this is related to the different mechanisms of cell uptake (free diffusion for Doxorubicin as compared to fluid phase endocytosis for P-GFLG-DOX). However, use of OV-TL16-targeted HPMA-copolymer-based delivery system for Doxorubicin, which internalizes by receptor-mediated endocytosis, increases the cytotoxicity 34-fold over the nontargeted conjugates and nearly restores the cytotoxicity to that of free Doxorubicin [28]. Although the cytotoxicity is slightly reduced as compared to the free drug, this disadvantage is outweighed by the decrease in the systemic side effects and the specificity afforded by this approach. Another advantage of targeted conjugates is the possibility to target tumor cells growing in ascitic fluid [28].

11.10.2 HPMA Copolymer-Based Delivery System Bearing HIV Tat Protein as a Transduction Moiety

The HIV Tat protein is known to have the ability to translocate across the cell membrane in a rapid, concentration-dependent manner. The energy dependence and the mechanism of transport in the case of Tat are currently being debated.

The conjugate synthesized consisted of a HPMA copolymer bearing a pendant FITC-labeled Tat protein. The HPMA copolymer conjugate was synthesized in a multistep procedure (Figure 11.10) [108]. This procedure serves to illustrate the multistep reactions and the series of reagents that may need to be used in order to introduce the required functionality in the desired polymeric delivery system.

Confocal microscopy experiments performed with live cells incubated with the polymer bearing the Tat protein (that was labeled with FITC) for 1 h demonstrated that this conjugate strongly associated with the plasma membrane. The conjugate is also localized in the cytoplasm and the nucleus [108]. Nuclear and cytoplasmic localization was corroborated using propidium iodide (PI) and chloromethyl-benzoylaminotetramethyl rhodamine (CMTMR) as nuclear and cytoplasmic markers, respectively. Punctate staining observed in the cytoplasm indicated that the polymer was also internalized by endocytosis, reflective of the macromolecular nature of the delivery system. Experiments performed at 4°C (designed to block the endocytotic route, which is an energy-dependent process) demonstrated continued internalization by a non-energy-dependent Tat-mediated pathway [108]. Internalization of the conjugate was observed to occur in a time- and concentration-dependent manner [108]. Another set of experiments performed with a similar polymer, where the backbone was labeled with Texas Red, demonstrated that the polymer translocated to the same sites as Tat [108]. It implies that the attachment of a drug to this

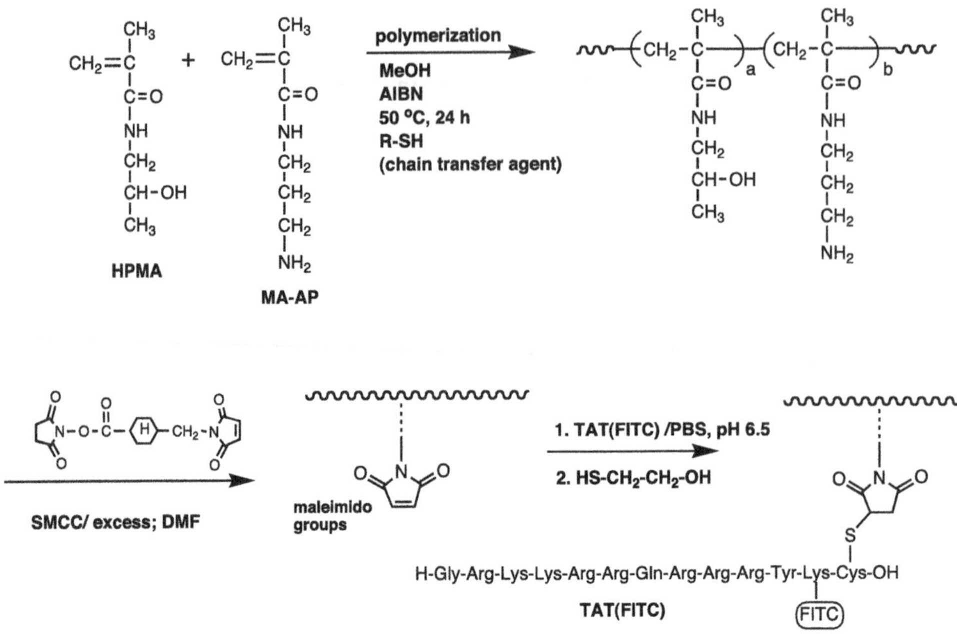

FIGURE 11.10 Synthetic scheme for HPMA copolymer bearing pendant HIV Tat peptide for cytoplasmic delivery. The first step involves the copolymerization of HPMA (*N*-(2-hydroxypropyl)methacrylamide) and MA–AP (*N*-(3-aminopropyl)methacrylamide hydrochloride) to form the polymer precursor. The polymer precursor is then reacted with SMCC (succinimidyl 4-(*N*-maleimidomethyl) cyclohexane-1-carboxylate) to produce HPMA copolymer bearing pendant maleimide groups, which were reacted with FITC labeled Tat protein to form a thioether linkage. The Tat sequence is modified at the N-terminal to enable the attachment of fluorescein isothiocyanate (FITC). The presence of the FITC label enables tracking the movement of the Tat sequence. The Tat protein as a protein transduction domain enhances the internalization of the polymer into the cells. (From Nori, A. et al., Tat-conjugated synthetic macromolecules facilitate cytoplasmic drug delivery to human ovarian carcinoma cells, *Bioconjugate Chem.*, 14(1), 44, 2003.)

polymer backbone (containing Tat) could potentially be used to deliver drugs and/or genes to the cytoplasm and the nucleus. Work is being carried out on developing such systems.

11.10.3 EFFICACY OF POLYMER–DRUG CONJUGATES IN OVARIAN CARCINOMA XENOGRAFTS *IN VIVO*

Ovarian carcinoma xenografts have been used to demonstrate the *in vivo* efficacy of polymer–drug conjugates in comparison with the free drug. These studies are precursor studies used to validate efficacy performed before the initiation of clinical trials.

11.10.3.1 HPMA Copolymer–DOX Conjugates for Anticancer Therapy

HPMA copolymer conjugates bearing Doxorubicin attached via a biodegradable GFLG spacer (P-GFLG-DOX) were synthesized using a polymer-analogous reaction as described in Figure 11.6. This conjugate was evaluated in solid tumor mice models of Doxorubicin-sensitive and Doxorubicin-resistant human ovarian carcinomas. Briefly, these models were generated by the subcutaneous transplantation of five million cells of A2780 (Doxorubicin–sensitive) or A2780/AD (Doxorubicin–resistant) human ovarian carcinoma cells into the flanks of female athymic nude mice [53]. One of the major mechanisms of drug resistance in A2780/AD cells is because of P-glycoprotein (P-gp), which is encoded by the *MDR1* gene. P-glycoprotein is an efflux pump that pumps several structurally unrelated drugs (including DOX) from the cell and leads to subtherapeutic intracellular concentrations. Presence of the *MDR1* gene and hence P-glycoprotein is a marker of multidrug resistance. After the grafts had achieved a consistent growth rate and defined volume, the mice were treated with the maximum tolerated dose of free Doxorubicin (5 mg/kg) and P-GFLG-DOX (25 mg/kg), as determined from preliminary experiments.

Free Doxorubicin demonstrated regression of the Doxorubicin-sensitive (A2780) human ovarian carcinoma xenografts 2.8-fold (as compared to the controls) after 32 days of treatment. However, no statistically significant decrease in the size of the Doxorubicin resistant (A2780/AD) human ovarian carcinoma xenografts was seen (Figure 11.11) [53]. In contrast, P-GFLG-DOX demonstrated a dramatic decrease in the size of both types of xenografts as compared to the controls. The size of the sensitive (A2780) ovarian carcinoma xenografts was decreased 28-fold, whereas the resistant (A2780/AD) ovarian carcinoma xenografts was decreased 18-fold after 32 days of treatment (Figure 11.11) [53]. Polymer–drug conjugates are thus proven to be more effective *in vivo* in both Doxorubicin-sensitive and Doxorubicin-resistant carcinoma xenografts.

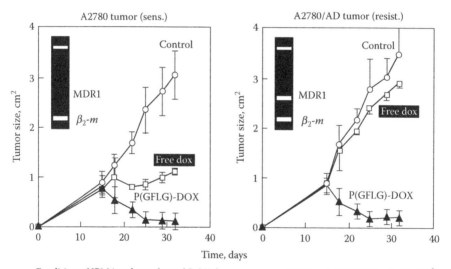

Conditions: HPMA polymer bound DOX; human ovarian A2780 and A2780/AD cells (5×10^6) transplanted s.c; treatment i.p. 6 times with max. dose DOX: 5mg/kg, P-DOX: 25 mg/kg

FIGURE 11.11 Efficacy of free DOX and P-GFLG-DOX on the growth of A2780 and A2780/AD human ovarian carcinoma xenografts in mice. Experiments were performed in Doxorubicin-sensitive (A2780) and Doxorubicin-resistant (A2780/AD) ovarian carcinoma xenografts in nude mice. Free Doxorubicin demonstrated tumor regression only in the Doxorubicin-sensitive (A2780) xenografts (as compared to the controls). No statistically significant decrease in Doxorubicin-resistant (A2780/AD) xenografts was seen after administration of free Doxorubicin. In contrast, P-GFLG-DOX demonstrated a dramatic decrease in the size of both types of xenografts as compared to the controls. (Adapted from Minko, T., Kopečková, P., and Kopeček, J., Efficacy of the chemotherapeutic action of HPMA copolymer-bound Doxorubicin in a solid tumor model of ovarian carcinoma, *Int. J. Cancer*, 86(1), 108, 2000.)

11.10.3.2 HPMA Copolymer–Drug Conjugates for Combination Chemotherapy and Photodynamic Therapy

Photodynamic therapy is a newer paradigm in anticancer therapy that involves activation of specific compounds called *photosensitizers* with specific wavelengths of light in order to induce cell death. Illumination of these compounds results in the generation of free radicals and singlet oxygen, which cause cell damage; accumulation of cell damage results in impairment of cellular processes and results in cell death. A combination of chemotherapy and photodynamic therapy may result in a synergistic response, resulting in a better cure rate than monotherapy. Combination therapy was evaluated with targeted macromolecular therapeutic agents (HPMA copolymer–Doxorubicin–OV-TL16 immunoconjugates for chemotherapy and HPMA copolymer–Mesochlorin e_6–OV-TL16 immunoconjugates for photodynamic therapy) *in vivo* [123]. Synthesis of these conjugates was performed using a polymer-analogous method and sequential attachment of drug and antibody (Figure 11.12) [123]. Targeted conjugates were used to achieve specific localization in the tumor and increased cell uptake, thereby enhancing the cytotoxic effect. The results of chemotherapy were compared with combination therapy with nontargeted conjugates.

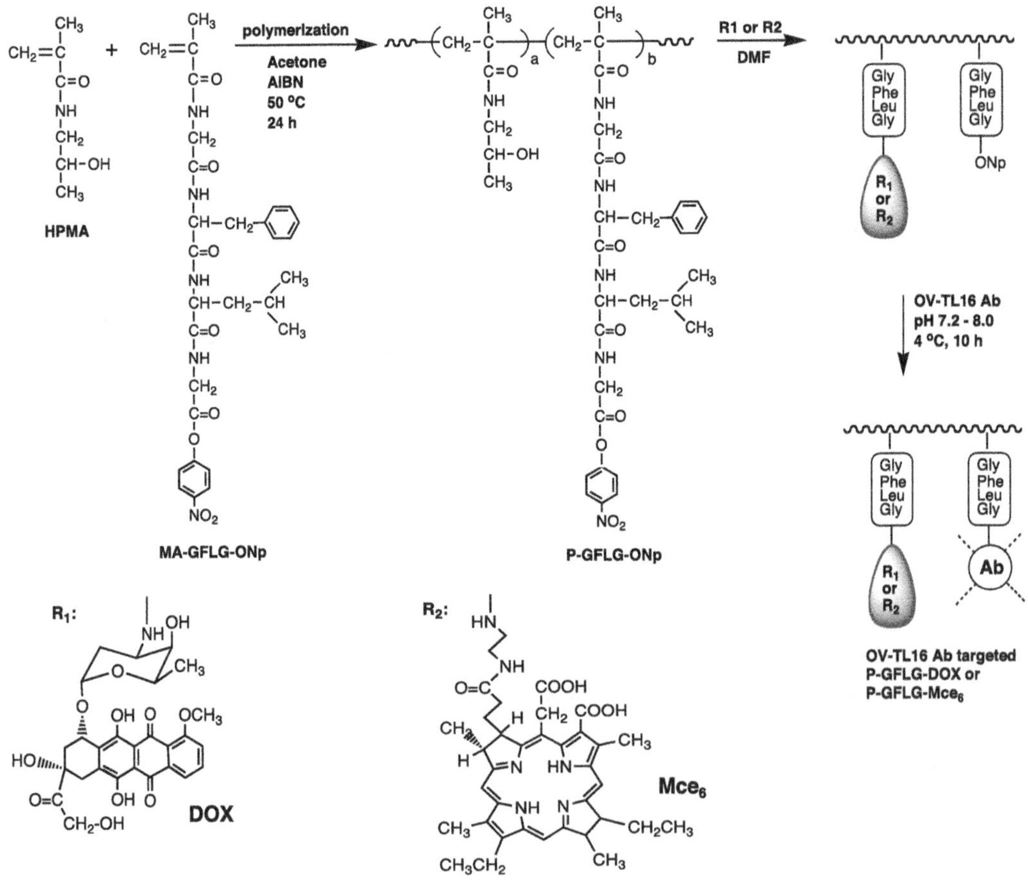

FIGURE 11.12 Synthetic procedure for targeted macromolecular conjugates for combination chemotherapy and photodynamic therapy. The first step involves the polymerization of HPMA and MA-GFLG-ONp to form the polymer precursor, P-GFLG-ONp. The polymer precursor is then serially aminolyzed with Doxorubicin or Mesochlorin e_6 (Mce$_6$) followed by OV-TL16 antibody to synthesize the two different types of targeted polymer–drug conjugates.

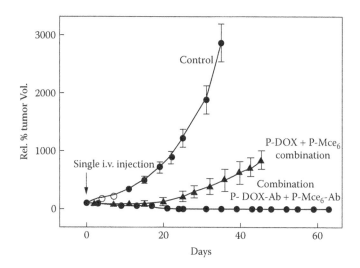

FIGURE 11.13 Efficacy of combination chemotherapy and photodynamic therapy of OVCAR-3 xenografts in nude mice with nontargeted and OV-TL16 antibody-targeted conjugates. Therapeutic efficacy of a combination therapy of HPMA copolymer-bound Mce$_6$ and DOX targeted with OV-TL16 antibodies toward OVCAR-3 xenografts was compared to nontreated xenografts and nontargeted combination chemotherapy and photodynamic therapy. Equivalent doses of targeted combination therapy enhanced the tumor-suppressive effect as compared to nontargeted combination therapy. Dose administered: 2.2 mg/kg DOX equivalent and 1.5 mg/kg Mce$_6$ equivalent. Irradiation for photodynamic therapy: 650 nm, 200 mW/cm^2, 18 h after administration. (Adapted from Shiah, J.-G. et al., Combination chemotherapy and photodynamic therapy of targetable N-(2-hydroxypropyl)methacrylamide copolymer-Doxorubicin/mesochlorin e$_6$-OV-TL 16 antibody immunoconjugates, *J. Controlled Release,* 74, 249, 2001.)

Mice bearing OVCAR-3 xenografts (which express OA-3 antigens specifically targeted by the OV-TL16 antibody) were developed by the subcutaneous implantation of OVCAR-3 cells. After the xenografts had reached a particular size with consistent growth rates, the conjugates were administered intravenously and efficacy was determined by serial monitoring over nine weeks.

Therapeutic results are summarized in Figure 11.13. Combination treatment with nontargeted conjugates inhibited tumor growth for approximately 20 days [123]. Antibody-targeted conjugates were able to inhibit the growth of the xenografts for more than 60 days in equivalent doses [123]. Active targeting using antibodies was thus demonstrated to dramatically increase the tumor accumulation with a concomitant-enhanced therapeutic effect. However, it must be pointed out that the increase in molecular weight following attachment of antibodies could also play a role in the increased accumulation, resulting in an enhanced therapeutic effect.

11.11 POLYMER–DRUG CONJUGATES IN CLINICAL TRIALS AND APPROVED POLYMER–DRUG CONJUGATES

Macromolecular therapeutics have developed considerably in the last 20 years; more than ten polymer–drug conjugates have entered clinical trials for therapeutic validation in the last decade. A poly(styrene-*co*-maleic acid) conjugated neocarzinostatin (SMANCS) is currently approved for clinical application in Japan [124,125].

Table 11.10 lists some of the conjugates that are currently undergoing clinical trials. HPMA copolymers are the most common polymer backbones in the conjugates being currently evaluated. Results from some of these conjugates are promising — FDA approval will undoubtedly speed the process of development of newer conjugates and their clinical evaluation.

TABLE 11.10
Polymer–Drug Conjugates in Clinical Trials

Polymer Backbone	Polymer–Drug Conjugate	Phase of Clinical Trials	References
N-(2-hydroxypropyl) methacrylamide copolymer	HPMA copolymer–Doxorubicin (PK1)	II	126,127
	HPMA copolymer–Doxorubicin-Galactosamine (PK2)	I/II	128
	HPMA copolymer–Paclitaxel (PNU166945)	I	129
	HPMA copolymer–Camptothecin (PNU166148, MAG-CPT)	I	130–132
	HPMA copolymer–cis–Platinate (AP5280)	I/II	133
Polyglutamic acid	Polyglutamic acid–Paclitaxel (CT-2103, XYOTAX)	III	134–138
	Polyglutamic acid–Camptothecin (CT–2106)	I	139
Polyethylene glycol (PEG)	PEG–Camptothecin (PEG-CPT)	II	140

11.12 CONCLUDING REMARKS AND OUTLOOK FOR THE FUTURE

Current research in the field of polymer–anticancer drug conjugates is directed towards the identification of the mechanism of action of free and polymer-bound drugs at the cellular and subcellular levels. The information gained from this research will enable the development of second-generation macromolecular therapeutics using a rational design strategy, which draws on the knowledge of predetermined cellular and subcellular mechanisms and targets. Clinical trials based on the first generation of macromolecular anticancer therapeutics are also actively under way — approval for clinical use for this first generation of macromolecular anticancer drugs is expected soon. Such agents will surely prove to be a valuable addition to the armamentarium that is currently available to oncologists.

Newer applications for polymer–drug conjugates are also being explored [141,142]. Inflammatory diseases are characterized by an increase in the vascular permeability (similar to tumors). Though there may be lesser amounts of retention as the lymphatics are not blocked, there may still be a therapeutic advantage offered by the conjugation of drugs to polymer backbones. These represent new and exciting avenues of research for polymeric drug delivery scientists.

Continued research and understanding of the principles of polymeric drug delivery will enable us to achieve the goal of efficacious and specific drug treatment for a vast array of clinical disorders — the "magic bullet" concept, espoused by Paul Ehrlich [143]. A holistic approach, drawing on advances made in several scientific disciplines such as polymer chemistry, pharmaceutics, pharmacology, and molecular biology, will be invaluable in this regard.

REFERENCES

1. Jatzkewitz, H., Peptamin (glycyl-L-leucyl-mescaline) bound to blood plasma expander (polyvinylpyrrolidone) as a new depot form of a biologically active primary amine (mescaline), *Z. Naturforsch.*, 10b, 27, 1955.
2. Shumikhina, K.I., Panarin, E.F., and Ushakov, S.N., [Experimental study of polymer salts of penicillins], *Antibiotiki*, 11(9), 767, 1966.

3. Givental, N.I. et al., [Experimental studies on penicillin polymer derivatives], *Antibiotiki*, 10(8), 701, 1965.

4. De Duve, C. et al., Commentary: lysosomotropic agents, *Biochem. Pharmacol.*, 23(18), 2495, 1974.

5. Ringsdorf, H., Structure and properties of pharmacologically active polymers, *J. Polym. Sci. Polym. Symp.*, 51, 135, 1975.

6. Matsumura, Y. and Maeda, H., A new concept for macromolecular therapeutics in cancer chemotherapy: mechanism of tumoritropic accumulation of proteins and the antitumor agent SMANCS, *Cancer Res.*, 46(12 pt. 1), 6387, 1986.

7. Shaunak, S. et al., Reduction of the viral load of HIV-1 after the intraperitoneal administration of dextrin 2-sulphate in patients with AIDS, *Aids*, 12(4), 399, 1998.

8. Thornton, M. et al., Anti-Kaposi's sarcoma and antiangiogenic activities of sulfated dextrins, *Antimicrob. Agents Chemother.*, 43(10), 2528, 1999.

9. Stafford, M.K. et al., A placebo-controlled, double-blind prospective study in healthy female volunteers of dextrin sulphate gel: a novel potential intravaginal virucide, *J. Acquir. Immune Defic. Syndr. Hum. Retrovirol.*, 14(3), 213, 1997.

10. Teitelbaum, D., Arnon, R., and Sela, M., Cop 1 as a candidate drug for multiple sclerosis, *J. Neural Transm. Suppl.*, 49, 85, 1997.

11. Teitelbaum, D., Sela, M., and Arnon, R., Copolymer 1 from the laboratory to FDA, *Isr. J. Med. Sci.*, 33(4), 280, 1997.

12. Aharoni, R. et al., Copolymer 1 induces T cells of the T helper type 2 that crossreact with myelin basic protein and suppress experimental autoimmune encephalomyelitis, *Proc. Natl. Acad. Sci. USA.*, 94(20), 10821, 1997.

13. Brenner, T. et al., Humoral and cellular immune responses to Copolymer 1 in multiple sclerosis patients treated with Copaxone, *J. Neuroimmunol.*, 115(1–2), 152, 2001.

14. Bleyer, A.J. et al., A comparison of the calcium-free phosphate binder sevelamer hydrochloride with calcium acetate in the treatment of hyperphosphatemia in hemodialysis patients, *Am. J. Kidney Dis.*, 33(4), 694, 1999.

15. Slatopolsky, E.A., Burke, S.K., and Dillon, M.A., RenaGel, a nonabsorbed calcium- and aluminum-free phosphate binder, lowers serum phosphorus and parathyroid hormone. The RenaGel Study Group, *Kidney Int.*, 55(1), 299, 1999.

16. Goldberg, D.I. et al., Effect of RenaGel, a non-absorbed, calcium- and aluminium-free phosphate binder, on serum phosphorus, calcium, and intact parathyroid hormone in end-stage renal disease patients, *Nephrol. Dial. Transplant.*, 13(9), 2303, 1998.

17. Burke, S.K., Slatopolsky, E.A., and Goldberg, D.I., RenaGel, a novel calcium- and aluminium-free phosphate binder, inhibits phosphate absorption in normal volunteers, *Nephrol. Dial. Transplant.*, 12(8), 1640, 1997.

18. Thorling, E.B., Larsen, B., and Nielsen, H., Inhibitory effect of DEAE-dextran on tumour growth. 3. Effect of charge density and molecular size, *Acta Pathol. Microbiol. Scand. [A]*, 79(2), 81, 1971.

19. Larsen, B. and Thorling, E.B., Inhibitory effect of DEAE-dextran on tumour growth. (1). Action of dextran sulphate after in vitro incubation, *Acta Pathol. Microbiol. Scand.*, 75(2), 229, 1969.

20. Thorling, E.B. and Larsen, B., Inhibitory effect of DEAE-dextran on tumour growth. (2). (A) Effect of DEAE-dextran in vivo on the transplantable ascites tumour JBI in C3H/A mice. (B) Action of dextran sulphate administered after inoculation of DEAE-dextran inhibited tumour cells, *Acta Pathol. Microbiol. Scand.*, 75(2), 237, 1969.

21. Saiki, I. et al., Inhibition of lung metastasis by synthetic and recombinant fragments of human fibronectin with functional domains, *Jpn. J. Cancer Res.*, 81(10), 1003, 1990.

22. Duncan, R. et al., Tyrosinamide residues enhance pinocytic capture of N-(2-hydroxypropyl)methacrylamide copolymers, *Biochim. Biophys. Acta*, 799(1), 1, 1984.

23. McCormick, L. et al., Interaction of a cationic N-(2-hydroxypropyl)methacrylamide copolymer with rat visceral yolk sac cultured in vitro and rat liver in vivo, *J. Bioact. Comp. Polym.*, 1, 755, 518, 1986.

24. Říhová, B. et al., Antibody-directed affinity therapy applied to the immune system: in vivo effectiveness and limited toxicity of daunomycin conjugated to HPMA copolymers and targeting antibody, *Clin. Immunol. Immunopathol.*, 46(1), 100, 1988.

25. Duncan, R. et al., Pinocytic uptake and intracellular degradation of N-(2-hydroxypropyl)meth-acrylamide) copolymers. A potential drug delivery system, *Biochim. Biophys. Acta.*, 678, 143, 1981.

26. O'Hare, K.B. et al., Effect of galactose on interaction of N-(2-hydroxypropyl)methacrylamide copol-ymers with hepatoma cells in culture: preliminary application to an anticancer agent, daunomycin, *Hepatology*, 10(2), 207, 1989.

27. Omelyanenko, V. et al., Targetable HPMA copolymer-adriamycin conjugates: recognition, internal-ization, and subcellular fate, *J. Controlled Release*, 53(1–3), 25, 1998.

28. Omelyanenko, V. et al., HPMA copolymer-anticancer drug-OV-TL16 antibody conjugates. II. Pro-cessing in epithelial ovarian carcinoma cells in vitro, *Int. J. Cancer*, 75(4), 600–608, 1998.

29. Foster, S. and Lloyd, J.B., Solute transport across the mammalian lysosome membrane, *Biochim. Biophys. Acta*, 947, 465, 1988.

30. Willner, D. et al., (6-Maleimidocaproyl)hydrazone of Doxorubicin — a new derivative for the prep-aration of immunoconjugates of Doxorubicin, *Bioconjugate Chem.*, 4(6), 521, 1993.

31. Shen, W.C. and Ryser, H.J., cis-Aconityl spacer between daunomycin and macromolecular carriers: a model of pH-sensitive linkage releasing drug from a lysosomotropic conjugate, *Biochem. Biophys. Res. Commun.*, 102(3), 1048, 1981.

32. Shen, W.C., Ryser, H.J., and LaManna, L., Disulfide spacer between methotrexate and poly(D-lysine): a probe for exploring the reductive process in endocytosis, *J. Biol. Chem.*, 260(20), 10905, 1985.

33. Kopeček, J. and Rejmanová, P., Enzymatically degradable bonds in synthetic polymers, in *Controlled Drug Delivery*, Bruck, S.D., Ed., Vol. I, CRC Press, Boca Raton, FL, 1983, p. 81.

34. Duncan, R. et al., Polymers containing enzymatically degradable bonds. 7. Design of oligopeptide side-chains in poly[N-(2-hydroxypropyl)methacrylamide] copolymers to promote efficient degrada-tion by lysosomal enzymes, *Makromol. Chem.*, 184, 1997, 1983.

35. Rejmanová, P. et al., Polymers containing enzymatically degradable bonds. 8. Degradation of oli-gopeptide sequences in N-(2-hydroxypropyl)methacrylamide copolymers by bovine spleen cathepsin B, *Makromol. Chem.*, 184, 2009, 1983.

36. Rejmanová, P. et al., Stability in rat plasma and serum of lysosomally degradable oligopeptide sequences in N-(2-hydroxypropyl)methacrylamide copolymers, *Biomaterials*, 6(1), 45, 1985.

37. Maeda, H., Seymour, L.W., and Myamoto, Y., Conjugates of anticancer agents and polymers: advan-tages of macromolecular therapeutics in vivo, *Bioconjugate Chem.*, 3(5), 351, 1992.

38. Baban, D.F. and Seymour, L.W., Control of tumour vascular permeability, *Adv. Drug Delivery Rev.*, 34(1), 109, 1998.

39. Maeda, H. et al., Vascular permeability enhancement in solid tumor: various factors, mechanisms involved and its implications, *Int. Immunopharmacol.*, 3(3), 319, 2003.

40. Maeda, H. et al., Bradykinin and nitric oxide in infectious disease and cancer, *Immunopharmacology*, 33(1–3), 222, 1996.

41. Doi, K. et al., Excessive production of nitric oxide in rat solid tumor and its implication in rapid tumor growth, *Cancer*, 77(Suppl. 8), 1598, 1996.

42. Maeda, H. et al., Enhanced vascular permeability in solid tumor is mediated by nitric oxide and inhibited by both new nitric oxide scavenger and nitric oxide synthase inhibitor, *Jpn. J. Cancer Res.*, 85(4), 331, 1994.

43. Maeda, H. et al., Kallikrein-kinin in infection and cancer, *Immunopharmacology*, 43(2–3), 115, 1999.

44. Matsumura, Y. et al., Kinin-generating cascade in advanced cancer patients and in vitro study, *Jpn. J. Cancer Res.*, 82(6), 732, 1991.

45. Suzuki, M., Takahashi, T., and Sato, T., Medial regression and its functional significance in tumor-supplying host arteries. A morphometric study of hepatic arteries in human livers with hepatocellular carcinoma, *Cancer*, 59(3), 444, 1987.

46. Skinner, S.A., Tutton, P.J., and O'Brien, P.E., Microvascular architecture of experimental colon tumors in the rat, *Cancer Res.*, 50(8), 2411, 1990.

47. Yamaoka, T., Tabata, Y., and Ikada, Y., Distribution and tissue uptake of poly(ethylene glycol) with different molecular weights after intravenous administration to mice, *J. Pharm. Sci.*, 83(4), 601, 1994.

48. Yamaoka, T., Tabata, Y., and Ikada, Y., Fate of water-soluble polymers administered via different routes, *J. Pharm. Sci.*, 84(3), 349, 1995.

49. Yamaoka, T., Tabata, Y., and Ikada, Y., Comparison of body distribution of poly(vinyl alcohol) with other water-soluble polymers after intravenous administration, *J. Pharm. Pharmacol.*, 47(6), 479, 1995.

50. Říhová, B. and Říha, I., Immunological problems of polymer-bound drugs, *Crit. Rev. Ther. Drug Carrier Syst.*, 1(4), 311, 1985.

51. Kopeček, J. et al., HPMA copolymer-anticancer drug conjugates: design, activity, and mechanism of action, *Eur. J. Pharm. Biopharm.*, 50(1), 61, 2000.

52. Germann, U.A., P-glycoprotein: a mediator of multidrug resistance in tumour cells, *Eur. J. Cancer*, 32A(6), 927, 1996.

53. Minko, T., Kopečková, P., and Kopeček, J., Efficacy of the chemotherapeutic action of HPMA copolymer-bound Doxorubicin in a solid tumor model of ovarian carcinoma, *Int. J. Cancer*, 86(1), 108, 2000.

54. Putnam, D. and Kopeček, J., Polymer conjugates with anticancer activity, *Adv. Polym. Sci.*, 122, 55, 1995.

55. Crepon, B. et al., Enzymatic degradation and immunogenic properties of derivatized dextrans, *Biomaterials*, 12(6), 550, 1991.

56. Chiu, H.C. et al., Lysosomal degradability of poly(alpha-amino acids), *J. Biomed. Mater. Res.*, 34(3), 381, 1997.

57. Chiu, H.C. et al., Enzymatic degradation of poly(ethylene glycol) modified dextrans, *J. Bioact. Comp. Polym.*, 9, 388, 1994.

58. Krinick, N.L. and Kopeček, J., Soluble polymers as targetable drug carriers, in *Targeted Drug Delivery, Handbook of Experimental Pharmacology*, Juliano, R.L., Ed., Springer-Verlag, Berlin, 1991, p. 105.

59. Duncan, R., The dawning era of polymer therapeutics, *Nat. Rev. Drug Discovery*, 2(5), 347, 2003.

60. Rizzardo, E. et al., Tailored polymers by free radical processes, *Macromolecular Symposia*, 143 (World Polymer Congress, 37th International Symposium on Macromolecules, 1998), 291, 1999.

61. Chiefari, J. et al., Living free-radical polymerization by reversible addition-fragmentation chain transfer: the RAFT process, *Macromolecules*, 31(16), 5559, 1998.

62. Wang, J.S. and Matyjaszewski, K., Controlled/living radical polymerization. atom transfer radical polymerization in the presence of transition-metal complexes, *J. Am. Chem. Soc.*, 117(20), 5614, 1995.

63. Matyjaszewski, K. and Xia, J., Atom transfer radical polymerization, *Chem. Rev.*, 101(9), 2921, 2001.

64. *IUPAC Compendium of Chemical Terminology*, The Gold Book, 2nd ed., McNaught, A.O. and Wilkinson, A. Eds., Blackwell Science, 1997.

65. Dvořák, M., Kopečková, P., and Kopeček, J., High-molecular weight HPMA copolymer-adriamycin conjugates, *J. Controlled Release*, 60(2–3), 321, 1999.

66. Shiah, J.G. et al., Biodistribution and antitumour efficacy of long-circulating N-(2-hydroxypropyl)methacrylamide copolymer-Doxorubicin conjugates in nude mice, *Eur. J. Cancer*, 37(1), 131, 2001.

67. Omelyanenko, V. et al., HPMA copolymer-anticancer drug-OV-TL16 antibody conjugates. 1. Influence of the method of synthesis on the binding affinity to OVCAR-3 ovarian carcinoma cells in vitro, *J. Drug Target.*, 3(5), 357, 1996.

68. Lee, R.J. and Low, P.S., Delivery of liposomes into cultured KB cells via folate receptor-mediated endocytosis, *J. Biol. Chem.*, 269(5), 3198, 1994.

69. Gabizon, A. et al., Targeting folate receptor with folate linked to extremities of poly(ethylene glycol)-grafted liposomes: in vitro studies, *Bioconjugate Chem.*, 10(2), 289, 1999.

70. Iinuma, H. et al., Intracellular targeting therapy of cisplatin-encapsulated transferrin-polyethylene glycol liposome on peritoneal dissemination of gastric cancer, *Int. J. Cancer*, 99(1), 130, 2002.

71. Eavarone, D.A., Yu, X., and Bellamkonda, R.V., Targeted drug delivery to C6 glioma by transferrin-coupled liposomes, *J. Biomed. Mater. Res.*, 51(1), 10, 2000.

72. Tsuruo, T. et al., Molecular targeting therapy of cancer: drug resistance, apoptosis and survival signal, *Cancer Sci.*, 94(1), 15, 2003.

73. Sobolev, A.S. et al., Internalizable insulin-BSA-chlorin e_6 conjugate is a more effective photosensitizer than chlorin e_6 alone, *Biochem. Int.*, 26(3), 445, 1992.

74. Akhlynina, T.V. et al., Insulin-mediated intracellular targeting enhances the photodynamic activity of chlorin e_6, *Cancer Res.*, 55(5), 1014, 1995.

75. Backer, M.V. et al., Molecular vehicles for targeted drug delivery, *Bioconjugate Chem.*, 13(3), 462, 2002.

76. Lanciotti, J. et al., Targeting adenoviral vectors using heterofunctional polyethylene glycol FGF2 conjugates, *Mol. Ther.*, 8(1), 99, 2003.

77. Vega, J. et al., Targeting Doxorubicin to epidermal growth factor receptors by site-specific conjugation of C225 to poly(L-glutamic acid) through a polyethylene glycol spacer, *Pharm. Res.*, 20(5), 826, 2003.

78. Gijsens, A. et al., Epidermal growth factor-mediated targeting of chlorin e_6 selectively potentiates its photodynamic activity, *Cancer Res.*, 60(8), 2197, 2000.

79. Gijsens, A. and De Witte, P., [Targeting of chlorin e_6 by EGF increasing its photodynamic activity in selective ways], *Verh. K. Acad. Geneeskd Belg.*, 62(4), 329, 2000.

80. Ogris, M. et al., Tumor-targeted gene therapy: strategies for the preparation of ligand-polyethylene glycol-polyethylenimine/DNA complexes, *J. Controlled Release*, 91(1–2), 173, 2003.

81. Blessing, T. et al., Different strategies for formation of pegylated EGF-conjugated PEI/DNA complexes for targeted gene delivery, *Bioconjugate Chem.*, 12(4), 529, 2001.

82. David, A. et al., Enhanced biorecognition and internalization of HPMA copolymers containing multiple or multivalent carbohydrate side-chains by human hepatocarcinoma cells, *Bioconjugate Chem.*, 12(6), 890, 2001.

83. Duncan, R. et al., Fate of N-(2-hydroxypropyl)methacrylamide copolymers with pendent galactosamine residues after intravenous administration to rats, *Biochim. Biophys. Acta*, 880(1), 62, 1986.

84. Mammen, M., Choi, S.-K., and Whitesides, G.M., Polyvalent interactions in biological systems: implications for design and use of multivalent ligands and inhibitors, *Angew. Chem. Int. Ed.*, 37, 2754, 1998.

85. Kalderon, D. et al., A short amino acid sequence able to specify nuclear location, *Cell*, 39 (3 pt. 2), 499, 1984.

86. Beven, L. et al., Effects on mollicutes (wall-less bacteria) of synthetic peptides comprising a signal peptide or a membrane fusion peptide, and a nuclear localization sequence (NLS) — a comparison with melittin, *Biochim. Biophys. Acta*, 1329(2), 357, 1997.

87. Richardson, W.D., Roberts, B.L., and Smith, A.E., Nuclear location signals in polyoma virus large-T, *Cell*, 44(1), 77, 1986.

88. Moreland, R.B. et al., Amino acid sequences that determine the nuclear localization of yeast histone 2B, *Mol. Cell Biol.*, 7(11), 4048, 1987.

89. Chida, K. and Vogt, P.K., Nuclear translocation of viral Jun but not of cellular Jun is cell cycle dependent, *Proc. Natl. Acad. Sci. USA*, 89(10), 4290, 1992.

90. Robbins, J. et al., Two interdependent basic domains in nucleoplasmin nuclear targeting sequence: identification of a class of bipartite nuclear targeting sequence, *Cell*, 64(3), 615, 1991.

91. Kleinschmidt, J.A. and Seiter, A., Identification of domains involved in nuclear uptake and histone binding of protein N1 of Xenopus laevis, *EMBO. J.*, 7(6), 1605, 1988.

92. Jans, D.A. et al., Cyclin-dependent kinase site-regulated signal-dependent nuclear localization of the SW15 yeast transcription factor in mammalian cells, *J. Biol. Chem.*, 270(29), 17064, 1995.

93. Chen, G.L. et al., Import of human bifunctional enzyme into peroxisomes of human hepatoma cells in vitro, *Biochem. Biophys. Res. Commun.*, 178(3), 1084, 1991.

94. Swinkels, B.W. et al., A novel, cleavable peroxisomal targeting signal at the amino-terminus of the rat 3-ketoacyl-CoA thiolase, *EMBO. J.*, 10(11), 3255, 1991.

95. Schröder, S. et al., The Golgi-localization of yeast Emp47p depends on its di-lysine motif but is not affected by the ret1-1 mutation in alpha-COP, *J. Cell Biol.*, 131(4), 895, 1995.

96. Mathew, E.C. et al., The effects of targeting the vaccinia virus B5R protein to the endoplasmic reticulum on virus morphogenesis and dissemination, *Virology*, 265(1), 131, 1999.

97. Calvert, M.E. et al., Oolemmal proteomics--identification of highly abundant heat shock proteins and molecular chaperones in the mature mouse egg and their localization on the plasma membrane, *Reprod. Biol. Endocrinol.*, 1(1), 27, 2003.

98. Hurt, E.C. et al., The first twelve amino acids (less than half of the pre-sequence) of an imported mitochondrial protein can direct mouse cytosolic dihydrofolate reductase into the yeast mitochondrial matrix, *EMBO. J.*, 4(8), 2061, 1985.

99. Kurz, M. et al., Biogenesis of Tim proteins of the mitochondrial carrier import pathway: differential targeting mechanisms and crossing over with the main import pathway, *Mol. Biol. Cell.*, 10(7), 2461, 1999.

100. Dice, J.F. and Chiang, H.L., Peptide signals for protein degradation within lysosomes, *Biochem. Soc. Symp.*, 55, 45, 1989.

101. Dice, J.F. and Terlecky, S.R., Targeting of cytosolic proteins to lysosomes for degradation, *Crit. Rev. Ther. Drug Carrier Syst.*, 7(3), 211, 1990.

102. Schwarze, S.R. et al., In vivo protein transduction: delivery of a biologically active protein into the mouse, *Science*, 285(5433), 1569, 1999.

103. Levchenko, T.S. et al., Tat peptide-mediated intracellular delivery of liposomes, *Methods Enzymol.*, 372, 339, 2003.

104. Torchilin, V.P. and Levchenko, T.S., TAT-liposomes: a novel intracellular drug carrier, *Curr. Protein Pept. Sci.*, 4(2), 133, 2003.

105. Torchilin, V.P. et al., TAT peptide on the surface of liposomes affords their efficient intracellular delivery even at low temperature and in the presence of metabolic inhibitors, *Proc. Natl. Acad. Sci. USA*, 98(15), 8786, 2001.

106. Polyakov, V. et al., Novel Tat-peptide chelates for direct transduction of technetium-99m and rhenium into human cells for imaging and radiotherapy, *Bioconjugate Chem.*, 11(6), 762, 2000.

107. Astriab-Fisher, A. et al., Conjugates of antisense oligonucleotides with the Tat and antennapedia cell-penetrating peptides: effects on cellular uptake, binding to target sequences, and biologic actions, *Pharm. Res.*, 19(6), 744, 2002.

108. Nori, A. et al., Tat-conjugated synthetic macromolecules facilitate cytoplasmic drug delivery to human ovarian carcinoma cells, *Bioconjugate Chem.*, 14(1), 44, 2003.

109. Elliott, G. and O'Hare, P., Intercellular trafficking of VP22-GFP fusion proteins, *Gene Ther.*, 6(1), 149, 1999.

110. Suzuki, K. et al., Enhanced effect of myocardial gene transfection by VP22-mediated intercellular protein transport, *J. Mol. Cell Cardiol.*, 36(4), 603, 2004.

111. Satchi, R., Connors, T.A., and Duncan, R., PDEPT: polymer-directed enzyme prodrug therapy. I. HPMA copolymer-cathepsin B and PK1 as a model combination, *Br. J. Cancer*, 85(7), 1070, 2001.

112. Satchi-Fainaro, R. et al., PDEPT: polymer-directed enzyme prodrug therapy. 2. HPMA copolymer-beta-lactamase and HPMA copolymer-C-DOX as a model combination, *Bioconjugate Chem.*, 14(4), 797, 2003.

113. Bagshawe, K.D., Antibody directed enzymes revive anti-cancer prodrugs concept, *Br. J. Cancer*, 56, 531, 1987.

114. Flanagan, P.A. et al., Immunogenicity of protein-N-(2-hydroxypropyl)methacrylamide copolymer conjugates measured in A/J and B10 mice, *J. Bioact. Comp. Polym.*, 5, 151, 1990.

115. Sharma, S.K. et al., Human immune response to monoclonal antibody-enzyme conjugates in ADEPT pilot clinical trial, *Cell Biophys.*, 21, 109, 1992.

116. Ulbrich K. et al., Polymeric drugs based on conjugates of synthetic and natural macromolecules I. Synthesis and physico-chemical characterization, *J. Controlled Release*, 64, 63, 2000.

117. Lu, Z.R., Kopečková, P., and Kopeček, J., Polymerizable Fab' antibody fragments for targeting of anticancer drugs, *Nat. Biotechnol.*, 17(11), 1101, 1999.

118. Lu, Z.R. et al., Preparation and biological evaluation of polymerizable antibody Fab' fragment targeted polymeric drug delivery system, *J. Controlled Release*, 74(1–3), 263, 2001.

119. Tanaka, M. and Yoshida, S., Mechanism of the inhibition of calf thymus DNA polymerases alpha and beta by daunomycin and adriamycin, *J. Biochem. (Tokyo)*, 87(3), 911, 1980.

120. Facchinetti, T. et al., Intercalation with DNA is a prerequisite for daunomycin, adriamycin and its congeners in inhibiting DNAase I, *Chem. Biol. Interact.*, 20(1), 97, 1978.

121. Marco, A. and Arcamone, F., DNA complexing antibiotics: daunomycin, adriamycin and their derivatives, *Arzneimittelforschung*, 25(3), 368, 1975.

122. Plumbridge, T.W. and Brown, J.R., The interaction of adriamycin and adriamycin analogues with nucleic acids in the B and A conformations, *Biochim. Biophys. Acta*, 563(1), 181, 1979.

123. Shiah, J.-G. et al., Combination chemotherapy and photodynamic therapy of targetable N-(2-hydroxypropyl)methacrylamide copolymer-Doxorubicin/mesochlorin e_6-OV-TL 16 antibody immunoconjugates, *J. Controlled Release*, 74, 249, 2001.

124. Abe, S. and Otsuki, M., Styrene maleic acid neocarzinostatin treatment for hepatocellular carcinoma, *Curr. Med. Chem. Anti-Cancer Agents*, 2(6), 715, 2002.

125. Tsuchia, K. et al., Tumor-targeted chemotherapy with SMANCS in lipiodol for renal cell carcinoma: longer survival with larger size tumors, *Urology*, 55, 495, 2000.

126. Duncan, R., Coatsworth, J.K., and Burtles, S., Preclinical toxicology of a novel polymeric antitumour agent: HPMA copolymer-Doxorubicin (PK1), *Hum. Exp. Toxicol.*, 17(2), 93, 1998.

127. Vasey, P.A. et al., Phase I clinical and pharmacokinetic study of PK1 [N-(2-hydroxypropyl)methacrylamide copolymer Doxorubicin]: first member of a new class of chemotherapeutic agents-drug-polymer conjugates, Cancer Research Campaign Phase I/II Committee, *Clin. Cancer Res.*, 5(1), 83, 1999.

128. Hopewel, J.W. et al., Preclinical evaluation of the cardiotoxicity of PK2: a novel HPMA copolymer-Doxorubicin-galactosamine conjugate antitumour agent, *Hum. Exp. Toxicol.*, 20(9), 461, 2001.

129. Meerum Terwogt, J.M. et al., Phase I clinical and pharmacokinetic study of PNU166945, a novel water-soluble polymer-conjugated prodrug of paclitaxel, *Anticancer Drugs*, 12(4), 315, 2001.

130. Wachters, F.M. et al., A phase I study with MAG-camptothecin intravenously administered weekly for 3 weeks in a 4-week cycle in adult patients with solid tumours, *Br. J. Cancer*, 90(12), 2261, 2004.

131. Sarapa, N. et al., Assessment of normal and tumor tissue uptake of MAG-CPT, a polymer-bound prodrug of camptothecin, in patients undergoing elective surgery for colorectal carcinoma, *Cancer Chemother. Pharmacol.*, 52(5), 424, 2003.

132. Schoemaker, N.E. et al., A phase I and pharmacokinetic study of MAG-CPT, a water-soluble polymer conjugate of camptothecin, *Br. J. Cancer*, 87(6), 608, 2002.

133. Rademaker-Lakhai, J.M. et al., A Phase I and pharmacological study of the platinum polymer AP5280 given as an intravenous infusion once every 3 weeks in patients with solid tumors, *Clin. Cancer Res.*, 10(10), 3386, 2004.

134. Singer, J.W. et al., Poly-(L)-glutamic acid-paclitaxel (CT-2103) [XYOTAX], a biodegradable polymeric drug conjugate: characterization, preclinical pharmacology and preliminary clinical data, *Adv. Exp. Med. Biol.*, 519, 81, 2003.

135. Sludden, A.V. et al., Phase I and pharmacologic study of CT-2103, a poly(L-glutamic acid)-paclitaxel conjugate, *Proc. Am. Assoc. Cancer Res.*, 42, 2883, 2001.

136. Sabbatini, P. et al., A phase I/II study of PG-paclitaxel (CT-2103) in pts with recurrent ovarian, fallopian tube or peritoneal cancer, *Proc. Am. Soc. Clin. Oncol.*, 871, 2002.

137. Kudelka, A.P. et al., Preliminary report of a phase I study of escalating dose PG-paclitaxel (CT-2103) and fixed dose cisplatin in patients with solid tumors, *Proc. Am. Soc. Clin. Oncol.*, 2146, 2002.

138. Schulz, J. et al., Phase II study of CT-2103 in patients with colorectal cancer having recurrent disease after treatment with a 5-fluorouracil-containing regimen, *Proc. Am. Soc. Clin. Oncol.*, 2330, 2002.

139. De Vries, P. et al., Optimisation of CT-2106: a water soluble poly-L-glutamic acid (PG)-camptothecin conjugate with enhanced in vivo antitumor efficacy, *Proc. AACR-NCI-EORTC Int. Conf.*, 100, 2001.

140. Rowinsky, E.K. et al., A phase I and pharmacokinetic study of pegylated camptothecin as a 1-hour infusion every 3 weeks in patients with advanced solid malignancies, *J. Clin. Oncol.*, 21(1), 148, 2003.

141. Wang, D. et al., Cathepsin K inhibitor-polymer conjugates: potential drugs for the treatment of osteoporosis and rheumatoid arthritis, *Int. J. Pharm.*, 277(1–2), 73, 2004.

142. Wang, D. et al., Synthesis and evaluation of water-soluble polymeric bone-targeted drug delivery systems, *Bioconjugate Chem.*, 14(5), 853, 2003.

143. Ehrlich, P., *Studies in Immunity*, Plenum Press, New York, 1906.

12 Polymers Used for the Delivery of Genes in Gene Therapy

Pei Lee Kan, Andreas G. Schätzlein, and Ijeoma F. Uchegbu

CONTENTS

12.1 INTRODUCTION

The completion of the Human Genome Project [1] has moved us closer to understanding the genetic basis of disease and will doubtless provide more information on the interplay between genes and ill health. Genes are storage facilities, which serve as repositories for the amino acid sequences of the cell's workhorses — the proteins. Proteins, in turn, control cell physiology and cell biochemistry. Mutated genes can give rise to nonfunctional proteins or pathogenic proteins and ultimately disease. Such disease-causing genes may be used as therapeutic targets in gene therapy. Gene therapy is important not just because it is an alternative means of treating disease but also because it offers the hope of treatments for currently incurable diseases such as cystic fibrosis, sickle cell anemia, and cancer. Such diseases are either hereditary or acquired and can be either monogenetic in origin (due to the mutation of a single gene) or can originate from the malfunctioning of more than one gene. Examples of monogenetic diseases are cystic fibrosis [2], sickle cell anemia [3], and severe combined immune deficiency [4]; the exact genetic basis of diseases such as cancer is more complex and is typically the result of multiple mutations. In gene therapy, the therapeutic exogenous gene encodes for the replacement copy of a missing or faulty gene. Alternatively, as in the treatment of certain cancers, the therapeutic gene may encode for an enzyme capable of specific activation of a prodrug [5]. Another aspect of gene therapy is the use of genes as vaccines. Genes used in the prevention of infectious diseases are genes encoding for specific antigens that will ultimately produce prophylactic antibodies [6,7].

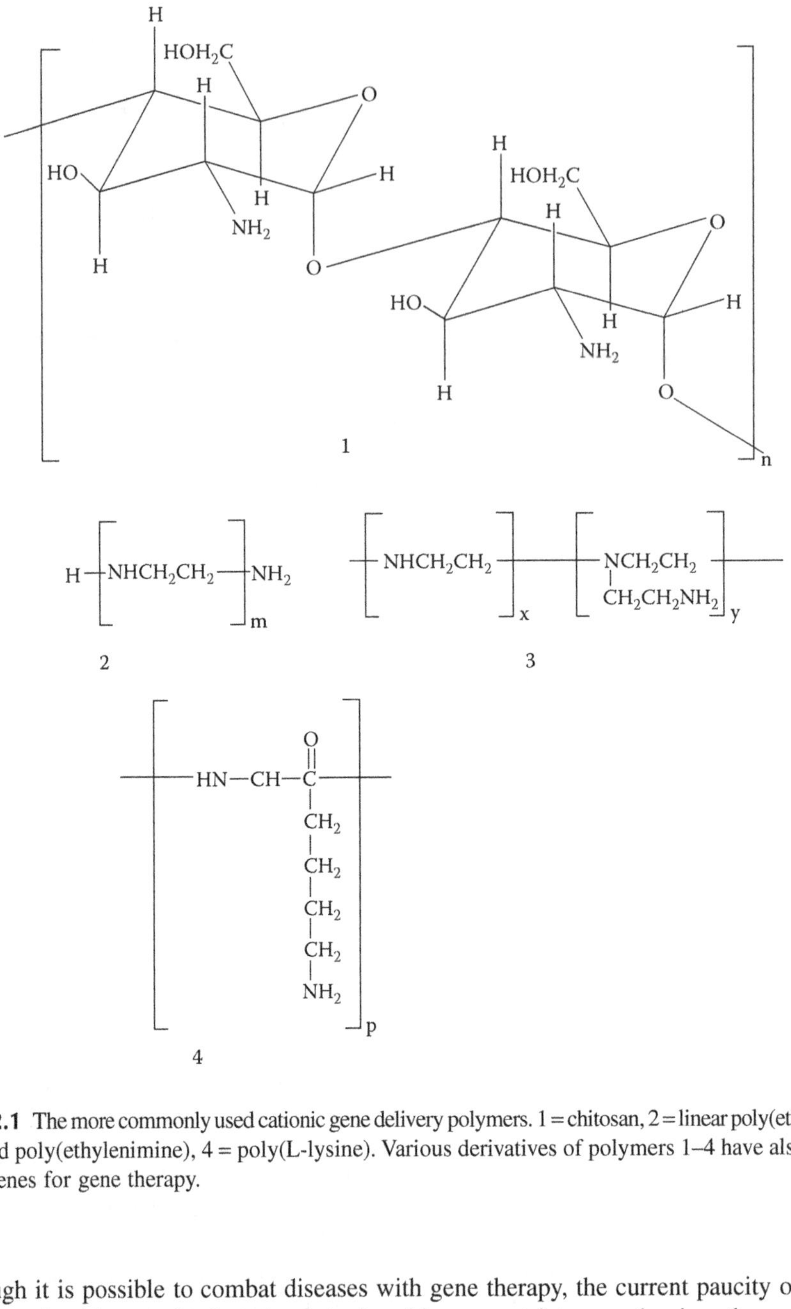

FIGURE 12.1 The more commonly used cationic gene delivery polymers. 1 = chitosan, 2 = linear poly(ethy lenimine), 3 = branched poly(ethylenimine), 4 = poly(L-lysine). Various derivatives of polymers 1–4 have also been used to deliver genes for gene therapy.

Although it is possible to combat diseases with gene therapy, the current paucity of marketed gene therapeutics hints at the fact that bringing this concept into practice is rather problematic. One key difficulty lies in the delivery of the therapeutic gene. The gene therapeutic, if administered for the treatment of a disease such as cancer or cystic fibrosis must evade degradation by extracellular nucleases, resist deactivation by other extracellular components, and traverse both the plasma and nuclear membranes intact in order to access the transcription machinery and produce the therapeutic protein. Each of these stages is fraught with a huge potential for failure, and to achieve effective gene therapy, these transport barriers must be overcome with the aid of delivery systems. It is in the delivery of genes that polymers are applied. Delivery systems fall into two main classes: viruses and synthetic compounds (nonviral systems). Nonviral gene delivery systems may be prepared from either polymers, lipids, or dendrimers [8].

Gene therapy is not a brand new concept; the first gene therapy clinical trial took place in May 1989 [9]. The trial involved cancer patients and gene transfer into human somatic cells using retroviruses as delivery systems in an *ex vivo* approach. Cells infected with the gene of interest were harvested and then reconstituted back into the patients. This clinical trial signaled the start of a long journey, and two years later the first nonviral gene therapy clinical trial was conducted [10]. Generally viral vectors are thought to have superior transfection efficiencies over that seen with nonviral vectors [11,12], and as such the former have been most frequently investigated in clinical trials [13]. However, serious safety issues have been associated with the use of viral vectors over the last five years, such as insertional mutagenesis with retroviral vectors [14] and a fatal response to the use of adenoviral gene delivery [15]. These events make the hunt for safe, effective and preferably nonviral gene-transfer systems even more important than was previously thought, especially as polymers, lipids, and dendrimers are envisaged to offer a superior safety profile to the use of viruses. That notwithstanding, the commercial launch of the viral gene medicine — Gendicine — in China is highly encouraging [16]. This gene therapeutic agent comprises an adenovirus carrying the p53 apoptosis causing gene that is injected locally into the tumor for the treatment of head and neck cancers. At the time of writing, this particular form of gene therapy is only licensed for use in China.

Currently gene therapy research is focused on achieving biodegradable gene delivery options that offer specificity of targeting to the desired cells on systemic administration, transfection efficiencies on par with viruses, and long-term gene expression by sustained-release mechanisms. In short, viral mimetics are sought. This chapter will focus on the role of polymers in achieving this aim.

Polymeric gene delivery systems (cationic) are usually positively charged at physiological pH [8], and the most commonly used polymers are shown in Figure 12.1. Cationic polymers, by virtue of their possession of protonable groups at physiological pH (amine groups), are able to undergo electrostatic interactions with DNA, the latter of which is anionic at physiological pH [8]. DNA is compacted within the electrostatic complex, a process termed DNA condensation, and the colloidal particles that result from this process are known as *polyplexes* (Figure 12.2). It is these polyplexes that enable the transport of DNA across the various biological barriers to its nuclear destination.

It is now appreciated that although the employment of polyplexes does aid the delivery of genes, the polyplexes themselves encounter a number of hurdles en route to the delivery of genes

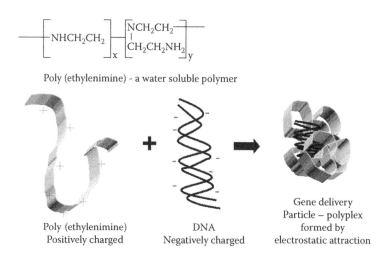

Poly (ethylenimine) - a water soluble polymer

| Poly (ethylenimine) Positively charged | DNA Negatively charged | Gene delivery Particle – polyplex formed by electrostatic attraction |

FIGURE 12.2 Polyplex formation on electrostatic binding of genes and polymers.

to target nuclei. Before considering the various polymers in detail, it is thus pertinent to first review the biological barriers to delivery encountered by DNA and its polymeric carriers.

12.2 BIOLOGICAL BARRIERS TO POLYMERIC GENE TRANSFER

Polymeric gene delivery systems carrying an exogenous gene payload face a number of biological barriers that hamper cellular entry of the therapeutic gene [5]. Biological barriers may be broadly classed as being of an extracellular (Figure 12.3a) and intracellular nature (Figure 12.3b). Examples of the extracellular barriers to gene delivery include: susceptibility to enzymatic degradation by nucleases in the serum and extracellular fluid [17], the presence of a mucus coat on certain cell surfaces [18], vulnerability to inactivation by interactions with blood components [19], the possibility of recognition and elimination by immunological defense systems [20], and the possibility of uptake by nontarget organs and tissues [21]. Once inside the cell the intracellular barriers to gene expression come into play, and these include: entrapment and degradation within the endosomes and lysosomes [22,23], vulnerability to cytoplasmic nuclease enzymatic attack [24], and the relative impenetrability of the nuclear membrane [25,26]. Once safely inside the nucleus the genes are transcribed to produce messenger RNA, which is, in turn, transported to the cytoplasm and eventually translated into the therapeutic protein. The biological barriers described here must be overcome in order to achieve a clinically relevant level of gene expression.

12.2.1 EXTRACELLULAR BARRIERS TO THE DELIVERY OF GENES IN GENE THERAPY

12.2.1.1 Interactions with Plasma and Blood Components

Upon entering the systemic circulation, the injected exogenous gene will be enzymatically degraded by the nucleases present in the serum [17]. However, upon incorporation of the gene within polyplexes, the gene does acquire some resistance to degradation by serum nucleases [27]. The polyplexes then need to travel to their target site of action. One factor that is crucial in allowing the polyplexes to travel unhindered to their target site is their particle size [28]. A colloidal (<1 µm) particle size is ideal. On intravenous injection of colloidal polyplexes, there is an interaction with serum proteins that leads to polyplex aggregation and an increase in particle size [19,21,29]. This size increase is believed to hinder transport through the fine capillaries and tissues, and results in polyplexes being entrapped within the first capillary bed encountered — that of the lung [19,21]. Exogenous gene expression is predominantly observed in the lung following intravenous administration of polyplexes [19,21]. It is clear that polyplexes must resist aggregation prior and subsequent to *in vivo* application [19,21,30]. However, most polyplexes tend to aggregate at physiological salt concentrations and are also bound by electrostatic attractions to negatively charged blood components such as serum proteins and blood cells [19,21]. Specifically, when negatively charged serum proteins are bound to the polyplexes, charge neutralization occurs, leading to an increase in polyplex particle size [21]. Such an increase in the size of the polyplex not only results in gene expression occurring predominantly in the lung but also ultimately reduces the level of gene transfer in the target region [19]. One other possible consequence of polyplexes interacting with serum proteins is that polyplexes may then be cleared along with other intravenously injected particulates from the blood by the macrophages of the reticuloendothelial system (in the liver, spleen, and bone marrow) [20]. Polyplex aggregation may be suppressed by the covalent attachment of poly(ethylene oxide) (poly(ethylene glycol) – PEG) moieties to the polyplex [19].

12.2.1.2 Uptake by the Target Cell

Even if the uncomplexed and naked therapeutic gene manages to evade devastation by the serum nucleases, it still needs to gain entry to the cell, the first barrier to penetration into the cell being posed by the inherent nature of the gene. DNA faces significant difficulty in entering the cells

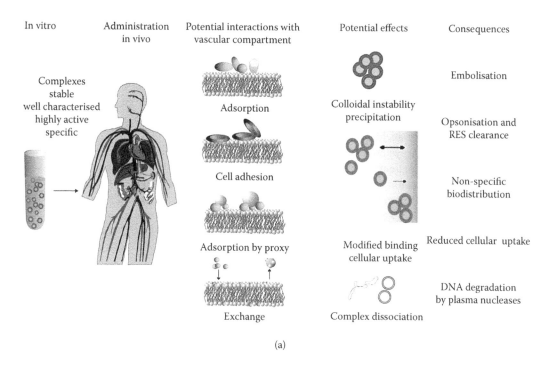

In vitro   Administration in vivo   Potential interactions with vascular compartment   Potential effects   Consequences

Complexes stable well characterised highly active specific

Adsorption

Cell adhesion

Adsorption by proxy

Exchange

Colloidal instability precipitation

Modified binding cellular uptake

Complex dissociation

Embolisation

Opsonisation and RES clearance

Non-specific biodistribution

Reduced cellular uptake

DNA degradation by plasma nucleases

(a)

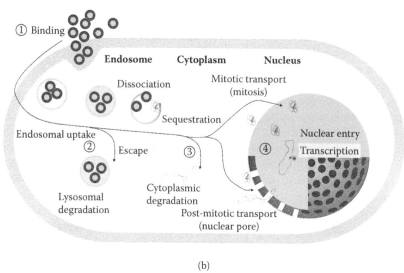

① Binding

Endosome   Cytoplasm   Nucleus

Dissociation

Mitotic transport (mitosis)

Sequestration

Endosomal uptake
②   Escape   ③

Nuclear entry
④ Transcription

Lysosomal degradation

Cytoplasmic degradation

Post-mitotic transport (nuclear pore)

(b)

FIGURE 12.3 Barriers to the delivery of therapeutic genes: (a) extracellular, (b) intracellular.

owing to its hydrophilic nature, large size, and polyanionic character. The surface charge of the cell membrane is negative [31], and it is envisaged that this cell surface will repel the approach of the large anionic DNA molecule. Polyplexes can assist in facilitating DNA uptake because they usually carry a positive charge due to the excess of positively charged polymer components they carry [8]. Via this positive charge, the polyplexes are able to interact with the anionic surface charge of the cells and facilitate endosomal uptake into the cell [32]. However, the electrostatic binding to the anionic cell surfaces is of a nonspecific nature, and can often lead to inefficiency in transfection because of electrostatic interactions with nontargeted cells when polyplexes are given by an intravenous route. These nonspecific interactions must be suppressed if gene expression with the exogenous gene is to be targeted to particular cells.

In order to increase the specificity of uptake into the target cells, homing devices are incorporated in the vector–DNA complex. Examples of such homing devices that are used to increase the specificity of recognition by the desired target cells include ligands such as galactose [33], antibodies [34], and transferrin [35]. These ligands will obviously be more efficient if the nonspecific interactions with blood components and cells are reduced. A commonly used strategy to reduce nonspecific interactions is the shielding of cationic surface charges using poly(ethylene oxide) moieties [19].

Additionally, certain systemic barriers to gene transfer are disease specific, e.g., in cystic fibrosis [36]. In cystic fibrosis patients, the thick mucus that coats the cystic fibrosis lung epithelium and the lack of specific receptors that may be exploited for receptor-mediated uptake has been cited as one of the key barriers to transfection, with mucus being a formidable barrier for the gene delivery particle to traverse [37]. Generally, although not specifically applied to polyplexes, strategies to overcome these barriers, such as the use of mucolytic agents, have had limited success [38].

12.2.2 INTRACELLULAR BARRIERS TO GENE TRANSFER

Upon arrival in the cell, the exogenous gene is once again faced with a number of hurdles that prevent it reaching the nucleus, which is the site of transcription. The polyplex is usually taken up by endocytosis, and DNA must escape from the endosome in order to avoid degradation, traverse the cytoplasm intact, and in turn cross the nuclear membrane to gain entry to the nucleus (Figure 12.3b).

12.2.2.1 Endosomal Escape

If the gene fails to escape from the endosome, the net result is a reduction in gene expression [28]. Some polyplexes can facilitate endosomal escape [39,40]. Cationic polyplexes prepared from cationic polymers such as poly(ethylenimine), by virtue of their high level of amino groups, are believed to act by buffering the acidic contents of these vacuoles [39–41]. The accompanying increase in the pH prevents the action of the degradative enzymes and eventually enables a rupture of the endosome by an increase in the ionic and latterly water content of the endosome [22,39–43]. The ionic content of the endosome is increased by an energy-driven influx of chloride ions and protons in response to the intraendosomal buffering by the polymer. This hypothesised mechanism of action by polyamines is termed *the proton sponge hypothesis*.

Peptides, although not strictly polymers, are also able to promote endosomal escape of gene-transfer systems, and a description of their actions is included here for completeness. Fusogenic peptides undergo a pH-triggered conformational change on entering the endosomes, which leads to membrane destabilisation and the release of entrapped DNA [23,44]. Examples of endosomolytic peptides are the viral peptides such as the amino-terminal domain of the influenza virus hemagglutinin HA2 subunit [23] and the synthetic mimics of amphiphilic anionic viral peptides [44].

12.2.2.2 Stability in the Cytoplasm

After escaping from the endosomes, DNA may be sequestered in the cytoplasm and subjected to the onslaught of cytoplasmic nucleases [24]. Microinjected plasmid DNA injected into the cytoplasm undergoes rapid degradation by cytoplasmic nucleases with an apparent half-life of 50 to 90 min [24]. The cytoplasm is a hostile environment for the exogenous gene, as exemplified by one study that reported that transgene expression was observed in 13% of the cells when 10000 copies of naked DNA were microinjected into the cytoplasm, whereas less than 10 copies of naked DNA were needed to induce the same level of gene expression when DNA was microinjected into the nucleus [45]. It is possible that polymeric gene delivery systems which protect DNA from nuclease degradation [46,47], may protect DNA from intracytoplasmic degradation.

12.2.2.3 Nuclear Import

Assuming that DNA remains stable within the cytoplasm, there is still a requirement for DNA to enter the nucleus for transcription to occur, and breaching the nuclear barrier is undoubtedly the most formidable challenge of all. The transport of DNA from the cytoplasmic medium into the nucleus is limited by the presence of the nuclear envelope. In dividing eukaryotic cells, nucleocytoplasmic transfer of DNA can occur when the nuclear envelope breaks down during mitosis [11]. Cells in the nondividing phase, however, are normally resistant to nucleocytoplasmic transfer of plasmid DNA [11]. In nondividing cells, the nucleocytoplasmic exchange of molecules occurs through the nuclear pore complexes (NPC) that span the nuclear envelope [48,49]. Hence, the nuclear envelope acts as a molecular sieve, enabling small aqueous molecules of up to 9 nm in diameter (<17-kDa) to diffuse freely through the NPC [49–52]. However, larger molecules of up to 25 nm (>41 kDa) such as plasmid DNA and larger DNA fragments undergo a sequence-specific active transport process involving multiple cellular components [49–52].

There is very little direct evidence that polymers actually assist the translocation of DNA or oligonucleotides to the nucleus. More common strategies include exploiting the nucleocytoplasmic transport machinery by modifying the plasmid DNA with specific sequences so that it can be recognized by cellular factors as a nuclear import substrate [53,54]. A common example of such modification is to attach a DNA nuclear localization signal (NLS), e.g., the simian virus 40 (SV40) enhancer domain, to the plasmid construct, aiding the recognition of these plasmid DNA constructs by transcription factors with subsequent nuclear import of the resultant complex [55]. The use of an SV40 enhancer sequence improves nuclear delivery *in vivo* and, in turn, gene transfer [53].

Furthermore, oligopeptide sequences known as NLS peptides, which direct transport to the nucleus, may be linked to plasmid DNA by the use of electrostatic attractions or covalent bonds [56–60]. The site for covalent attachment of NLS peptides to plasmid DNA has to be chosen with care, and the golden rule in this matter is to prevent binding of the NLS peptides to the expression cassette in order to ensure that the transcription ability of the transgene is preserved [61]. These NLS peptides are mainly composed of positively charged oligopeptides made up of sequences of lysine or arginine residues.

12.3 OVERCOMING THE BIOLOGICAL BARRIERS TO GENE TRANSFER

As can be appreciated from the foregoing account, some of the biological barriers highlighted above may be overcome with the aid of polymers. Although viruses are considered to be more efficient gene-transport systems than synthetic systems, the safety concerns associated with viral gene delivery [14,15] still mean that gene therapy would be best served by the use of synthetic materials that are as efficient as viruses. Desirable elements of such a vector would include: a polymer (cationic) sequence for DNA condensation, a stealth-type coating to evade detection by the macrophages of the reticuloendothelial system — preferably one that may be shed at the site of cell entry, a colloidal stabilizing entity to prevent colloidal instability in the blood and accumulation in lung capillaries, ligands facilitating cell-specific entry or the site-specific uncovering of a cationic surface to facilitate cell entry, an endosomolytic component that could also be a polycation, and finally NLS. Although synthetic viruses such as the ideal system described in the preceding text do not exist at present, various polymers have been evaluated for their ability to protect and deliver genes across the barriers outlined here, and these individual polymers are treated in the following text.

12.4 POLY(L-LYSINE)

The first cationic polymer-based gene delivery vehicle was poly(L-lysine), the use of which was first reported in 1987 [62]. In this pioneering effort, poly(L-lysine) was conjugated to asialoorosomucoid for targeted gene delivery to liver hepatocytes [62]. Since then a number of targeting ligands have been used to enable tissue- or pathology-specific gene expression, e.g., galactose for hepatocyte targeting [63,64], artery-wall-binding peptide for targeting the arteries [65], and both transferrin [35,66] and folate [67] for tumor targeting. A great deal of the knowledge gained early by working on poly(L-lysine) served to elucidate the problems confronting nonviral gene delivery and paved the way for the development of the more efficient systems that followed. This first-generation polymer can be said to have provided researchers with a valuable learning experience, although it is unlikely to feature as a gene delivery system in a marketed product. There are a number of reasons why poly(L-lysine) has not yet resulted in a synthetic gene therapeutic agent, some of which are detailed in the following text.

On its own, poly(L-lysine), although able to efficiently bind DNA, is not an effective gene-transfer agent [68] with adenovirus particles [69], histidyl residues [70], or lysomotropic agents such as chloroquine [71] being required for gene transfer to be observed. Additionally poly(L-lysine)-based polyplexes are associated with their own intrinsic cytotoxicity, and although this characteristic may be alleviated somewhat by glycosylation [73] or by converting the polymer to an amphiphile [68,72]; unnecessary cytotoxicity baggage associated with an intrinsic poor activity makes this polymer an unlikely first-choice material.

12.5 POLY(ETHYLENIMINE)

Poly(ethylenimine) (PEI; Figure 12.1) is one of the most efficient cationic polymer gene-transfer systems available, and although it has not yet been approved for clinical use, PEI anticancer gene formulations are able to achieve tumour regression through a combination of gene transfer [74] and an intrinsic antiproliferative activity [75]. PEI's *in vivo* gene-transfer ability has been proven on both local (intraventricular [76], intratracheal [77], and intratumoural [29]) and systemic [78] administration.

PEI exists in a number of molecular weight formats (0.42 to 800 kDa), and transfection efficiency is highest at a molecular weight of between 12 and 70 kDa [79,80] the most commonly used PEI molecular weight being 22 to 25 kDa [77,78]. Both linear and branched formats of the polymer exist (Figure 12.1); the linear molecule is a more efficient gene-transfer agent than the branched material [77,78,81], although the reason for this is unclear at present. Despite the fact that PEI is a successful gene-transfer agent for experimental animal studies, there have been reports of unacceptable toxicity with the use of this polymer [19,41,77,82]. Toxicity is undoubtedly modulated by reducing the quantity of protonable amine groups per molecule either through the attachment of poly(ethylene oxide) chains to PEI [83,84] or by the methylation of secondary and tertiary amines to give quaternary ammonium groups [84]. However, an improved biocompatibility with these two methods usually comes at the expense of a reduction in activity. Recently, low-molecular-weight (<2 kDa) cross-linked PEI, incorporating biodegradable cross-links holding individual molecules together, was shown to result in improved biocompatibility without the loss of gene-transfer activity [85], and the high-molecular-weight cross-linked material are believed to facilitate gene transfer into the cell with the degraded low-molecular-weight fragments resulting thereafter believed to be less toxic because of their low molecular weight.

Every third atom of the PEI molecule is nitrogen, resulting in a densely charged backbone composed of 25% primary, 50% secondary, and 25% tertiary amines. These amine groups are important for DNA binding and enabling the therapeutic transgene escape from the endosome on uptake into the cell [42]. The proton sponge hypothesis (see Subsection 12.2.2) has been put forward to explain the mechanism by which PEI enables escape of the exogenous gene from the endosome subsequent to cellular uptake.

Gene therapeutics may be administered locally or systemically but one of the problems associated with the systemic (intravenous) administration of cationic lipids and cationic polymers such as PEI is the fact that gene transfection occurs predominantly in the lung endothelium [78]. Among the nonviral systems, very few systems, such as the polypropylenimine dendrimers, have been found not to predominantly transfect the lung and instead to transfect the liver in mouse models [86]. This passive targeting to the lung is believed to follow aggregation of the polyplexes in the blood and their entrapment within the lung capillaries (see Subsection 12.2.1) [19]. Although transfection of the lung endothelial cells may sometimes be welcome, it is sometimes necessary to achieve gene expression in other areas such as tumors located at sites remote from the lung or the site of injection. To reduce the likelihood of passive lung targeting, poly(ethylene oxide) has been grafted on to PEI [83,87]. Conjugation of poly(ethylene oxide) units to PEI reduces the surface charge of the polyplexes and prevents their aggregation and localization within the lung capillaries [19,88,89]. However, although poly(ethylene oxide) chains improve the colloidal stability of these particulate formulations by providing a steric hindrance to particle aggregation [19,83], this strategy is often accompanied by diminished polyplex gene-transfer activity largely due to poor cellular uptake of the poly(ethylene oxide)-covered polyplex by cells [83,88]. It is thus necessary to apply a poly(ethylene oxide) coating as well as a ligand, promoting receptor mediated uptake, to counteract the poor cellular uptake problems (Figure 12.4a). Such a strategy has been used to produce a tumor necrosis factor-alpha gene medicine [74], with the iron transporter transferrin serving as the receptor-mediated uptake ligand. This targeted gene medicine was able to produce gene expression in tumors distant to the injection site and ultimately delay tumor progression (Figure 12.4b).

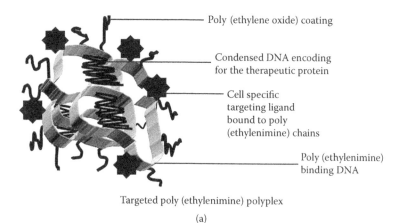

Poly (ethylene oxide) coating

Condensed DNA encoding for the therapeutic protein

Cell specific targeting ligand bound to poly (ethylenimine) chains

Poly (ethylenimine) binding DNA

Targeted poly (ethylenimine) polyplex

(a)

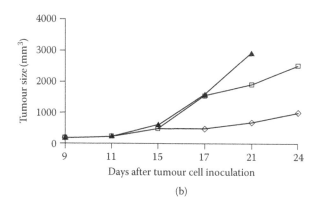

(b)

FIGURE 12.4 (a) Gene expression targeting after administration of a therapeutic gene may be achieved by coating polyplexes with covalently bound poly(ethylene oxide) and the use of targeting ligands; (b) the inhibition of tumour growth after the intravenous administration of PEI polyplexes to A/J mice bearing Neuro2a neuroblastoma. PEI polyplexes contained a plasmid coding for murine tumour necrosis factor-α ($\diamond$) or β-galactosidase ($\square$) and tumour growth was compared to that seen in an untreated group ($\blacktriangle$). (Reproduced with permission from Kircheis, R., Wightman, L., Kursa, M., Ostermann, E., and Wagner, E., Tumor-targeted gene delivery: an attractive strategy to use highly active effector molecules in cancer treatment, *Gene Ther.*, 9, 731–735, 2002.)

A variety of other PEI derivatives have been employed in an effort to improve the gene-transfer ability of PEI polyplexes. One such modification that has proved successful is the attachment of the NLS D-mellitin to PEI [90]. Other modifications, including the use of amphiphilic PEIs, have had limited success, with improvements in toxicity sometimes being observed but with no simultaneous improvements in gene-transfer efficiency [84,91–93]. In summary, it can be concluded that PEI is an efficient gene-transfer polymer that has proved its mettle in the pioneering work described by Kircheis et al. [74]; however, it appears that the cytotoxicity of this molecule is yet to be ameliorated to the extent that it may be considered as a suitable excipient candidate in the clinical development of gene therapeutics. What the field requires are derivatives that are orders of magnitude less cytotoxic than the current crop of PEIs but which also maintain the *in vivo* gene-transfer activity of the current molecules. Although improved biocompatibility has been demonstrated, very few studies have demonstrated improved biocompatibility with this polymer in conjunction with the preservation of the polymer's gene-transfer efficiency.

12.6 CHITOSAN

Chitosan (Figure 12.1) is a carbohydrate polymer, derived from chitin; the latter a by-product of the shellfish industry and was first reported as a gene delivery tool in the mid-1990s [94,95]. Chitosan is also one of the few agents, according to one report, that is capable of gene transfer via the oral route [7]. Chitosan is composed of N-acetyl-D-glucosamine and D-glucosamine monomers linked by $\beta(1,4)$glycosidic bonds. The presence of amino groups in chitosan gives it the ability to condense DNA. Chitosan is attractive as a gene delivery tool because of its good biocompatibility profile when compared to cationic liposomes [96–99], polyamine polymers [100], and polyamine dendrimers [98]. Chitosan is not as amine dense as poly(ethylenimine) or poly(L-lysine) (Figure 12.1), and this property could be responsible for its good biocompatibility and also possibly for its relatively poor gene-transfer ability [97,99,101–103]. Its favorable biocompatibility has prompted researchers to find ways to optimize gene transfer with this agent — controlling molecular weight appears to be the key; an optimum gene-transfer activity lies between a degree of polymerisation of 7 and 635 [103–106]. Additionally, increasing the charge density by incorporating a permanent positive charge in the molecule in the form of a trimethyl quaternary ammonium group appears to offer some marginal benefit [99], and the incorporation of targeting groups such as galactose improves targeting to hepatocytes [95,97]. Urocanic acid groups have aided gene transfer, the latter possibly by aiding endosomal escape [100]. However, chitosan, although able to achieve gene transfer to some extent, appears to lack the required level of efficiency that would be needed to allow it to be developed for the clinical delivery of genes.

12.7 OTHER GENE DELIVERY POLYMERS

The cationic polymers discussed earlier have so far served as key players in the gene delivery field, with poly(L-lysine) being the most studied of the poly(amino acid) class. Other polyamino acids with protonable nitrogen atoms, necessary for DNA binding, have also been studied; these include poly(L-histidine) [107] and poly(L-ornithine) [72] derivatives. In addition, various other polymers have been studied as gene-transfer systems. Among these are a group of biodegradable polymers, e.g., poly[α-(4-aminobutyl)-L-glycolic acid] [108–110], designed to degrade subsequent to having performed their delivery function. This strategy is aimed at minimizing the cytotoxicity associated with the accumulation of such agents within the cell, and hence is aimed at improving the biocompatibility of the gene-transfer agent. Other polymers that have been developed are thermosensitive ones designed to form a gel *in situ* on administration and thus provide a depot system capable of sustained DNA delivery [111].

12.8 CONCLUSION

In conclusion, a number of polymers by virtue of possessing a cationic charge at physiological pH have been found to be suitable candidates for the transfer of genes across the various biological barriers outlined in the preceding text. Although PEI and a few others have demonstrated the ability to bring about a therapeutic response in preclinical models, the search for efficient and safe gene delivery systems is far from over. We have achieved a modicum of success with these first-generation agents, although not to the degree warranted for the initiation of a clinical development program. The promise offered by gene therapy is so great that it is not possible to abandon hope just yet. It is feasible that a licensed nonviral gene therapeutic agent will emerge with a carrier drawn from the cationic lipid or cationic dendrimer class of agents; however, what has been learnt from these early studies on polymeric systems will continue to assist in the development of more efficient agents no matter from where such agents originate. An ideal gene delivery system has to be able to shuttle the gene safely to the nuclei of its target tissue with the travelling gene having limited encounters with degradative influences. We know that a cationic macromolecule can achieve this, and so long as its own inherent toxicity can be curtailed, it is likely that the first class of synthetic gene delivery agent that makes the clinical development journey may be a cationic macromolecule with targeting ability.

REFERENCES

1. McIlwain, C., World leaders heap praise on human genome landmark, *Nature,* 405, 983–984, 2000.
2. Porteous, D.J. and Dorin, J.R., Gene therapy for cystic fibrosis- where and when? *Hum. Mol. Genetic,* 2, 211–212, 1993.
3. Pawliuk, R.J., Westerman, K., Fabry, M.E., Payan, E., London, I.M., Bouhassira, E.E., Eaves, C.J., Humphries, K., Beuzard, Y., Nagel, R.L., and Leboulch, P., Correction of Sickle Cell Disease in transgenic mouse models by hematopoietic stem cell gene therapy, *Blood,* 98, 3247, 2001.
4. Cavazzana-Calvo, M., Hacein-Bey, S., de Saint Basile, G., Gross, F., Yvon, E., Nusbaum, P., Selz, F., Hue, C., Certain, S., Casanova, J.-L., Bousso, P., Le Deist, F., and Fischer, A., Gene therapy of human severe combined immunodeficiency (SCID)-X1 disease, *Science,* 288, 669–672, 2000.
5. Schatzlein, A.G., Non-viral vectors in cancer gene therapy: principles and progress, *Anti-Cancer Drug.,* 12, 275–304, 2001.
6. Pandha, H.S., Martin, L., Rigg, A.S., Ross, P., and Dalgleish, A.G., Gene therapy: recent progress in the clinical oncology arena, *Curr. Opin. Mol. Ther.,* 2, 362–375, 2000.
7. Roy, K., Mao, H.Q., Huang, S.K., and Leong, K.W., Oral gene delivery with chitosan-DNA nanoparticles generates immunologic protection in a murine model of peanut allergy, *Nat. Med.,* 5, 387–391, 1999.
8. Brown, M.D., Schatzlein, A.G., and Uchegbu, I.F., Gene delivery with synthetic (non viral) carriers, *Int. J. Pharm.,* 229, 1–21, 2001.
9. Rosenberg, S.A., Aebersold, P., Cornetta, K., Kasid, A., Morgan, R.A., Moen, R., Karson, E.M., Lotze, M.T., Yang, J.C., and Topalian, S.L., Gene transfer into humans-immunotherapy of patients with advanced melanoma, using tumor-infiltrating lymphocytes modified by retroviral gene transduction, *New Engl. J. Med.,* 323, 570–578, 1990.
10. Nabel, G.J., Nabel, E.G., Yang, Z.Y., Fox, B.A., Plautz, G.E., Gao, X., Huang, L., Shu, S., and Chang, A.E., Direct gene transfer with DNA-liposome complexes in melanoma: Expression, biologic activity, and lack of toxicity in humans, *Proc. Natl. Acad. Sci. USA,* 90, 11307–11311, 1993.
11. Brunner, S., Sauer, T., Carotta, S., Cotten, M., Saltik, M., and Wagner, E., Cell cycle dependence of gene transfer by lipoplex, polyplex and recombinant adenovirus, *Gene Ther.,* 7, 401–407, 2000.
12. Verma, I.M. and Somia, N., Gene therapy-promises, problems and prospects, *Nature,* 389, 239–242, 1997.
13. *Journal of Gene Medicine*, Gene Therapy Clinical Trials, http://www.wiley.co.uk/genetherapy/clinical, 2005.
14. Marshall, E., Second child in French trial is found to have leukemia, *Science,* 299, 320, 2003.
15. Marshall, E., Gene therapy death prompts review of adenovirus vector, *Science,* 286, 2244–2245, 2000.

16. Zhenzhen, L., Jiuchun, Z., Ke, W., Thorsteindsdottir, H., Quach, U., Singer, P.A., and Daar, A., Health biotechnology in China - reawakening of a giant, *Nat. Biotechnol.,* 22, DC13–DC18, 2004.

17. Hashida, M., Mahoto, R.I., Kawabata, K., Miyao, T., Nishikawa, M., and Takakura, Y., Pharmacokinetics and targeted delivery of proteins and genes, *J. Controlled Release,* 41, 91–97, 1996.

18. Alton, E.W., Geddes, D.M., Gill, D.R., Higgins, C.F., Hyde, S.C., Innes, J.A., and Porteous, D.J., Towards gene therapy for cystic fibrosis: a clinical progress report, *Gene Ther.,* 5, 291–292, 1998.

19. Ogris, M., Brunner, S., Schuller, S., Kircheis, R., and Wagner, E., PEGylated DNA/transferrin-PEI complexes: reduced interaction with blood components, extended circulation in blood and potential for systemic gene delivery, *Gene Ther.,* 6, 595–605, 1999.

20. Patel, H.M., Serum opsonins and liposomes: their interactions and opsonophagocytosis, *Crit. Rev. Ther. Drug Carrier Syst.,* 9, 39–90, 1992.

21. Dash, P.R., Read, M.L., Barrett, L.B., Wolfert, M.A., and Seymour, L.W., Factors affecting blood clearance and in vivo distribution of polyelectrolyte complexes for gene delivery, *Gene Ther.,* 6, 643–650, 1999.

22. Behr, J.P., The proton sponge: a means to enter cells viruses never thought of, *Med. Sci.,* 12, 56–58, 1996.

23. Wagner, E., Plank, C., Zatloukal, K., Cotton, M., and Birnstiel, M.L., Influenza virus hemagglutinin HA-2-N terminal fusogenic peptides augment gene transfer by transferrin-polylysine-DNA complexes: Towards a synthetic virus-like gene transfer vehicle, *Proc. Natl. Acad. Sci. USA,* 89, 7934–7938, 1992.

24. Lechardeur, D., Sohn, K.J., Haardt, M., Joshi, P.B., Monck, M., Graham, R.W., Beatty, B., Squire, J., Brodovich, H.O., and Lukacs, G.L., Metabolic stability of plasmid DNA in the cytosol: a potential barrier to gene transfer, *Gene Ther.,* 6, 482–497, 1999.

25. Zabner, J., Fasbender, A.J., Moninger, T., Poellinger, K.A., and Welsh, M.J., Cellular and molecular barriers to gene transfer by a cationic lipid, *J. Biol. Chem.,* 270, 18997–19007, 1995.

26. Goldfarb, D.S., Gariepy, J., Schoolnik, G., and Kornberg, D., Synthetic peptides as nuclear localization signals, *Nature,* 322, 641–644, 1986.

27. Chiou, H.C., Tangco, M.V., Levine, S.M., Robertson, D., Kormis, K., Wu, C.H., and Wu, G.Y., Enhanced resistance to nuclease degradation of nucleic acids complexed to asialoglycoprotein-polylysine carriers, *Nucl. Acid. Res.,* 22, 5439–5446, 1994.

28. Nishikawa, M. and Huang, L., Nonviral vectors in the new millennium: delivery barriers in gene transfer, *Hum. Gene Ther.,* 12, 861–870, 2001.

29. Coll, J.L., Chollet, P., Brambilla, E., Desplanques, D., Behr, J.P., and Favrot, M., *In vivo* delivery of tumours of DNA complexed with linear polyethylenimine, *Hum. Gene Ther.,* 10, 1659–1666, 1999.

30. Kircheis, R., Wightman, L., and Wagner, E., Design and gene delivery activity of modified polyethylenimines, *Adv. Drug Delivery Rev.,* 53, 341–358, 2001.

31. Singh, A.K., Kasinath, B.S., and Lewis, E.J., Interactions of polycations with cell-surface negative charges of epithelial cells, *Biochim. Biophys. Acta,* 1120, 337–342, 1992.

32. Mislick, K.A. and Baldeschwieler, J.D., Evidence of the role of proteoglycans in cation-mediated gene transfer, *Proc. Natl. Acad. Sci. USA,* 93, 12349–12354, 1996.

33. Plank, C., Zatloukal, K., Cotton, M., Mechtler, K., and Wagner, E., Gene transfer into hepatocytes using a asialoglycoprotein receptor mediated endocytosis of DNA complexed with an artificial tetra-antennary galactose ligand, *Bioconjugate Chem.,* 3, 533–539, 1992.

34. Trubetskoy, V.S., Torchilin, V.P., Kennel, S.J., and Huang, L., Use of N-terminated modified poly(L-lysine)-antibody conjugate as a carrier for targeted gene delivery in mouse lung endothelial cells, *Bioconjugate Chem.,* 3, 323–327, 1992.

35. Wagner, E., Zenke, M., Cotten, M., Beug, H., and Birnstiel, M.L., Transferrin-polycation conjugates as carriers for DNA uptake into cells, *Proc. Natl. Acad. Sci. USA,* 87, 3410–3414, 1990.

36. Pilewski, J.M., Gene therapy for airway diseases-continued progress towards identifying and overcoming barriers to efficiency, *Am. J. Respir. Cell Mol. Biol.,* 27, 117–121, 2002.

37. Ferrari, S., Geddes, D.M., and Alton, E., Barriers to and new approaches for gene therapy and gene delivery in cystic fibrosis, *Adv. Drug Del. Rev.,* 54, 1373–1393, 2002.

38. Ferrari, S., Kitson, C., Farley, R., Steel, R., Marriott, C., Parkins, D.A., Scarpa, M., Wainwright, B., Evans, M.J., Colledge, W.H., Geddes, D.M., and Alton, E., Mucus altering agents as adjuncts for non viral gene transfer to airway epithelium, *Gene Ther.,* 8, 1380–1386, 2001.

39. Akinc, A., Thomas, M., Klibanov, A.M., and Langer, R., Exploring polyethylenimine-mediated DNA transfection and the proton sponge hypothesis, *J. Gene Med.,* 7, 657–663, 2005.

40. Boussif, O., Zanta, M.A., and Behr, J.P., Optimized galenics improve in vitro gene transfer with cationic molecules up to 1000-fold, *Gene Ther.*, 3, 1074–1080, 1996.

41. Boussif, O., Lezoualc'h, F., Zanta, M.A., Mergny, M.D., Scherman, D., Demeneix, B., and Behr, J.P., A versatile vector for gene and oligonucleotide transfer into cells in culture and in vivo: polyethylenimine, *Proc. Natl. Acad. Sci. USA*, 92, 7297–7301, 1995.

42. Remy, J.S., Bassima, A., Zanta, M.A., Boussif, O., Behr, J.P., and Demeneix, B., Gene transfer with lipospermine and polyethyleneimines, *Adv. Drug Del. Rev.*, 30, 85–95, 1998.

43. Sonawane, N.D., Szoka, F.C., and Verkman, A.S., Chloride accumulation and swelling in endosomes enhances DNA transfer by polyamine-DNA polyplexes, *J. Biol. Chem.*, 278, 44826–44831, 2003.

44. Murthy, N., Robinchaud, J.R., Tirrell, D.A., Stayton, P.S., and Hoffman, A.S., The design and synthesis of polymers for eukaryotic membrane disruption, *J. Controlled Release*, 61, 137–143, 1999.

45. Pollard, H., Remy, J.S., Loussouarn, G., Demolombe, S., Behr, J.P., and Escanade, D., Polyethylenimine but not cationic lipids promotes transgene delivery to the nucleus in mammalian cells, *J. Biol. Chem.*, 273, 7507–7511, 1998.

46. Goh, S.L., Murthy, N., Xu, M.C., and Frechet, J.M.J., Cross-linked microparticles as carriers for the delivery of plasmid DNA for vaccine development, *Bioconjugate Chem.*, 15, 467–474, 2004.

47. Brus, C., Petersen, H., Aigner, A., Czubayko, F., and Kissel, T., Efficiency of polyethylenimines and polyethylenimine-graft-poly (ethylene glycol) block copolymers to protect oligonucleotides against enzymatic degradation, *Eur. J. Pharm. Biopharm.*, 57, 427–430, 2004.

48. Kreiss, P., Cameron, B., Rangara, R., Mailhe, P., Aguerre-Charriol, O., Airiau, M., Scherman, D., Crouzet, J., and Pitard, B., Plasmid DNA size does not affect the physicochemical properties of lipoplexes but modulates gene transfer efficiency, *Nucl. Acid Res.*, 27, 3792–3798, 1999.

49. Ludtke, J.J., Zhang, G., Sebestyen, M.G., and Wolff, J.A., A nuclear localization signal can enhance both the nuclear transport and expression of 1 kb DNA, *J. Cell Sci.*, 112, 2033–2041, 1999.

50. Nigg, E.A., Nucleocytoplasmic transport: signals, mechanism and regulation, *Nature*, 386, 779–787, 1997.

51. Ohno, M., Fornerod, M., and Mattaj, I.W., Nucleocytoplasmic transport: the last 200 nanometers, *Cell*, 92, 327–336, 1998.

52. Peters, R., Lang, I., Scholz, M., Schulz, B., and Kayne, F., Fluorescence microphotolysis to measure nucleocytoplasmic transport in vivo and in vitro, *Biochem. Soc. Trans.*, 14, 821–822, 1986.

53. Young, J.L., Benoit, J.N., and Dean, D.A., Effect of a DNA nuclear targeting sequence on gene transfer and expression of plasmids in the intact vasculature, *Gene Ther.*, 10, 1465–1470, 2003.

54. Vacik, J., Dean, B.S., Zimmer, W.E., and Dean, D.A., Cell-specific nuclear import of plasmid DNA, *Gene Ther.*, 6, 1006–1014, 1999.

55. Wilson, G.L., Dean, B.S., Wang, G., and Dean, D.A., Nuclear import of plasmid DNA in digitonin-permeabilized cells requires both cytoplasmic factors and specific DNA sequences, *J. Biol. Chem.*, 274, 22025–22032, 1999.

56. Aronsohn, A.I. and Hughes, J.A., Nuclear localization signal peptides enhance cationic liposome-mediated gene therapy, *J. Drug Target.*, 5, 163–169, 1998.

57. Schwartz, B., Innov, M.A., Pitard, B., Escriou, V., Rangara, R., Byk, G., Wils, P., Crouzet, J., and Scherman, D., Synthetic DNA-compacting peptides derived from human sequence enhance cationic lipid-mediated gene transfer in vitro and in vivo, *Gene Ther.*, 6, 282–292, 1999.

58. Zanta, M.A., Belguise-Valladier, P., and Behr, J.P., Gene delivery: a single nuclear localization peptide is sufficient to carry DNA to the cell nucleus, *Proc. Natl. Acad. Sci. USA*, 96, 91–96, 1999.

59. Adam, S.A. and Gerace, L., Cytosolic proteins that specifically bind nuclear localization signals are receptors for nuclear import, *Cell*, 66, 837–847, 1991.

60. Robbins, J., Dilworth, S.M., Laskey, R.A., and Dingwall, C., Two independent basic domains in nucleoplasmin nuclear targeting sequence: identification of a class of bipartite nuclear targeting sequence, *Cell*, 64, 615–623, 1991.

61. Cartier, R. and Reszka, R., Utilization of synthetic peptides containing nuclear localization signals for non viral gene transfer systems, *Gene Ther.*, 9, 157–167, 2002.

62. Wu, G.Y. and Wu, C.H., Receptor-mediated in vitro gene transformation by a soluble DNA carrier system, *J. Biol. Chem.*, 262, 4429–4432, 1987.

63. Han, J. and Yeom, Y.I., Specific gene transfer mediated by galactosylated poly-L-lysine into hepatoma cells, *Int. J. Pharm.*, 202, 151–160, 2000.

64. Perales, J.C., Ferkol, T., Beegen, H., Ratnoff, O.D., and Hanson, R.W., Gene transfer in vivo: sustained expression and regulation of genes introduced into the liver by receptor-targeted uptake, *Proc. Natl. Acad. Sci. USA,* 91, 4086–4090, 1994.

65. Nah, J.-W., Yu, L., Han, S.O., Ahn, C.H., and Kim, S.W., Artery wall binding peptide-poly(ethylene glycol)-grafted-poly(L-lysine)-based gene delivery to artery wall cells, *J. Controlled Release,* 78, 273–284, 2002.

66. Cotten, M., Langle-Rouault, F., Kirlappos, H., Wagner, E., Mechtler, M., Zenke, M., Beug, H., and Birnstiel, M.L., Transferrin-polycation-mediated introduction of DNA into human leukemic cells: stimulation by agents that affect the survival of transfected DNA or modulate transferrin receptor levels, *Proc. Natl. Acad. Sci. USA,* 87, 4033–4037, 1990.

67. Mislick, K.A., Baldeschwieler, J.D., Kayyem, J.F., and Meade, T.J., Transfection of folate-polylysine DNA complexes: evidence for lysosomal delivery, *Bioconjugate Chem,* 6, 512–515, 1995.

68. Brown, M.D., Schatzlein, A., Brownlie, A., Jack, V., Wang, W., Tetley, L., Gray, A.I., and Uchegbu, I.F., Preliminary characterization of novel amino acid based polymeric vesicles as gene and drug delivery agents, *Bioconjugate Chem.,* 11, 880–891, 2000.

69. Curiel, D.T., Agarwal, S., Wagner, E., and Cotton, M., Adenovirus enhancement of transferrin-polylysine-mediated gene delivery, *Proc. Natl. Acad. Sci. USA,* 88, 8850–8854, 1991.

70. Midoux, P. and Monsigny, M., Efficient gene transfer by histidylated poly-L-Lysine/pDNA complexes, *Bioconjugate Chem.,* 10, 406–411, 1999.

71. Pouton, C.W., Lucas, P., Thomas, B.J., Uduehi, A.N., Milroy, D.A., and Moss, S.H., Polycation-DNA complexes for gene delivery: a comparison of the biopharmaceutical properties of cationic polypeptides and cationic lipids, *J. Controlled Release,* 53, 289–299, 1998.

72. Brown, M.D., Gray, A.I., Tetley, L., Santovena, A., Rene, J., Schatzlein, A.G., and Uchegbu, I.F., In vitro and in vivo gene transfer with polyamino acid vesicles, *J. Controlled Release,* 93, 193–211, 2003.

73. Boussif, O., Delair, T., Brua, C., Veron, L., Pavirani, A., and Kolbe, H.V., Synthesis of polyallylamine derivatives and their use as gene transfer vectors *in vitro, Bioconjugate Chem.,* 10, 877–883, 1999.

74. Kircheis, R., Wightman, L., Kursa, M., Ostermann, E., and Wagner, E., Tumor-targeted gene delivery: an attractive strategy to use highly active effector molecules in cancer treatment, *Gene Ther.,* 9, 731–735, 2002.

75. Dufes, C., Keith, N., Bisland, A., Proutski, I., Uchegbu, I.F., and Schatzlein, A.G., Synthetic anti-cancer gene medicine exploiting intrinsic anti-tumour activity of cationic vector to cure established tumours, *Cancer Res.,* 65, 8079–8084, 2005.

76. Goula, D., Remy, J.S., Erbacher, P., Wasowicz, M., Levi, G., Abdallah, B., and Demeneix, B.A., Size, diffusibility and transfection performance of linear PEI/DNA complexes in the mouse central nervous system, *Gene Ther.,* 5, 712–717, 1998.

77. Ferrari, S., Moro, E., Pettenazzo, A., Behr, J.P., Zacchello, F., and Scarpa, M., ExGen 500 is an efficient vector for gene delivery to lung epithelial cells in vitro and in vivo, *Gene Ther.,* 4, 1100–1106, 1997.

78. Bragonzi, A., Boletta, A., Biffi, A., Muggia, A., Sersale, G., Cheng, S.H., Bordignon, C., Assael, B.M., and Conese, M., Comparison between cationic polymers and lipids in mediating systemic gene delivery to the lungs, *Gene Ther.,* 6, 1995–2004, 1999.

79. Godbey, W.T., Wu, K.K., and Mikos, A.G., Size matters: molecular weight affects the efficiency of poly(ethylenimine) as a gene delivery vehicle, *J. Biomed. Mater. Res.,* 45, 268–275, 1999.

80. Fischer, D., Bieber, T., Li, Y., Elsasser, H.P., and Kissel, T., A novel non-viral vector for DNA delivery based on low molecular weight, branched polyethylenimine: effect of molecular weight on transfection efficiency and cytotoxicity, *Pharm. Res.,* 16, 1273–1279, 1999.

81. Wightman, L., Kircheis, R., Rossler, V., Carotta, S., Ruzicka, R., Kursa, M., and Wagner, E., Different behavior of branched and linear polyethylenimine for gene delivery in vitro and in vivo, *J. Gene Med.,* 3, 362–372, 2001.

82. Godbey, W.T., Wu, K.K., and Mikos, A.G., Poly(ethylenimine)-mediated gene delivery affects endothelial cell function and viability, *Biomaterials,* 22, 471–480, 2001.

83. Kichler, A., Chillon, M., Leborgne, C., Danos, O., and Frisch, B., Intranasal gene delivery with a polyethylenimine-PEG conjugate, *J. Controlled Release,* 81, 379–388, 2002.

84. Brownlie, A., Uchegbu, I.F., and Schatzlein, A.G., PEI based vesicle-polymer hybrid gene delivery system with improved biocompatibility, *Int. J. Pharm.,* 274, 41–52, 2004.

85. Thomas, M., Ge, Q., Lu, J.J., Chen, J.Z., and Klibanov, A.M., Cross-linked small polyethylenimines: While still nontoxic, deliver DNA efficiently to mammalian cells in vitro and in vivo, *Pharm. Res.*, 22, 373–380, 2005.

86. Schatzlein, A.G., Zinselmeyer, B.H., Elouzi, A., Dufes, C., Chim, Y.T.A., Roberts, C.J., Davies, M.C., Munro, A., Gray, A.I., and Uchegbu, I.F., Preferential liver gene expression with polypropylenimine dendrimers, *J. Controlled Release*, 101, 247–258, 2005.

87. Tang, G.P., Zeng, J.M., Gao, S.J., Ma, Y.X., Shi, L., Li, Y., Too, H.P., and Wang, S., Polyethylene glycol modified polyethylenimine for improved CNS gene transfer effects of PEGylation extent, *Biomaterials*, 24, 2351–2362, 2003.

88. Nguyen, H.K., Lemieux, P., Vinogradov, S.V., Gebhart, C.L., Guerin, N., Paradis, G., Bronich, T.K., Alakhov, V.Y., and Kabanov, A.V., Evaluation of polyether-polyethyleneimine graft copolymers as gene transfer agents, *Gene Ther.*, 7, 126–138, 2000.

89. Sung, S.-J., Min, S.H., Cho, K.Y., Lee, S., Min, Y.J., Yeom, Y.I., and Park, J.-K., Effect of polyethylene glycol on gene delivery of polyethylenimine, *Biol. Pharm. Bull.*, 26, 492–500, 2003.

90. Ogris, M., Carlisle, R.C., Bettinger, T., and Seymour, L.W., Melittin enables efficient vesicular escape and enhanced nuclear access of nonviral gene delivery vectors, *J. Biol. Chem.*, 276, 47550–47555, 2001.

91. Han, S.-O., Mahato, R.I., and Kim, S.W., Water-soluble lipopolymer for gene delivery, *Bioconjugate Chem.*, 12, 337–345, 2001.

92. Thomas, M. and Klibanov, A.M., Enhancing polyethylenimine's delivery of plasmid DNA into mammalian cells, *Proc. Natl. Acad. Sci. USA*, 99, 14640–14645, 2002.

93. Wang, D.-A., Narang, A.S., Kotb, M., Gaber, A.O., Miller, D.D., Kim, S.W., and Mahato, R.I., Novel branched poly(ethylenimine)-cholesterol water soluble lipopolymers for gene delivery, *Biomacromolecules*, 3, 1197–1207, 2002.

94. Mumper, R.J., Wang, J., Claspell, J.M., and Rolland, A.P., Novel polymeric condensing carriers for gene delivery, *Proceed. Int. Symp. Controlled Release Bioact. Mater.*, 22, 178–179, 1995.

95. Murata, J., Ohya, Y., and Ouchi, T., Possibility of application of quaternary chitosan having pendant galactose residues as gene delivery tool, *Carbohydr. Polymer.*, 29, 69–74, 1996.

96. Corsi, K., Chellat, F., Yahia, L., and Fernandes, J.C., Mesenchymal stem cells, MG63 and HEK293 transfection using chitosan-DNA nanoparticles, *Biomaterials*, 24, 1255–1264, 2003.

97. Gao, S.Y., Chen, J.N., Xu, X.R., Ding, Z., Yang, Y.H., Hua, Z.C., and Zhang, J.F., Galactosylated low molecular weight chitosan as DNA carrier for hepatocyte-targeting, *Int. J. Pharm.*, 255, 57–68, 2003.

98. Li, X.W., Lee, D.K.L., Chan, A.S.C., and Alpar, H.O., Sustained expression in mammalian cells with DNA complexed with chitosan nanoparticles, *Biochim. Biophys. Acta*, 1630, 7–18, 2003.

99. Thanou, M., Florea, B.I., Geldof, M., Junginger, H.E., and Borchard, G., Quaternized chitosan oligomers as novel gene delivery vectors in epithelial cell lines, *Biomaterials*, 23, 153–159, 2002.

100. Kim, T.H., Ihm, J.E., Choi, Y.J., Nah, J.W., and Cho, C.S., Efficient gene delivery by urocanic acid-modified chitosan, *J. Controlled Release*, 93, 389–402, 2003.

101. Leong, K.W., Mao, H.Q., Truong-Le, V., Roy, K., Walsh, S.M., and August, J.T., DNA-polycation nanospheres as non-viral gene delivery vehicles, *J. Controlled Release*, 53, 183–193, 1998.

102. Erbacher, P., Zou, S., Bettinger, T., Steffan, A.M., and Remy, J.S., Chitosan-based vector/DNA complexes for gene delivery: biophysical characteristics and transfection ability, *Pharm. Res.*, 15, 1332–1339, 1998.

103. MacLaughlin, F.C., Mumper, R.J., Wang, J.J., Tagliaferri, J.M., Gill, I., Hinchcliffe, M., and Rolland, A.P., Chitosan and depolymerized chitosan oligomers as condensing carriers for in vivo plasmid delivery, *J. Controlled Release*, 56, 259–272, 1998.

104. Ishii, T., Okahata, Y., and Sato, T., Mechanism of cell transfection with plasmid/chitosan complexes, *Biochim. Biophys. Acta*, 1514, 51–64, 2001.

105. Sato, T., Ishii, T., and Okahata, Y., In vitro gene delivery mediated by chitosan: effect of pH, serum, and molecular mass of chitosan on the transfection efficiency, *Biomaterials*, 22, 2075–2080, 2001.

106. Uchegbu, I.F., Sadiq, L., Pardakhty, A., El-Hammadi, M., Gray, A.I., Tetley, L., Wang, W., Zinselmeyer, B.H., and Schätzlein, A.G., Gene transfer with three amphiphilic glycol chitosans — the degree of polymerisation is the main controller of transfection efficacy, *J. Drug Target.*, 12, 527–539, 2004.

107. Putnam, D., Zelikin, A.N., Izumrudov, V.A., and Langer, R., Polyhistidine-PEG: DNA nanocomposites for gene delivery, *Biomaterials*, 24, 4425–4433, 2003.

108. Lim, Y.B., Han, S.O., Kong, H.U., Lee, Y., Park, J.S., Jeong, B., and Kim, S.W., Biodegradable polyester, poly alpha-(4 aminobutyl)-L-glycolic acid, as a non-toxic gene carrier, *Pharm. Res.,* 17, 811–816, 2000.

109. Lee, M., Ko, K.S., Oh, S., and Kim, S.W., Prevention of autoimmune insulitis by delivery of a chimeric plasmid encoding interleukin-4 and interleukin-10, *J. Controlled Release,* 88, 333–342, 2003.

110. Maheshwari, A., Han, S., Mahato, R.I., and Kim, S.W., Biodegradable polymer-based interleukin-12 gene delivery: role of induced cytokines, tumor infiltrating cells and nitric oxide in anti-tumor activity, *Gene Ther.,* 9, 1075–1084, 2002.

111. Hinrichs, W.L., Schuurmans-Nieuwenbroek, N.M.E., van de Wetering, P., and Hennink, W.E., Thermosensitive polymers as carriers for gene delivery, *J. Controlled Release,* 60, 249–259, 1999.

13 Dendrimers in Drug and Gene Delivery

Christine Dufès, Ijeoma F. Uchegbu,
and Andreas G. Schätzlein

CONTENTS

13.1 OVERVIEW

Herman Staudinger's realization that macromolecules consisted not, as previously thought, of aggregates but were in fact long, chain-like molecules, started a long journey of discovery, which has since led to a wide array of new polymeric materials that have affected every aspect of our lives (for a broad historical overview, see Reference 1). Compared to these linear polymers, which have for a long time been the main focus of polymer chemists, dendrimers are relative newcomers. Nevertheless, because of their special properties, these dendritic polymers have received widespread attention in the last two decades.

Dendrimers (from the Greek "dendron," meaning tree, and "meros," meaning part) are highly ordered, branched monodisperse macromolecules [3]. Such dendritic structures first emerged in a new class of polymers named *cascade molecules*, initially reported by Vögtle et al. at the end of the 1970s [4]. Further development by Tomalia et al. [5], as well as Newkome's group [6,7], gave rise to larger dendritic structures. These hyper-branched molecules were called *dendrimers* or *arborols* (from the Latin "arbor" for tree). For a historical perspective, see Reference 8.

Since their conception in the late 1970s and early 1980s, the unique properties of dendrimers have spawned a whole range of new research areas ranging from drug and gene delivery applications to processing, diagnostics, and nanoengineering [8]. Their unique molecular architecture means that dendrimers have a number of distinctive properties that differentiate them from other polymers; specifically, the stepwise synthesis approach means that they tend to be monodisperse with a well-defined size and structure. The chemistry of dendrimers is quite adaptable and allows synthesis of a broad range of molecules with different properties.

Therefore, dendrimers lend themselves to nanoengineering of a variety of materials that take advantage of these properties. Examples include applications in drug and gene delivery, imaging, boron neutron capture therapy, and various biotechnological diagnostics and sensing functions. This chapter will give an overview of the physical, chemical, and biological properties of the more important dendrimer materials and their use in drug and gene delivery applications. For more general reviews, see Reference 9 and Reference 10.

13.2 STRUCTURE AND SYNTHESIS

The classical polymerization processes used for the production of most of the conventional polymers produces molecules with a statistical distribution of the degree of polymerization and molecular weight, which is reflected in a high degree of polydispersity, i.e., $M_w/M_n > 2$–10.

By contrast, the chemistry of dendritic molecules is based on controlled, stepwise synthesis, which tends to create practically monodisperse macromolecules with well-defined size and molecular mass [2].

Dendrimers are three-dimensional macromolecules with a basic structure that resembles trees, i.e., they possess a "root" based on a core molecule with 2+ symmetry to which the dendritic trees ("dendrons") are attached (Figure 13.1). The tree architecture is based on a repeat sequence of simple branched monomer units. The synthetic approaches that lead to these structures fall into two classes, depending on whether the synthesis occurs from the root to the branches (divergent) or from the branches toward the root (convergent) (Figure 13.2).

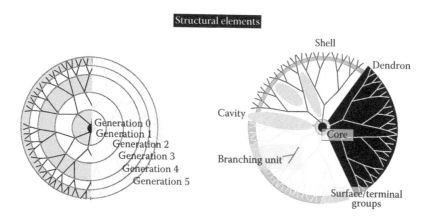

FIGURE 13.1 Dendrimer structure. The stepwise synthesis of dendrimers means that they have a well-defined hierarchical structure. This hypothetical dendrimer is based on a core with three covalent root attachment points, but other common cores have di- or tetracovalent cores. The valency of the core dictates the number of linked dendrons and the overall symmetry of the molecule. The dendrons are synthesized by covalent coupling of the branch units. For each additional layer or generation that is being added to the structure, the reaction sequence is repeated. In this case, the units have two new branching points at which additional units can be attached. (The generation count is not always consistent: normally generation 0 refers to the core, although sometimes it is used to describe the dendrimer after the first reaction cycle.) The number of branching points, branching angles, and the length of the branching units determine to what extent each generation increases molecular volume vs. surface area. For the higher generations, the density of the terminal groups reaches a point where, for steric reasons, no further groups can be added (starburst effect). Dendrimers of higher generation also have a typical molecular density profile under favorable conditions; the high peripheral molecular density establishes a steric outer shell and the lower density at the centre creates cavities that can accommodate guest molecules.

Mathematical description of dendrimer structure is as follows:

$$\text{Number of surface groups} \quad (Z) = N_c N_b^G$$

$$\text{Number of branched cells} \quad (BC) = N_c \left[\frac{N_b^G - 1}{N_b - 1} \right] = \text{ Number of bonds/generation}$$

$$\text{Molecular Weight} \quad (MW) = M_c + N_c \left[M_{RU} \left(\frac{N_b^G - 1}{N_b - 1} \right) + M_t N_b^G \right]$$

These equations are applicable to a PAMAM with EDA core, where N_c is the core cell multiplicity, N_b, the branch cell multiplicity, and G, the generation [2].

13.2.1 DENDRIMER CHEMISTRY

The basic building blocks for the dendrimers are based on a multivalent root or core to which two or more branches can be reacted with each generation. A large variety of dendrimer building blocks have been reported (reviewed more extensively in, e.g., Reference 9 and Reference 11) with different cores, branching units, and end groups of organic, inorganic, or organometallic origin.

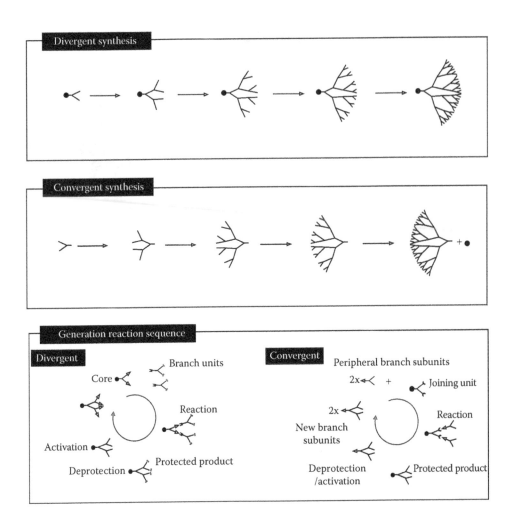

FIGURE 13.2 Dendrimer synthesis strategies. *Synthetic strategies for dendrimers are based on the conceptually different divergent and convergent approaches.* In the divergent method, the dendrimer is synthesized from the multifunctional core as the starting point and built up one monomer layer, or generation, at a time (see Reference 210, Tomalia, D.A. et al., Dendritic macromolecules — synthesis of starburst dendrimers, *Macromolecules*, 19(9): 2466–2468, 1986). The core molecule reacts with monomer molecules containing one reactive group and two (or more) inactive groups. The reactive group reacts with one of the roots of the core molecule, giving the first-generation dendrimer. After activation of the inactive groups at the periphery of the molecule, the reaction sequence is repeated with the next generation of monomers. The process is repeated for several generations until steric effects prevent further reactions of the end groups (starburst effect). In the convergent approach also, the dendrimer is built up layer after layer but, this time, starting from the end groups and terminating at the core (see Reference 211, Hawker, C.J. and Frechet, J.M.J., Preparation of polymers with controlled molecular architecture — a new convergent approach to dendritic macromolecules, *J. Am. Chem. Soc.*, 112(21): 7638–7647, 1990). Here two (or more) peripheral branch subunits are reacted with a single joining unit that has two (or more) corresponding active sites and a distal inactive site. The product is a new larger branch subunit that is again reacted with a joining unit. When the growing branched polymeric dendrons have reached target size they are, in turn, attached to a core molecule to yield the dendrimer. Dendrimers are generally highly symmetric.

13.2.1.1 Core

The reactivity and valency of the core and its structure determine the symmetry and number of dendrons rooted from that core. This choice also influences polarity and molecular density of the core and thus its microenvironment (*vide infra*). Among the most commonly used core molecules are ammonia, ethylenediamine, propyldiamine, and benzene tricarboxylic acid chloride.

Recently, a reactive triallyl chloride core has been developed for aliphatic polyether dendrons. The main advantage of this new core is that it contains three alkene functionalities that can be used after dendrimer formation for further dendritic growth. The resulting "dendrimer in dendrimer" would then allow covalent attachments of guest molecules at the surface of the dendrimer growing into the dendritic boxes [12].

Other dendrimer cores have been designed to perform a range of specific functions, such as light absorption, and energy or charge transfer, or catalysis of chemical reactions. For example, dendrimers containing a porphyrin core and terminal dimethoxybenzene or benzoquinone groups allow an efficient photoinduced electron transfer from the excited porphyrin to the benzoquinone end groups [13].

13.2.1.2 Linker/Base Unit

The most commonly used linker functionalities are amide, ether, ester, urethane, phosphorus, and silane, and the branch junctures are those derived from amine, benzyl, phosphorus, quaternary carbon, silane, and metal ions. Although the majority of dendrimers have organic backbones, a variety of dendrimers containing heteroatoms (Si, P, B, Ge, and Bi) have also been synthesized. In most of these cases, the heteroatoms were intercalated into the organic skeleton.

In addition to the chemical reactivity and microenvironment, the interplay between core and branch units also determines the steric characteristics of the dendrimer, i.e., the relationship between the increase in volume and surface area of the dendritic molecule. With each new layer the molecule size increases linearly, whereas the number of surface groups increases exponentially [2,14]. Shorter, highly branched subunits with limited conformational flexibility will, in principle, more rapidly lead to crowding and steric inhibition of the addition of further generations (*starburst effect*), whereas flexible longer branches will have a lower molecular density and can potentially support further growth. For example, Majoral et al. have shown that the use of divalent phosphorous-type branch junctures, able to react with a large variety of functional groups, leads to the synthesis of particularly high-generation dendrimers [15]. Overall, the steric limitation of dendrimer growth leads to relatively small molecular sizes, ranging from around 1 to 13 nm in diameter for generation 0 to generation 10 for polyamidoamine (PAMAM) dendrimers [2,14,16,17].

13.2.1.3 Surface

A consequence of the branched nature of dendritic polymers is that these molecules have a very high surface-to-volume ratio. Therefore, the surface groups determine to a large extent the properties and interactions of the material [14]. These groups can be lipophilic or hydrophilic, nonionic, cationic, or anionic depending on the specific chemistry. In addition, the terminal moieties can be functionalized with a number of groups, e.g., by the addition of carbohydrates (glycol dendrimer) or amino acids or peptides, and thus yield novel materials [9,18–22]. This flexibility can be taken a step further by reaction of the terminal groups in one dendrimer to give different functionalities. This approach has been applied to the tumor targeting of drug-loaded dendrimers, e.g., for cancer treatment by a nuclear capture reaction [23]: the irradiation of the isotope ^{10}B with low-energy or thermal neutrons results in the production of toxic and high energy particles and ^{7}Li ions. Thanks to their multivalency, dendrimers can carry many boron molecules while also bearing tumor-specific antibodies [24].

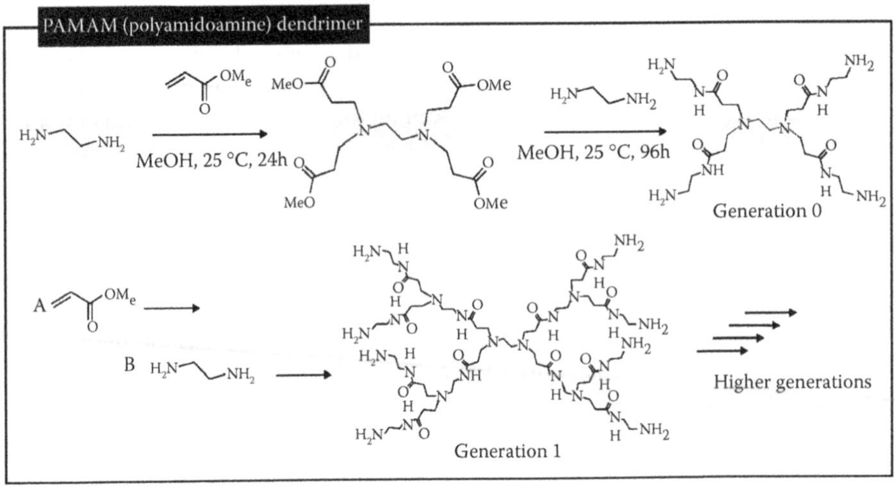

FIGURE 13.3 Synthesis of polyamidoamine (PAMAM) dendrimers. The PAMAM dendrimers are normally based on an ethylenediamine or ammonia core with four and three branching points, respectively (see Reference 5, Tomalia, D.A. et al., A new class of polymers — starburst-dendritic macromolecules, *Polym. J.*, 17(1): 117–132, 1985). Using a divergent approach, the molecule is built up iteratively from the core through addition of methylacrylate, followed by amidation of the resulting ester with ethylenediamine. Each complete reaction sequence results in a new "full" dendrimer generation (e.g. G3, G4, ...) with terminal amine functionality, whereas the intermediate "half" generations (e.g., G2.5, G3.5, ...) terminate in anionic carboxylate groups.

Although the chemistry of dendritic polymers is thus quite flexible, the concern for biocompatibility means that the range of chemical architectures for dendrimers used in biomedical applications is much more limited. It is, in particular, the commercially available PAMAM and PPI (polypropylenimine) dendrimers that have been explored widely (Figure 13.3 and Figure 13.4). Other biocompatible dendrimers employ chemistries that include, among others, polyaryl ether, poly(L-lysine) (PLL), polyester (2,2-*bis*(hydroxymethyl) propionic acid), polyesters of glycerol and succinic acid, and polyglycerol [24].

13.2.2 LIMITATIONS OF DENDRIMER CHEMISTRY

Conventional polymers are formed in a statistical polymerization process, which generally produces polydisperse molecules with a broader Mw/Mn ratio. By contrast, the size and molecular mass of the dendrimers are controlled during each step. Consequently, dendrimers can theoretically be considered to be monodisperse (Mw/Mn = 1).

In reality, however, the efficiency for the reactions used for the stepwise synthesis of dendrimers is less than 100%. This consideration is particularly important when dendrimers are being synthesized via the divergent approach, i.e., a stepwise build-up from the core, where a relatively large number of reactions are being performed on one molecule. Consequently, incomplete or side reactions will introduce defects, which accumulate with each generation. As the purification of these reaction products would be extremely challenging, dendrimers, although relatively monodisperse, tend not to be 100% pure. The exact proportion of defective molecules will depend on the specific nature of the synthetic approach. For example, the PPI$_{G5}$ (where the subscript denotes the dendrimer generation) requires 248 reactions; assuming 99.5% selectivity, only 29% of the dendrimers would be free of defects [25]. For a PAMAM$_{G4}$, it has been suggested that the amount of pure dendrimer would be on the order of 8% [25]. Despite the defects such dendrimers would still have a relatively narrow polydispersity with Mw/Mn close to unity.

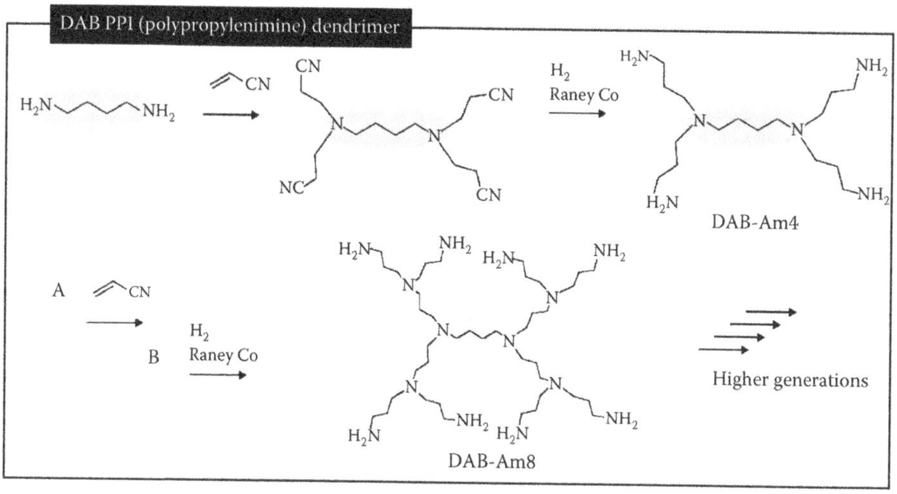

FIGURE 13.4 Synthesis of polypropylenimine (PPI) dendrimers. The other commercially available dendrimer with relevance for drug and gene delivery is based on polypropylenimine (PPI) units, with butylenediamine (DAB) used as the core molecule. The repetitive reaction sequence involves Michael addition of acrylonitrile to a primary amino group followed by hydrogenation of nitrile groups to primary amino groups (see References 212, 213, and 214, Worner, C. and Mulhaupt, R., Polynitrile-functional and polyamine-functional poly(trimethylene imine) dendrimers, *Angew. Chem. Int. Ed. Engl.*, 32(9): 1306–1308, 1993; Debrabandervandenberg, E.M.M. and Meijer, E.W., Poly(propylene imine) dendrimers — large-scale synthesis by heterogeneously catalyzed hydrogenations, *Angew. Chem. Int. Ed. Engl.*, 32(9): 1308–1311, 1993; and Debrabandervandenberg, E.M.M. et al., Large-scale production of polypropylenimine dendrimers, *Macromolecular Symposia*, 77: 51–62, 1994). These dendrimers are frequently referred to as DAB-*x*, or DAB-Am-*x*, with *x* giving the number of surface amines; depending on the source, DAB-Am 4 is sometimes referred to as G0 or G1.

In contrast to the divergent approach, the convergent strategy, starting from the periphery of the units, limits the number of side reactions at each step and lends itself better to purification of the intermediates, thus making the production of defect-free material more feasible.

13.3 PROPERTIES OF DENDRITIC MOLECULES

Because of their molecular architecture, dendrimers show some unique physical and chemical properties, which make them particularly interesting for drug and gene delivery applications. Direct comparison with linear or branched conventional polymers is, however, not trivial because of the difficulty of changing polymer architecture without affecting other parameters. Nevertheless, a comparative study of the properties exhibited by dendrimers and linear macromolecules of the same repeating unit $OC_6H_4P(Ph)_2 = N - P = S$ (including both $P = N$ and $P = S$ double bonds, and P-O and P-C single bonds) provides an acute insight into how their molecular features affect the structure–property relationship (i.e., the fact that phosphorus-based dendrimers are soluble in organic solvents, contrary to linear polymers) [26].

13.3.1 SHAPE

Owing to the steric effects, discussed earlier, dendrimers adopt different shapes, depending on the generation: at lower generations they tend to be planar and elliptical, but take on a more spherical shape at higher generations. Theoretically, the number of branches and the density of the molecule increase at the periphery until steric overcrowding prevents further reactions (the starburst effect). Consequently, schematic drawings of dendrimer structure suggest that the molecular density is significantly lower in the core than in the shell, where the increased number of branches leads to

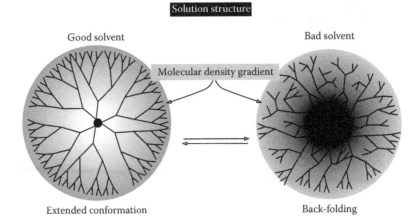

FIGURE 13.5 Molecular density and solution structure of a hypothetical dendrimer. The equilibrium between structures with dense shell vs. dense core depends on dendrimer chemistry and solvent properties (polarity, pH, salt, etc.); backfolding of peripheral groups into the centre modifies molecular density away from the outer shell and leads to a more even distribution of molecular density or a "dense core" dendrimer structure.

a generation dependent crowding. One must however bear in mind that these aesthetically pleasing, ordered structures are highly stylized and may not necessarily reflect the true shape of the molecules in solution (cf. Figure 13.5). Whereas the increased density in the shell has been supported by a number of models, some backfolding of the terminal branches toward the core has also been predicted under certain conditions [25,27].

The actual conformation of dendrimers in solution will ultimately depend on a number of factors, including the specific dendrimer chemistry and architecture, as well as on the interactions with the bulk solvent. For example, for the PPI_{G3} (DAB-Am16), NMR studies suggest a predominantly extended-chain conformation in a "good" solvent (chloroform), but a folded conformation when exposed to a "poor" solvent (benzene) [28]. PAMAM dendrimers are potentially less sensitive to such changes [29,30]. In a similar fashion, the low ionic strength of a solvent would lead to a more extended conformation, whereas in higher salt conditions shielding would promote a denser core conformation [25]. Furthermore, the dendrimer may be sensitive to changes in pH that may affect conformation, e.g., with the repulsion of positively charged amines at lower pH leading to more extended conformations [31,32].

13.3.2 Environment

From the principal dendrimer building blocks, a number of distinct environments are created within the macromolecule. The distinct characteristics will be less clearly defined for the lower-generation dendrimers, which tend to have a much more open and flexible conformation. For higher-generation dendrimers, the "outer shell" just beneath the surface molecule provides a barrier that separates the inside and outside environments, creating a well-defined microenvironment.

Thus, in particular, for higher-generation dendrimers, the core is somewhat protected from the exterior environment by the dendritic branches and surrounded by internal cavities, which potentially allows the encapsulation of guest molecules (*vide infra*). As mentioned earlier, the solvent interaction of the dendrimer will influence its conformation and therefore may also influence the specific properties of the intramolecular environment.

The crowding or starburst effect determines the permeability of the shell for guest or solvent molecules: generations G0–G3 are completely open and merely provide a flexible scaffold. With increase in generation, the number of external groups increases, leading to a semi-rigid type of container (G4–G6) and, finally, to a fairly rigid architecture with a highly restricted surface permeability [2]. This principle applies to symmetric dendrimers in general, but the specific generation at which this occurs will depend on the scaling of the specific branch cell parameters.

13.3.3 VISCOSITY

The intrinsic viscosity of linear polymers increases continuously with molecular mass and obeys the Kuhn–Mark–Houwink–Sakurada equation. By contrast, dendrimer solutions have significantly lower intrinsic viscosity [33], and as the molecular mass increases, the intrinsic viscosity goes through a maximum at a specific generation and then begins to decline [34]. This effect is likely to be related to a gradual transition of dendrimer shape, with a more open, extended conformation being dominant for the lower generations and a more compact shape being adopted for higher generations. The compact shape also reduces the likelihood of entanglement, which affects larger classical polymers.

13.3.4 MULTIVALENCY

In nature, tree-like structures have evolved to maximize the exposed surface area, e.g., to maximize the light exposure or the number of leaves of a tree. In a similar fashion, dendritic architecture creates molecules in which a large proportion of the groups are exposed at the surface. These groups, depending on their specific nature, will to a large degree determine the chemical and physical properties of the molecule [33]. The presence of numerous terminal groups in dendrimers facilitates multiple simultaneous interactions of surface groups with the solvent, surfaces, or other individual molecules. As a consequence, dendrimers tend to show increased solubility, reactivity, and binding [33]. Lower-generation dendrimers, which are large enough to be spherical but do not form a tightly packed surface, have enormous surface areas in relation to their molecular volume (up to 1000 m^2 g^1) [35].

Accordingly, dendrimer miscibility with various solvents is largely determined by the nature of the surface groups: dendrimers bearing hydrophilic groups on their surface are soluble in polar solvents, whereas those having hydrophobic groups on their surface are soluble in non-polar solvents [3].

The high reactivity of dendrimers comes into play when other molecules are being conjugated to dendrimers, which thus provide a high loading capacity per mole, e.g., for drugs or MRI contrast agents (*vide infra*) and in many technological uses of dendrimers such as their use as catalysts. The versatility of the dendrimers has been exploited to attach various ligands, such as transferrin, sugars, and antibodies for receptor-specific targeting, several drug molecules, and solubilizing groups to the periphery of the dendrimers [24].

Finally, the many terminal groups allow dendrimers not only to have a large number of potential binding sites per mole but also to have multivalent interactions. Multivalency is of general importance for biological interactions but may be of particular importance for biomedical applications, because multimeric binding through statistical and/or cooperative effects can increase affinity, avidity, and specificity of binding [36].

For example, the biologically important carbohydrate–protein interactions tend to be relatively weak. A specific cooperative increase in binding (glycoside effect) for this type of interaction has been emulated through multimeric glycodendrimers (for more detailed information, see Reference 21). Furthermore, multimeric binding of antibodies to dendrimer-linked antigenic peptides has been used to enhance the immune response using the so-called multiple antigen peptides (MAP) [22].

The multimeric surface groups are also important in the use of dendrimers as synthetic gene delivery vectors. The protonated amines, e.g., of PAMAM dendrimers, can interact with the anionic plasmid DNA by electrostatic means and thus form nanomeric complexes [37]. Efficient complex formation between dendrimer and DNA tends to favor the higher-generation cationic dendrimers (*vide infra*). Apart from other possible reasons, this is probably related to the fact that the larger dendrimers have a higher number of binding groups per molecule [11].

13.3.5 FUNCTIONALISATION

Thus, modification of reactive molecules at the dendrimer surface is a promising strategy for the creation of novel biomaterials with defined properties. Examples for this approach include the development of several peptide-based dendrimers, such as those based on PLL, as promising vaccine, antiviral, and antibacterial candidates [22]. In addition, dendrimers incorporating carbohydrate moieties at their core, branch points, or periphery seem to be promising immunological tools because of their multivalent binding capacity [19,38]. The introduction of stabilizing polyethylene oxide chains on the dendrimer periphery has allowed the incorporation of anticancer drugs such as 5-fluorouracil [39], methotrexate, and doxorubicin [40], and can slow the drug release rates in these systems. Drug release can also be controlled by attaching pH-sensitive hydrophobic acetal groups on the dendrimer periphery. Loss of the hydrophobic groups on acetal hydrolysis at acid pH disrupts the micelle and allows the release of the loaded drug [41].

13.3.6 INTERNAL CAVITIES

Clearly the terminal groups are of broad relevance for the use of dendrimers in drug and gene delivery. Yet, the fact that dendrimers can sustain a different environment in the periphery from that in the core, as well as their specific molecular architecture, does offer additional functionality. In particular, the globular shape and the outer shell mean that internal cavities may potentially be used to encapsulate guest molecules in the interior of the macromolecular host (Figure 13.6).

The core itself can provide an environment with a solubility different from that of the shell or bulk. Fréchet and colleagues report unimolecular micelles that accommodate apolar guest molecules in the core via hydrophobic interactions [42]. The so-called "dendrophanes," dendritic molecules

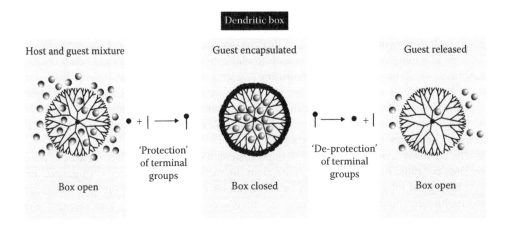

FIGURE 13.6 Dendritic box encapsulation. Guest molecules can be retained within the cavities of a dendrimer by the creation of a steric shell. (From Reference 48, Jansen, J., Debrabandervandenberg, E.M.M., and Meijer, E.W., Encapsulation of guest molecules into a dendritic box, *Science*, 266(5188): 1226–1229, 1994.) The box was constructed through synthesis of a chiral shell of protected amino acids on DAB-Am 64. Owing to the dense packing, the shell physically locks guest molecules inside the core ("dendrimer box"). The small guest molecules are unable to escape from the core even after exhaustive dialysis. The encapsulation capacity of the dendrimer is proportional to the volume of the internal dendrimer cavity and could accommodate up to four large molecules (rhodamine B) or 8 to 10 smaller molecules. The release of the guest molecules is triggered through hydrolysis of the outer shell (see Jansen, J., Debrabandervandenberg, E.M.M., and Meijer, E.W., Encapsulation of guest molecules into a dendritic box, *Science*, 266(5188): 1226–1229, 1994). Although this model would not be useful for drug delivery under physiological conditions, it elegantly demonstrates the principle of steric encapsulation.

with a "cylophane" core, bind aromatic compounds and act as carriers for steroids [43]. Accommodation of polar guests was demonstrated by the "dendroclefts," designed by Diederichs and colleagues; these molecules are based on water-soluble dendrimers with an optically active core that accommodates glycosides in a diastereoselective fashion [44].

Modification of PAMAM surface amines with TRIS (tris(hydroxymethyl)amino methane) creates highly-water-soluble dendrimers that are capable of solubilization of acidic aromatic antibacterial compounds with triggered release at a low pH [45]. The ability of PAMAM dendrimers to accommodate the hydrophobic dye Nile red was shown to be generation dependent, thus reflecting the functional consequences of increased core size [46]. Furthermore, through interaction with anionic surfactants, supramolecular assemblies were formed, which were even more efficient in solubilizing the dye [46]. Through reaction of the terminal amines with epoxyalkanes, Tomalia and colleagues created hydrocarbon-soluble dendrimers that could act as reverse micelles [47].

An encapsulation strategy that is unique to dendrimers is based on the idea of the "dendritic box" [48]. The principle behind this is the idea that the high number of terminal groups in the higher-generation dendrimers produce a steric shell that separates the dendrimer core from the bulk and thus can retain suitable molecules as "guests" within the host molecule (cf. Figure 13.6).

13.4 GENERAL BIOLOGICAL PROPERTIES

13.4.1 *IN VITRO*-CELL CULTURE

When considering the general biocompatibility of dendrimer-based drug and gene delivery systems, one needs to be careful to distinguish between interactions and effects of the free dendrimer and those related to the delivery system as a whole, i.e., when the dendrimer is part of a supramolecular assembly. Dendrimers with suitable properties (i.e., appropriate hydrophile–lipophile balance (HLB), size, and topology) can self-assemble into higher-order structures, thus increasing their potential for use as drugs and gene carriers [49–51]. Self-assembling dendrimers with a variety of structures have been reported by several groups as recently described in Reference 52. Other supramolecular assemblies can be formed by interaction with other molecules, e.g., by complexation with drugs or DNA. The biological properties of such supramolecular structures may differ considerably from that of the free molecule. Although the complexation of a potentially toxic polymer can change its biological interaction profile and limit its toxicity, particulate materials may show distinct biodistribution or cellular trafficking characteristics, which can modify the toxicity profile.

Initial *in vitro* biological evaluations of PAMAM dendrimers reported them to be relatively nontoxic [53]. In particular, in cytotoxicity assays they compare favorably with some of the other transfection agents, especially against cationic polymers of higher molecular weight, such as PEI (poly(ethylenimine) of molecular weight 600 to 1000 kDa) and PLL (36.6 kDa) or DEAE-dextran (diethylaminoethyl-dextran, 500 kDa), which in these assays are around three orders of magnitude more toxic [54]. In contrast to the large-molecular-weight PEI and PLL, the PAMAM dendrimer toxicity did not seem to stem from membrane damage as assayed by LDH release or hemolysis [54].

Nevertheless, dendrimers interact effectively with cell membranes, and the electrostatic interactions of cationic polymers and anionic cell surfaces are very important for the cellular uptake of charged DNA complexes [55]. In fact, studies of membrane interactions of PAMAM dendrimers with dimyristoyl phoshphatidyl choline (DMPC) and its phosphatidyl cholate salt (DMPA-Na) vesicles suggested that vesicles can in fact wrap around larger dendrimers [56]. The interaction of PAMAM dendrimers with membranes has also recently been shown to induce the formation of transient holes (G7) or enlarge existing holes (G5) [57]. Membrane interactions are thought to be important for toxicity because damage to cell membranes can directly damage cells; furthermore, such interactions may pose a problem on systemic injection when erythrocyte lysis or aggregation can lead to fatal toxicity.

Similar to other polymers, dendrimer size or molecular weight appears to be a key determinant of dendrimer cytotoxicity. This has been established for PAMAM [58] and PPI dendrimers [59].

The cytotoxicity of PAMAM dendrimers increases with generation for both whole-generation cationic dendrimers (G2–G4) and the "half-generation" anionic intermediates (G2.5, G3.5) [60,61], clearly demonstrating molecular weight as a key parameter independent of surface charge. Nevertheless, charge is one of the other determinants of dendrimer toxicity: cationic charges appear to be overall more toxic, although the toxicity also depends on the specific groups involved, i.e., for amines it has been proposed that primary amines are relatively more toxic than secondary or tertiary amines [54]. A concentration-dependent tendency to cause hemolysis and changes in erythrocyte morphology has been linked to the presence of primary amine groups [62]. In contrast to PAMAM dendrimers, PPI dendrimers with DAB (diaminobutane) and DAE (diaminoethane) cores did not show a generation-dependent hemolytic effect [62]. In general, the dendrimers were found to interact significantly less with erythrocytes than PEI but were nevertheless hemolytic at concentrations above 1 mg ml^1. Effects such as hemolysis clearly depend on membrane interactions, and studies on dendrimer membrane interactions suggest that it may be difficult to separate charge-dependent toxicity from membrane toxicity.

We have previously used the quaternization of amines as a strategy to reduce the toxicity of polymers [63,64]. The approach also seems to be beneficial for the higher-generation PPI dendrimers used in synthetic gene delivery systems [65], but the effects of quaternization on nanoparticles may be complex and can include changes of complex morphology and physicochemistry that would be difficult to deconvolute.

In contrast to the cationic dendrimers, anionic dendrimers, e.g., bearing a carboxylate surface, have been reported to be generally non-cytotoxic over a broad concentration range [66], although even for anionic dendrimers (e.g., half-generation PAMAM), a correlation exists between toxicity and molecular weight [61].

The modification of surface amines and the shielding of charges through attachment of hydrophilic polymers reduce the number of primary amines and create a steric barrier that limits interactions. Poly(ethylene glycol) (PEG) is widely used for this purpose in other delivery systems [67,68] and also seems to be efficient in conjunction with dendrimers [39,61,69].

On the other hand, the attachment of a limited number of C_{12} lauroyl groups also appears to be beneficial [69]. It has been suggested that for higher generations, nontoxic surface groups may be more effective because access to a potentially toxic core is diminished for steric reasons [62].

13.4.2 *In Vivo*

Because of the multitude of potential cellular and macromolecular interactions, the step from cell culture and *in vitro* models to *in vivo* administration of dendrimers and dendrimer-based delivery systems adds several layers of complexity, particularly when intravascular administration is being considered.

13.4.2.1 Oral Uptake

Dendrimers have sizes in the range between conventional particulate drug carriers, macromolecules, and small molecules. It has been suggested that particles of the appropriate size may be taken up by the gut more effectively [70]. A study of the oral uptake of lipidic peptide-based dendrons found around 3% of the administered dose in the blood 6 h after administration [71,72]. This is lower than that for larger types of particles and could suggest that the optimum size for uptake of macromolecules or particulates in the gut is larger than the size of most dendritic polymers [73].

This observation is also supported by an *in vitro* study using an inverted intestinal sac system. Here, relatively high serosal transfer of anionic dendrimers was observed with the uptake of anionic dendrimers of generation G5.5 being higher than for G2.5. Serosal transfer for the cationic species (G3, G4) was found to be around 30% lower, but these molecules also exhibited extensive non-specific binding [74].

13.4.2.2 Biodistribution

[125]I-labeled cationic PAMAM dendrimers (G3–G4) are rapidly eliminated from the circulation (around 99% in 1h) but are accumulated in the liver (more than 60%) [66]. A similar pattern was found for the anionic half-generation PAMAM dendrimers (G2.5, G3.5, and G5.5), although clearance was somewhat slower and accumulation in the liver less pronounced [62]. An earlier study by Roberts and colleagues [60] reported kidney accumulation for PAMAM$_{G3}$ and accumulation in the pancreas for the PAMAM$_{G5}$ and PAMAM$_{G7}$. A high level of kidney excretion was observed for G7, but studies with PAMAM dendrimers with varying degrees of terminal biotinylation suggest that retention may increase with size and charge density [75].

13.4.2.3 Conjugates and Delivery Systems

Clearly these observations do not necessarily hold true when dendrimers are being used as part of a delivery system. Dendrimer conjugates or particulate systems will have a different way of interacting with cells and macromolecules, which will affect their pharmacokinetics, biodistribution, and metabolism.

Although dendrimers tend to be of no or very low immunogenicity [60,76], their use as scaffolds for the presentation of multiple antigenic peptides [22,77] demonstrates that conjugation can dramatically change their biological properties. An example of how the combination of a compound with a dendrimer alters the activity of the compound is the complexation of dendrimers with DNA: in general the toxicity of cationic polymers bound to DNA decreases in *in vitro* assays, but the particulate nature of the complexes is likely to have a major influence on complex biodistribution e.g., by exploiting the enhanced permeability and retention effect, which can lead to an accumulation of particulate or macromolecular drugs in a tumor [78,79]. Charge-ratio-dependent complement activation has been observed for PAMAM$_{G5}$ complexes [80], which may lead to problems on intravenous injection or administration to the lung [81].

13.5 APPLICATIONS

Many potential applications of dendrimers are based on their unparalleled molecular uniformity, multifunctional surface, and presence of internal cavities. Areas of biomedical research in which dendrimers have already demonstrated their utility are dominated by drug and gene delivery but other applications including imaging (MRI) or radiotherapy are also relevant.

Properties of an ideal macromolecular drug delivery or biomedical vector [2] are as follows:

- Structural control over size and shape of drug or imaging-agent cargo space
- Biocompatible, nontoxic polymer/pendant functionality
- Precise, nanoscale container and/or scaffolding properties with high-drug- or high-imaging-agent-capacity features
- Well-defined scaffolding and/or surface modifiable functionality for cell-specific targeting moieties
- Lack of immunogenicity
- Appropriate cellular adhesion, endocytosis, and intracellular trafficking to allow therapeutic delivery or imaging in the cytoplasm or nucleus
- Acceptable bioelimination or biodegradation
- Controlled or triggerable drug release
- Molecular-level isolation and protection of the drug against inactivation during transit to target cells
- Minimal nonspecific cellular and blood-protein-binding properties
- Ease of consistent, reproducible, clinical-grade synthesis

13.5.1 DRUG DELIVERY

In order for the dendrimer to be able to act as a drug delivery system some form of drug "packaging" or loading has to create an association between the carrier and drug. In principle, dendrimers can act as exoreceptors or endoreceptors for the drug or plasmid [82], i.e., loading can occur through interaction sites located on the molecule's surface or in the core of the molecule (*vide supra*). The interaction can be of a covalent or a noncovalent nature: covalent binding of drugs creates drug–dendrimer conjugates similar to other polymer–drug conjugates [79], whereas noncovalent interaction, such as electrostatic, hydrophobic, or hydrogen-bonding type of interactions, bind the drug in a nonspecific, metastable fashion. The multiplicity of dendrimer groups tends to stabilize these weaker interactions through cooperation [36]. For larger dendrimers, the differential solubility of the drug between the bulk phase and dendrimer core may also contribute to drug encapsulation. In addition, strategies such as coprecipitation may then further stabilize such complexes. Proof of concept has been demonstrated for various encapsulation strategies in model systems [83], but the number of applications in which dendrimer-based systems are being applied to drug delivery challenges *in vivo* is more limited (cf. Table 13.1–Table 13.3).

13.5.1.1 Unmodified Polymers as Carriers

Unmodified dendrimers such as PAMAM can interact with drug molecules based on the nature of the surface groups, e.g., via electrostatic interactions or, alternatively, via the advantageous drug solubilization in a more favorable microenvironment. The latter would be expected to be most pronounced for the higher-generation dendrimers (*vide supra*), but, interestingly, most studies exploring the use of unmodified dendrimers only use low- to medium-generation dendrimers, i.e., G1–G5. This suggests that for the majority of examples the interaction with the surface groups, e.g., electrostatic complexation, may be the predominant means of association. In this case, the stability of such complexes may be insufficient to withstand pronounced changes in the bulk, e.g., with increase in ionic strength and extensive buffering. It is also unclear to what extent supramolecular assemblies between dendrimers or between multiple dendrimers and drug molecules play a role, in particular at higher concentrations [84,85].

13.5.1.2 Graft- and Copolymers

The conjugation of either hydrophilic or hydrophobic groups to the dendrimer "surface" is a strategy to create better-defined favorable microenvironments and, effectively, monomolecular micelles (cf. Table 13.2 top). In particular, the combination of lower-generation PAMAM dendrimers with poly(ethylene glycol) of various molecular weights (5000) has been used frequently. Drug loading in these systems can be quite reasonable, but as for the unmodified dendrimers, the stability of the encapsulation in a biological environment is uncertain.

13.5.1.3 Supramolecular Systems

Supramolecular assemblies (cf. Table 13.2 bottom) can be used to stabilize the interaction of dendrimer and drug, e.g., by sequestration of these complexes into liposomes. PAMAM dendrimers grafted with fatty acid residues can also efficiently encapsulate drugs when particles are formed in the presence of phospholipids. These structures are sufficiently stable to allow oral administration and have been shown to increase the bioavailability of the encapsulated drug [86]. Supramolecular systems can also be formed from dendrimers or amphiphilic dendrons that interact with liposomes or can form vesicles in the presence of cholesterol [52,87]. Dendrimer-based microcapsules have been formed by coprecipitation of dendrimers onto a core which is subsequently dissolved [88].

TABLE 13.1
Unmodified Dendrimers as Carrier Systems

Dendrimer/Modification	Drug/Model Compound	Model	Results	Reference
PAMAM G4	Ibuprofen	*In vitro*	Ibuprofen solubility increased linearly with PAMAM G4 concentration	215
PAMAM G4, G4.5	Nonsteroidal anti-inflammatory drug indomethacin	*In vivo* (rat paw model), transdermal for inflamed regions	Transdermal flux of indomethacin increased by factor 2.27 (PAMAM G4) and 1.95 (PAMAM G4.5) compared to the free drug. Anti-inflammatory effect increased by 1.6 and 1.5 times in rat paw model	216,217
Polyglycerol dendrimers G4, G5	Anticancer drug paclitaxel (PTX)	*In vitro*	The PTX solubility increased by up to 10,000; dependent on the dendrimer generation. Dendritic structure supports solubilization at low dendrimer concentrations	218, 219
Generation 4 carboxylated poly(glycerol succinic acid) dendrimer	Anticancer drug 10-hydroxycamptothecin (10HCPT)	*In vitro*/cells	Cytotoxicity assays with human breast cancer cells showed 10HCPT retains activity upon encapsulation.	220
PAMAM G3–G4 and Perstorp polyol (G5 hyperbranched polyester with OH)	Nonsteroidal anti-inflammatory drug Ibuprofen	*In vitro*/cells	PAMAM G4 encapsulates up to 78 molecules via electrostatic interactions; retarded *in vitro* release; accelerated uptake in A549 cells; polyol only encapsulates 24 molecules	221
PAMAM G0–G3 and G0.5–G2.5	Calcium channel blocking agent nifedipine	*In vitro*	Increased aqueous solubility maximum at pH7; aqueous solubility enhancement ranking: G2.5 > G3 > G1.5 > G2 > or = G0.5 > G1 > G0	222
Dendrimer citric acid-polyethylene–citric acid G1–G3	Antibacterial 5-aminosalicylic acid, pyridine, nonsteroidal anti-inflammatory mefenamic acid and diclofenac	*In vitro*	Stability of drug or dendrimer and release studied	223
PAMAM G1.5, G2, G3, G3.5, G4	Miotic drug pilocarpine nitrate, mydriatic drug tropicamide	Ocular delivery/*in vivo* rabbit	Increased residence time on cornea to prolong exposure to drugs; prolonged for carboxyl and hydroxyl surface groups independent of concentration (0.25–2%)	224

TABLE 13.2
Dendrimer Graft- and Copolymers, Supramolecular Systems

Dendrimer/Modification	Drug/Model Compound	Model	Results	Reference
Dendrimer Copolymers and Graft Polymers				
Copolymer of hydrophobic core (with 6, 12, 24, and 48 phenolic end groups, based on 4, 4-*bis* (4'-hydroxyphenyl) pentanol) and hydrophilic shell poly(ethylene glycol) [PEG] mesylate	Pyrene, indomethacin	*In vitro*	Dendritic unimolecular micelles solubilizing pyrene; indomethacin 11 wt.% loading level, sustained release	225
PAMAM G3, G4 poly(ethylene glycol) 550 MW, 2000 MW copolymer	Anticancer drugs doxorubicin and methotrexate (MTX)	*In vitro*	Encapsulation of doxorubicin, MTX increases with generation and chain length of poly(ethylene glycol) grafts; G4 with PEG2000 could retain 6.5 adriamycin molecules or 26 methotrexate molecules; sustained release in low ionic strength but rapid in isotonic solutions	40
Star block copolymer: block copolymer linked to PAMAM core; inner hydrophobic block poly (e-caprolactone), outer hydrophilic block poly(ethylene glycol) (PEG)	Non-steroidal anti-inflammatory drug indomethacin, anticancer drugs doxorubicin and etoposide	*In vitro*/cells	Loading capacity of up to 22% (w/w) was achieved with etoposide; a cytotoxicity assay demonstrated that the star-PCL-PEG copolymer is nontoxic in cell culture	226
PAMAM G3 PEG (MW 750, 2000, 5000) copolymer	Pyrene	*In vitro*	No obvious correlation with dissolved pyrene and micelle, but concentrated micelles tended to dissolve more pyrene.	227
Supramolecular Systems				
Dendrimer in liposome	Anticancer drug methotrexate	*In vitro*	Dendrimer retains methotrexate (MTX) inside liposomes	228
PAMAM fatty acid dendrimer graft with phospholipid	Anticancer drug 5-fluorouracil (5-FU)	*In vivo* oral bioavailability (rat)	53% w/w 5-FU loading and improved oral bioavailability in rats	86

TABLE 13.2
Dendrimer Graft- and Copolymers, Supramolecular Systems (Continued)

Dendrimer/Modification	Drug/Model Compound	Model	Results	Reference
PAMAM-polystyrenesulfonate microcapsule	Anticancer drug doxorubicin	*In vitro*	Encapsulation of doxorubicin	88
Dendrisome: lysine-derived amphiphilic dendron aggregates with cholesterol to form vesicles	Radiolabeled antibiotic penicillin G (model of negatively-charged water-soluble compound)	*In vitro*	Cationic vesicles (zeta potential = +50 mV) with higher encapsulation efficiencies and slower release rates compared to the liposomes; cholesterol leads to size increase (310 nm – > 560 nm), shape irregularities, and increases leakage	52

TABLE 13.3
Dendrimer Conjugates

Dendrimer/Modification	Drug/Model Compound	Model	Results	Reference
Polyether dendrimers conjugates	Ligand folic acid, anticancer drug methotrexate	*In vitro*	G2 dendrimer with 16 residues conjugated with 12.6 folate	89
PAMAM G0.5–G5.5	Anticancer drug 5-fluorouracil	*In vitro*	Release of 5-FU by hydrolysis in a phosphate buffer solution (pH 7.4) at 37°C dependent on generation	229
PAMAM G3.5	Anticancer drug cisplatin (Pt)	*In vivo* murine xenograft (L1210, B16F10)	20–25% w/w load and sustained release *in vitro*; equiactive to free drug given intraperitoneally against intraperitoneal L1210, in contrast to free Pt active against i.p. B16F10; and given intravenously against subcutaneous B16F10 xenografts; selective accumulation of the dendrimer Pt in solid tumor tissue by the EPR effect (a 50-fold increase in area under curve compared with cisplatin) and reduced toxicity.	92
PAMAM G5 conjugate	Ligand folic acid, fluorescein, anticancer drug methotrexate	*In vitro*/cells	Cytotoxicity in KB cells improved by 100 × over free drug	90

(Continued)

TABLE 13.3
Dendrimer Conjugates (Continued)

Dendrimer/ Modification	Drug/Model Compound	Model	Results	Reference
Polyester dendrimer 2,2-*bis* (hydroxymethyl) propanoic acid units	Anticancer drug doxorubicin	*In vitro*/cells/*in vivo* pharmacokinetics	Drug release at acidic pHs; reduced *in vitro* toxicity or activity; increased plasma half-life of coupled doxorubicin	230, 231
PAMAM conjugate 5 aminosalycilic acid with *p*-aminobenzoic acid (PABA) and *p*-aminohippuric acid (PAHA) spacers	Prodrug sulfasalazine (releasing antibacterial 5-aminosalicylic acid)	*In vitro*	45.6% (PABA) and 57.0% (PAHA) of the dose released in 24 h; sustained release compared to commercial prodrugs	232
Antibody–Dendrimer–FITC conjugate	Fluorescein (FITC)	*In vitro*/cells	*In vitro* studies of these conjugates show that they specifically bind to cells expressing PSMA	91
Conjugate with PAMAM G3 and lauroyl-PAMAM G3	Propanolol	*In vitro*/cells (Caco2)	Improved uptake when conjugated to G3 dendrimers, further with lauroyl-G3 dendrimers; suggested uptake via endocytosis avoiding P-gp pump	233
Methylprednisolone polyamido dendrimer	Corticosteroid methylprednisol-one	*In vitro*/cells	Payload of 32% w/w; rapid cellular uptake (A549) with conjugate mostly localized in cytosol; conjugate showed comparable pharmacological activity to free MP, as measured by inhibition of prostaglandin secretion	234

13.5.1.4 Dendrimer Conjugates

Covalent conjugation strategies utilize a large number of terminal functional groups to achieve relatively high drug loading per dendrimer molecule. The density of reactive groups and the well-defined molecular structure represent potential advantages over other polymers used in polymer–drug conjugates [79]. Covalent conjugation chemistry is also the method of choice for the introduction of targeting moieties [89–91]. Dendrimer conjugates, as well as other macromolecular drugs and particulate drug carriers, can also take advantage of the enhanced permeability and retention (EPR) effect to achieve accumulation in tumors [78]; a dendrimer–cisplatin conjugate achieved a 50-fold increase in drug concentration in murine xenograft models area under the curve (AUC) compared to the free drug [92]. A key issue for dendrimer–drug conjugates is the issue of activity, i.e., is the conjugated drug active or is it necessary to ensure release of the drug in its free form? In general, a conjugate will need to be relatively stable until the site of action has been reached, and then efficient release of the free drug will be required. This can be achieved either through non-specific hydrolysis or potentially in a site-specific fashion, e.g., through specific enzyme-cleavable bonds.

In summary, the complexity of biological systems means that although dendrimers have a number of properties that make them, in principle, particularly suited as materials for drug delivery, it remains a challenge to translate these advantages into workable delivery solutions.

13.5.2 GENE THERAPY

Genetic therapy is based on the use of therapeutic nucleic acids (NA), either in the form of genes (i.e., double-stranded plasmid DNA), short interfering RNA (siRNA), or antisense oligonucleotides [93]. The potential of these approaches to transform the therapy of many diseases is evident; however, delivery, and in particular systemic delivery, remains a major obstacle.

A variety of viral and synthetic vector systems are in preclinical and clinical development, all of which have distinct advantages and disadvantages [94,95]. The recent licensing of a locally (into the tumor) injected adenoviral therapy for head and neck cancer demonstrates the continuing progress in the field [96], although other reports serve as a reminder of the potential risks of viral gene therapy [97,98]. In contrast to viral vectors, the nonviral (synthetic) systems are in general reputed to lack efficiency, yet they offer flexibility and safety. However, we will see that dendrimers have in fact recently been demonstrated to provide a promising alternative to viral systems (*vide infra*). Ultimately, the suitability of any gene delivery system will need to be carefully matched with the clinical situation, the specific disease, and the chosen therapeutic strategy [99–101]. For a detailed review on the use of dendrimers in gene delivery, also see Reference 102.

13.5.2.1 The Challenges of Gene Delivery — Introduction

Nucleic acids, unless significantly chemically modified, tend to be rapidly degraded in tissues or in the systemic circulation [103], therefore they need to be "packaged" in synthetic vectors. These are commonly based on cationic carrier molecules such as lipids or polymers [99,101], which complex the nucleic acid (NA) into nanoparticles. In the complexation process an excess of the cationic carrier is used to create nanoparticles carrying a positive charge. This improves colloidal stability, facilitates cell adsorption, and mediates efficient endosomal uptake into cells [104].

Unless they have been administered locally, the complexes need to travel in the vascular compartment to reach the appropriate organ or site of action. If the target site lies in the parenchyma, the particles need to extravasate and travel through the interstitium to finally reach the target cells.

This is obviously not easy to achieve; further challenges exist: when the positively charged synthetic vector systems are administered *in vivo*, the nonspecific nature of electrostatic interactions leads to promiscuous interaction of the particles with biological surfaces, macromolecules, and cells. In the process, complexes may be destabilized and their biodistribution altered [105]. These effects may partly explain the strong bias toward specific organs, in particular the lung and to some extent also the liver, that has frequently been observed after intravenous administration of positively charged lipoplexes and polyplexes [106–110].

Once the complexes have been taken up into cells by endocytosis, they need to escape from the endosome to avoid degradation by lysosomal enzymes. This is one of the bottlenecks of intracellular trafficking, and efficient synthetic vectors have specific mechanisms (e.g., "proton sponge," *vide infra*) that allow them to disrupt the endosomal membrane and reach the cytoplasm. In order to express therapeutic genes, it is then necessary for the DNA to reach the nucleus to gain access to the cellular transcription machinery [99].

13.5.2.2 Complex Formation

The complexation process between dendrimers and nucleic acids is fundamentally the same as that for other cationic polymers with high charge density: dendrimers interact with various forms of nucleic acids such as plasmid DNA or antisense oligonucleotides to form complexes that protect the nucleic acid from degradation [111,112]. The interaction between dendrimer and nucleic acid is based on electrostatic interaction [53,111,113] and lacks any sequence specificity [114]. The nature of the resulting complex is not only dependent on the stoichiometry and concentration of the DNA phosphates and dendrimer amines but also on the bulk solvent properties (e.g., pH, salt concentration, buffer strength) and even the dynamics of mixing (for a more detailed review, see Reference 102). Because of the need for cationic charge and the need to buffer endosomal pH changes (*vide infra*), dendrimers used as synthetic gene therapy vectors tend to contain protonable amines. Both commercially available dendrimers, PAMAM and PPI, have these properties and, in particular, complexes of PAMAM dendrimers and DNA have been studied widely.

PAMAM dendrimers bind DNA at a 1:1 stoichiometry of primary amine to phosphate, but it is only at higher ratios that more stable and efficient complexes are formed [113]. Although, in principle, large and small dendrimers can bind to DNA, it appears that only the higher generations are able to produce the soluble charged complexes suitable for transfection [59,115–117].

The complexes formed at different dendrimer to DNA ratios can have quite different physico-chemical properties [59,117,118] and morphologies [112,113,119,120]. Interestingly, there is some evidence to suggest that at least for some of the dendrimer-based systems there is considerable heterogeneity among the complexes formed under specific conditions [37]. Although this in itself is not surprising, the observation that for the formulation of PAMAM G7–DNA complexes, more than 90% of transfection resulted from 10 to 20% of complexes (found in the low-density aqueous-soluble fraction) demonstrates that the formation of nanoparticles needs to be finely tuned to optimize transfection efficiency.

13.5.2.3 Mechanism

In mechanistic terms, it appears that dendrimers behave very similar to other polymeric transfection agents, and differences between specific systems appear to be subtle by nature rather than profound. Nevertheless, a number of interesting observations that give some insight into the mechanism of dendrimer-mediated transfection have been reported.

Binding and uptake of the PAMAM dendrimer Superfect™ depend on cholesterol [121], as does the binding of lipoplexes [122]. It is currently not clear whether the ability of the uncomplexed dendrimer to interact with membranes [57,123,124] is relevant for the uptake and intracellular processing of dendrimer DNA complexes.

There is now good evidence supporting the notion that dendrimers such as PAMAM and PPI exploit their inherent buffering capacity to disrupt endosomes [125]. Polymers with such high buffering capacity act as a "proton sponge" [58,126], i.e., they buffer the drop in endosomal pH, which leads to an increased accumulation of osmotically active Cl and thus induces endosome swelling and rupture [125].

The transfer from the cytoplasm to the nucleus is a critical step in the transfection process. Fluorescence microscopy of dendrimer–antisense complexes (Oregon-green-conjugated PAMAM G5 and TAMRA-labeled antisense oligonucleotide) suggest that the dendrimer itself has the ability to accumulate to some extent to the nucleus [127] in a similar manner to that reported for PEI [128].

One potentially intriguing difference between polymeric and lipidic delivery systems seems to lie in their intracellular processing: for lipid-based systems, dissociation of the complex at the level of the endosome seems to be obligatory, whereas this does not necessarily hold true for polymeric systems that appear to have at least some activity even when still complexed. Specifically, PAMAM G5 dendrimer–antisense oligonucleotide complexes seemed to be active, although a large proportion of antisense oligonucleotide in the nucleus seemed to be still complexed [127]. However, an early study suggested that PAMAM dendrimers inhibit the initiation of transcription *in vitro*, but the elongation of the RNA transcript would not be affected [111].

13.5.2.4 Dendrimers as Cellular Transfection Agents

Dendrimers in the guise of commercially available transfection kits have become familiar tools for many scientists working with cells, and PAMAM- or PPI-based agents have been shown to be able to efficiently deliver nucleic acids ranging from small oligonucleotides [53,127,129–133] to plasmids and artificial chromosomes [134].

Although dendrimers can form complexes with DNA over a broad range of ratios, it is the higher-generation dendrimers (e.g., PAMAM G5–G10) that more efficiently transfect cells [116]. For these higher-generation dendrimers, a near-exponential increase in efficiency with generation has been observed [116]. On the other hand, toxicity has been shown to be molecular weight dependent. Thus, a balance needs to be struck between the transfection enhancements and the related toxic effects. Our own observations with the DAB-PPI dendrimers show that the ability of DAB-PPI dendrimers to bind DNA, as well as their cytotoxicity, is generation dependent [59]. Physicochemical characterization of complexes and molecular-modeling studies support the notion that an optimal size, i.e., dendrimer generation, for DNA binding exists, which also shows some correlation with the efficiency of transfection. In this study the lower-generation PPI dendrimers, specifically PPI$_{G3}$ (DAB-AM16), strike a favorable balance, with transfection efficiencies being similar to that of the cationic lipid DOTAP [59].

The first report of the use of starburst PAMAM dendrimers as transfection agents demonstrated efficient transgene expression in adherent and suspension cell cultures, with the PAMAM G6 (NH$_3$) dendrimer DNA being most efficient at charge ratios of 6:1 [135]. However, the realization that degradation of the dendrimer had contributed to these results led to the discovery of the fractured or activated dendrimers [115]. The process decreases the molecular density in the centre of the molecule and probably increases conformational flexibility. These changes improve the efficiency of the complexes, with enhancements on the order of > 50 × [115]. These significant differences in biological effects between almost identical compounds highlight the importance of the effects of even subtle changes in the complex's physicochemistry on the transfection efficiency of complexes.

Another indicator of the importance of polymer structure comes from comparisons between linear, branched, and dendritic polymers, where the transfection efficiency may vary by three orders of magnitude [136]. The ranking of transfection efficiency was 22kD linear PEI (Exgen500™) > activated PAMAM dendrimer (Superfect™) >> 25kD branched PEI > P123-g-PEI(2k), a Pluronic PEI graft block copolymer; the polymer-based systems were also found to be more active than some of the commercial cationic lipid systems [136]. A PPI$_{G5}$ dendrimer with DAB core (DAB-Am64, Astramol™), despite having an architecture similar to that of the PAMAM dendrimer, appeared to be the least efficient agent, and its application was also hampered by signs of toxicity at higher N/P ratios, an issue that had previously been highlighted [66]. The correlation between changes in chemical and physical properties and transfection efficiency is, however, not always clear, as the same study highlights: other factors such as specific cell line, incubation time of the complexes with the cells, and cell density were also shown to modulate results by up to three orders of magnitude [136].

13.5.2.5 *In Vivo* Gene Expression and Experimental Therapy

The transition from cell-based transfection experiments to *in vivo* studies is the logical next step in the development of gene delivery systems. However, it is difficult to extrapolate the *in vitro* results obtained with these systems to *in vivo* performance. When one considers the added levels of complexity *in vivo*, i.e., the multitude of macromolecular and cellular components that can potentially interact with the nanoparticles before they reach the target cells, this it is not surprising. Most of the applications of dendrimers for gene delivery have so far focused on their local or *ex vivo* administration, thus highlighting the particular challenge that the systemic delivery of genetic material presents. Despite these challenges there is some evidence that dendrimer-based delivery systems have a significant potential for the delivery of genetic therapies *in vivo*.

13.5.2.6 Localized or *Ex Vivo* Administration

13.5.2.6.1   Eye

Direct application of activated PAMAM (Superfect™)–gene complexes *ex vivo* on human and rabbit corneas resulted in 6 to 10% of cells being transfected (18:1 ratio) [137], intravitreal injection of complexes with antisense oligonucleotides, and a lipid lysine dendrimer inhibits neovascularization of the choroidea by downregulation of vascular endothelial growth factor (VEGF) over a period of up to two months [138].

13.5.2.6.2   Tumor

Intratumoral injection of 100 μg HSV-tk suicide vector complexed with Superfect™ PAMAM dendrimer at a 3:1 ratio (w/w) led to a pronounced growth delay [139]. The plasmid contained Epstein–Barr virus (EBV) sequences with the ability to replicate and persist in the nucleus of the transfected cells (carrying the EBV nuclear antigen, EBNA1, and oriP). The animals received up to four weekly cycles (single injection of complex followed by 100 mg/kg/d of the prodrug ganciclovir for 6 d) [139]. Measuring levels of β-gal expression for the plasmid employing the EBNA1/oriP system were found to be eight times higher than in a conventional plasmid, and/or in conjunction with a vector expressing *Fas* ligand the injection of a 10-μg plasmid complexed with dendrimer (Superfect™) at a ratio of 10:1 (w/w) also led to a pronounced tumor growth delay [140].

A growth delay was also demonstrated after intratumoral injection of plasmids coding for the antiangiogenic peptide angiostatin or the tissue inhibitor of metalloproteinase (TIMP)-2 in special dendrimer–plasmid–oligonucleotide complexes [141,142]. The formulation was based on a mixture of 5 μg of plasmid, 60 μg of activated PAMAM dendrimer (Superfect™), and 20 μg of a 36-mer oligonucleotide complexing the plasmid coding for the therapeutic gene.

Efficient local delivery of an ^{111}In-labeled oligonucleotide to tumor cells in an intraperitoneal model has been demonstrated when complexes with PAMAM$_{G4}$ were injected [143].

13.5.2.6.3   Heart

Following direct injection in a murine cardiac transplant model, PAMAM$_{G5}$ dendrimer complexes demonstrated more widespread and prolonged expression compared to the naked plasmid and, when combined with a viral interleukin 10 gene, were able to prolong graft survival [144]. The efficiency of the procedure was improved at a higher charge ratio of 20:1 [145] and in combination with electroporation [146].

On direct local administration to the adventitia of the rabbit aorta, Superfect™ was also found to be more efficient (4.4%) than branched PEI 25kD (2.8%), branched PEI 800kD (1.8%), or naked DNA (0.5%) [147].

13.5.2.6.4   Lung

Gene expression after intratracheal instillation of fractured PAMAM dendrimer (Superfect™) complexes with a N/P ratio of 4.7 (32.1 μg dendrimer/20 μg plasmid, 50 μL) was found to be 130-fold lower than for the branched PEI 25kD formulation (N/P = 10:1) [148].

13.5.2.7 Systemic Administration

Intravascular administration of complexes with PAMAM$_{G9}$ (200 μg of DNA complexed with 650 μg of dendrimer) led to expression mainly in the lung parenchyma but not in other organs [149].

The systemic administration of dendrimers was also investigated for a PAMAM$_{G3}$ and conjugates of α-cyclodextrin (aCD) with the terminal amines of PAMAM$_{G3}$ [150]. After 12 h the spleen was clearly the preferred organ for gene expression, and gene expression here was at least one order of magnitude higher than the next highest organ, the liver [150]. The modified dendrimer led to a shift in the expression pattern that depended on the level of substitution and significantly improved the expression in some organs [150].

The aim of our own work has been the development of delivery systems for the systemic treatment of diseases and, specifically, of solid tumors. Cancer therapy is currently limited by the difficulty of efficiently delivering therapeutic molecules or genes to remote tumors and metastases by systemic administration [100,105,151].

We have previously developed a number of systems suitable for the *in vivo* delivery of genes [64,152,153]. We have also reported that the lower-generation PPI dendrimers are promising delivery systems that strike a good balance between binding or stability and toxicity [59]. Furthermore, we have demonstrated that these systems are potentially useful for systemic gene therapy: PPI dendrimers of G1–G4 (DAB-Am 4/8/16/32) were characterized and compared with their quaternized counterparts [65]. The quaternization improved DNA binding of the lower generations and the cytotoxicity of the higher generations that were tested. In particular, for PPI_{G2} quaternization proved advantageous as it rendered the previously systemically toxic complex safe. *In vivo* the formulations based on PPI_{G3} (DAB-Am16) and the quaternised PPI_{G2} (QDAB-Am8) efficiently expressed transgenes, predominantly in the liver rather than the lung [65].

We have recently been able to demonstrate that an intravenously administered gene medicine consisting of the PPI_{G3} complexes is able to induce intratumoral transgene expression [154]. When murine xenografts are treated by intravenous injection of PPI_{G3} complexes with a tumor necrosis factor-α (TNF-α) expression plasmid under control of a tumor-specific promoter, regression of established tumors has been observed in 100% of the animals. The treatment (5 injections over 10 d) also led to an excellent long-term response (at 17 weeks: 80% complete and 20% partial response). The antitumor activity is the result of a combination of the effects of the tumor-specific expression of TNF and an intrinsic antiproliferative effect of the dendrimer. This novel antiproliferative effect was also observed with other cationic polymers. The lack of apparent toxicity and significant weight loss compared to untreated controls suggests that the treatment is relatively well tolerated and safe [154].

13.5.3 IMAGING

13.5.3.1 Contrast Agents for Magnetic Resonance Imaging

Magnetic resonance imaging (MRI) is a diagnostic method that can noninvasively provide a wealth of information regarding tumor metabolism, pathophysiology [155], etc. The deconvolution of nuclear resonance signals of water in an induced inhomogeneous field allows anatomical imaging of organs and blood vessels. By introduction of contrast agents, the relaxation time of the water molecules is shortened, which leads to an increased signal-to-noise ratio and imaging sensitivity [156]. Paramagnetic inorganic ion chelates, such as gadolinium diethylenetriaminepentaacetic acid (Gd-DTPA), are widely used in the clinic, but because of their low molecular weight they have the disadvantage of rapid extravascularization [156]. Alternative contrast agents, i.e., stable organic free radicals such as nitroxides are potentially useful for specifically targeted clinical uses, but their use is restricted by the relatively high doses required [157].

Owing to their defined structure and large number of available terminal functional groups, dendrimers seem particularly suited for use as macromolecular contrast agents for MRI [158]. The high density of surface groups means that the chelated Gd reaches a high local concentration with increased sensitivity. For example, the conjugation of the chelator 2-(4-isothiocyanatobenzyl)-6-methyl-diethylenetriaminepentaacetic acid to $PAMAM_{G6}$ leads to a metal–chelate conjugate carrying 170 Gd(III) ions [159]. For this conjugate the enhancement of relaxivity was twice that of other protein- or polymer-based macromolecular agents, and the enhancement half-life was also significantly increased [159].

Their defined structure and the wide range of molecular weights mean that these macromolecular agents can be tuned to image specific structures, e.g. larger dendrimers are particularly suited for imaging the blood pool because they avoid extravasation. The ability of specific dendrimer-based contrast agents to image specific organs or structures seems to depend primarily on their molecular weight and dendrimer hydrophilicity.

13.5.3.1.1   Kidney Imaging

Changes in size of the dendrimer-based macromolecular contrast agent altered the route of excretion [160]. It has been demonstrated that a generation 4 dendrimer-based contrast agent could efficiently detect renal injury caused by administration of cisplatin in mice [161]. Following this discovery, numerous PAMAM and PPI dendrimers having less than 60-kDa molecular weight were compared in order to find an efficient contrast agent for imaging early renal tubular damage [162]. All the dendrimer agents tested allowed the visualization of the renal functional anatomy of the mice. PPI-dendrimer-based agents were cleared more rapidly from the body than PAMAM-dendrimer-based agents with the same number of branches. PPI_{G2} was found to be the best candidate for functional kidney imaging as it was excreted most rapidly, yet it enabled visualization of mild renal tubular injury very early after injury. $PAMAM_{G2}$- and PPI_{G3}-dendrimer-based contrast agents were also relatively quickly excreted, making them potentially useful in clinical applications [163,162].

13.5.3.1.2   Lymphatic Imaging

Larger hydrophilic agents seem to be more suitable for lymphatic imaging [160]. A PAMAM-G8-based MRI contrast agent allowed visualization of the entire lymphatic system by micro-magnetic resonance lymphangiography. When comparing the efficiency of different dendrimers in lymphatic imaging in mice, $PAMAM_{G8}$ seems to give an optimal visualization of lymphatic vessels, whereas PPI_{G5} was found better suited for identification of lymph nodes [164].

13.5.3.1.3   Blood Pool Imaging

Less hydrophilic and larger-sized dendrimer-based contrast agents allow a better imaging of blood vessels [160]. Thanks to their prolonged retention in the circulation compared to Gd-DTPA, this was the first application of dendrimers in MRI [159]. When using contrast agents with PAMAM dendrimer cores smaller than generation 7 but with a molecular weight higher than 60 kDa, the larger molecules (from generation 5) are retained in the blood longer because of less excretion by the kidneys, thus enhancing MRI visualization of the heart and blood vessels, allowing a high level of anatomic detail to be observed [165–167].

But the use of these systems for the exclusive visualization of blood vessels is limited by their concomitant accumulation in the liver. In order to increase the hydrophilicity of the dendrimer-based contrast agent, which would result in a longer half-life in the circulation $PAMAM_{G4}$ dendrimers have been conjugated to polyethylene glycol. This resulted in a prolonged retention in the circulation and a decreased accumulation in the organs [168].

13.5.3.1.4   Liver Imaging

The more hydrophobic dendrimer-based contrast agents of larger molecular weight quickly accumulate in the liver and thus are potentially useful as liver MRI contrast agents [160]. A more hydrophobic PPI-G5-dendrimer-based contrast agent was compared with a $PAMAM_{G4}$ dendrimer for liver imaging. The PPI-based contrast agents accumulate significantly more in the liver and less in the blood than PAMAM-based contrast agents. A PPI-dendrimer-based contrast agent was used to visualize the liver parenchyma and both portal and hepatic veins of 0.5-mm diameter in mice [169].

13.5.3.1.5   Tumor Diagnostics

Targeted dendrimer-based contrast agents could work as tumor-specific contrast agents and could also be used as therapeutic drugs in gadolinium neutron capture therapy or with radioimmunother-apy [160]. PAMAM-G6-and PAMAM-G4-dendrimer-based contrast agents have been targeted to ovarian tumor cells expressing high-affinity folate receptors, by conjugation of folate to the dendrimer. These conjugates have been shown to enhance the visualization of tumor cells overexpressing the folate receptor (33% increase by contrast enhancement) compared with that of a nonspecific contrast agent [170–172]. More recent studies also used nonionic (surface amines capped with acetic anhydride) folate-conjugated PAMAM dendrimers labeled with fluorescein isothiocyanate (FITC) for targeting tumor cells expressing folate receptors [173].

Although the contrast media used in most of the dendrimer-based contrast agents was Gd-DTPA, PPI and PAMAM dendrimers were also conjugated with other contrast agents, such as nitroxides, in an attempt to increase the dose delivered to the organ to be visualized and thus achieve efficacy. PPI-G4- and PAMAM-G3-dendrimer-linked nitroxides were found to increase relaxivity compared to Gd-DTPA, and thus decrease the dose required to achieve MR image enhancement [157].

Another area in which the high number of terminal groups available for conjugation has proven important is in radiotherapy and, specifically, in boron neutron capture therapy (BNCT).

13.5.4 RADIOTHERAPY

BNCT is a cancer treatment based on the selective uptake of high amounts of nonradioactive boron ^{10}B by tumor cells (at least 10^9 atoms per cell), followed by irradiation with low-energy thermal neutrons (<0.025 eV) [174]. The resulting nuclear capture and fission reactions result in the production of highly energetic particles and ^{7}Li nuclei, both of which are highly toxic.

The main limitation of this technique is the inability to achieve selective and sufficiently high accumulation of ^{10}B in the tumor while sparing the normal cells. In theory, targeting of ^{10}B to tumors can be achieved using a number of strategies [151]. One example would be the use of antibodies to recognize surface membrane antigens highly expressed on tumor cells, but with conventional carrier systems the competition or steric hindrance between the boron-containing moieties and the antibodies can impair the targeting efficiency of the antibodies [175]. Here dendrimers have a potential advantage due to their multivalency. The first dendritic BNCT systems prepared by Barth et al. [176] was based on $PAMAM_{G2}$ and $PAMAM_{G4}$ dendrimers conjugated to isocyano polyhedral borane [Na(CH$_3$)$_3$ N ^{10}B H$_8$NCO] and to the monoclonal antibody IB16-6 directed at the murine B16 melanoma. However, one of the limitations of this system has been the accumulation in the liver and spleen [176].

Other studies describe the use of boronated PAMAM G5 conjugated to cetuximab (IMC-C225), a monoclonal antibody specific to the epidermal growth factor (EGF) receptor often overexpressed in brain tumors [177,178]. Following intratumoral administration of boronated cetuximab dendrimer, the mean boron concentration in the brain of rats bearing gliomas was almost ten-fold greater than in normal brain tissue. Furthermore, the antibody cetuximab is particularly attractive as a boron delivery agent as it can also lead by itself to cell cycle arrest by blocking the binding of EGF and transforming growth factor-β (TGF-β), which are involved in cell signaling pathways [179].

Hydrophilic polymer chains have frequently been used to increase circulation times and reduce the interaction of proteins and particulate delivery systems with the blood components [67,68]. As such, conjugation of boronated PAMAM dendrimers to poly(ethylene oxide) chains (to provide steric shielding in an attempt to reduce the liver uptake observed previously) and to folic acid moieties (in order to target folate receptors expressed on the tumor surface) has been carried out [180]. Biodistribution studies in mice bearing 24JK-FBP tumors expressing the folate receptor showed an increased uptake of the dendritic system in the tumors and in the liver and kidneys [180].

Other radiotherapy approaches using dendrimers involve the conjugation of chelators in combination with other radioisotopes along the lines established for MRI contrast agents (vide supra). In order to treat intraperitoneally disseminated tumors internally using a radionuclide, a $PAMAM_{G4}$ dendrimer has been conjugated with ^{111}In, emitting Auger and conversion electrons with very high specific activity [181]. The dendrimer was first biotinylated and then conjugated with 2-(p-isothiocyanatobenzyl)-6-methyl-diethylenetriaminepentaacetic acid (1B4M), a derivative of DTPA. The biotinylated chelate was loaded with ^{111}In and, finally, with avidin to facilitate its binding and internalization into cancer cells by interaction with glycoprotein-binding receptors present on the surface of the cancer cells. The complex showed efficient internalization into cancer cells and tumors after intraperitoneal administration [181].

Another type of radiometal-containing dendrimer with potential radiotherapeutic applications has been described by van Bommel et al. [182]. Here, an adamantine-terminated dendrimer was synthesized with two dendritic wedges around a rhenium core. Although rhenium is widely used as a nonradioactive model for technetium, rhenium itself has the potential to serve as a nuclide in radiotherapy because its isotopes [186]Re and [188]Re emit radiation [182].

13.5.5 Dendrimers as Drugs

Dendrimers have also been shown to be active drugs in their own right. Their activity can be described as antiproliferative in the broadest sense; this includes the inhibition of proliferation of microorganisms or unwanted cellular growth in wound healing or cancer.

13.5.5.1 Anti-Infective and Antimicrobial Dendrimers

The ability of dendrimers to carry multiple terminal groups can be exploited to create multivalent ligands [36] that can act as competitors of natural binding processes such as the binding of a pathogen to cell surfaces. In general, antiviral dendrimers work as artificial mimics of the anionic cell surfaces, thus the dendrimers are generally designed to have anionic surface groups such as carbohydrates and glycopeptides. These molecules are normally present at the mammalian cell surface and can be exploited for the binding of pathogens such as viruses. The competing dendrimers act as "nano decoys," thus preventing or reducing infection.

The binding of heat-labile E. coli enterotoxin and cholera toxin to the respective ganglioside receptor on the surface of intestinal epithelial cells could be reduced by multivalent glycodendrimers [183,184], and a similar strategy with mannosylated dendrimers also reduces binding of E. coli [185].

The first step in the infection of a cell by the influenza virus is the attachment of the virion to the cell membrane through the binding of a virus receptor hemagglutinin to cell surface sialic acid groups. Multivalent sialylic-acid-conjugated dendrimers (sialodendrimers) have been shown to be potent inhibitors of the hemagglutination of human erythrocytes by the influenza viruses [186]. The PAMAM G4–sialic acid conjugate was also able to completely prevent influenza pneumonitis in a murine model in a subtype-dependent fashion [187].

Multivalent polysulfonate dendrimers (phenyldicarboxylic acid, naphthyldisulfonic acid, and sulfated galactosyl ceramide) inhibit cellular adsorption of various HIV-1 strains [188,189]. When internalized, some inhibited virus replication (transcriptase/integrase) further [188]. The disruption of the binding of Tat peptide to the transacting responsive element (TAR) has also been described [190].

PAMAM- and PLL-based polysulfonate dendrimers were also active against herpes simplex virus (type 1 and type 2) in in vitro and in vivo models of genital herpes infection [191,192]. PLL-based dendrimers have also been shown to inhibit late-stage virus replication, probably through inhibition of DNA synthesis [193]. A small dendrimer-like compound was described, which inhibits respiratory syncytial virus (RSV) by interaction with a viral fusion protein [194].

In contrast to the aforementioned strategies based on the inhibition of binding, dendrimers have also been shown to be directly active against bacteria, specifically through interactions with bacterial membranes. The antibacterial dendrimers generally contain cationic surface functionalities such as amines [195,196] or cationic peptides [197]. The general mode of action is through membrane damage and subsequent bacterial lysis.

13.5.5.1.1 Prion Disease

PAMAM and PPI dendrimers have been shown to reduce the prion protein load in scrapie-infected neuroblastoma cells [198]. Exposure of these cells to PPI G4 (3 μg/ml over 4 weeks) also eradicates prion infectivity in a murine bioassay, probably by making the prion protein aggregates susceptible to proteolysis [199,200]. This activity of dendrimers has been related to their ability to act as chaotropic agents that through disruption of the hydrophobic interactions induce destabilization of normal protein tertiary structure [11].

13.5.5.2 Antiproliferative Activity of Dendrimers

13.5.5.2.1 Photodynamic Therapy

Using the ability of dendrimers to accommodate a high density of peripheral groups, dendritic molecules that contain in the branches light-absorbent groups that efficiently harvest light and transfer the energy to the core have been constructed. In polydynamic therapy (PDT) [201] this property is exploited to allow the formation of singlet oxygen upon irradiation with the appropriate light. The highly reactive singlet oxygen acts as a cytotoxic drug that is being produced only in regions where the light of appropriate frequency is focused with sufficient intensity. Crucial parameters for the safety of these photoactivated "prodrugs" are that they should lack any activity under normal light conditions and it should be possible to control their biodistribution. Dendrimers that contained the photosensitizer 5-aminolevulinic acid (ALA) as terminal functions in first- and second-generation dendrimers were synthesized and tested against tumor cells [202].

Third-generation aryl ether dendrimer porphyrins with quaternary ammonium or carboxylic terminal groups were used as supramolecular photosensitizers [203]. The light-harvesting dendrimer porphyrins differ in their cell interaction, depending on the dendrimer surface charge; they were shown to be associated with intracellular membranes where they induced photodamage [203]. Aryl ether porphyrins were also used as part of a micellar system for the delivery of PDT [204].

The activity of dendrimers against unwanted growth and proliferation is again based on the multiplicity of interactions. The interaction of some cytokines depends on the presence of heparin and heparin sulfate proteoglycan (HSPG), which act as their coreceptors. An antiangiogenic dendrimer was synthesized that would bind or compete for these Heparin- or HSPG-type binding sites on endothelial cells. This endostatin peptide mimic was able to inhibit angiogenesis in a chicken embryo chorioallantoic membrane assay [205].

The polyvalency of dendrimer glucosamine conjugates is also thought to be responsible for the ability of these molecules to efficiently inhibit scar-tissue formation [206]. The dendrimer–D(+)-glucosamine (DG) conjugate was found to reversibly modulate the immune response to lipopolysaccharide-induced synthesis of cytokines, whereas the D(+)-glucosamine 6-sulfate–dendrimer conjugate (DGS) was active as an inhibitor of angiogenesis. The DG conjugate was found to downregulate specific elements of dendritic cell function in the pathway of the toll-like receptor 4 (TLR4), which led to a subsequent reduced release of proinflammatory cytokines. The DGS conjugate inhibited proliferation of human umbilical vein endothelial cells (HUVEC), which is normally mediated by fibroblast growth factor-2 (FGF2). In combination, the dendrimer conjugates were able to prevent scar-tissue formation in a rabbit model of glaucoma filtration surgery, leading to a concomitant increase in the long-term success rate from 30 to 80% [206]. Another example for immune modulation using conjugates of the hapten 2,4 dinitrophenyl (DNP) [207] is described in the literature. Interestingly, larger dendrimer–DNA conjugates were found to trigger mast cell degranulation, whereas smaller conjugates were found to be inhibitory [207]. Dendrimer-mediated antiproliferative activity through immune stimulation has also been reported for a PAMAM dendrimer conjugated with N-acetyl-glucosamine, which was found to delay tumor growth in a dose-dependent fashion on intraperitoneal administration [208].

In the report by Shaunak et al., the unmodified PAMAM G3.5 was found not to have any activity [206]. Our own observations suggest that cationic dendrimers such as Superfect™ or PPI$_{G3}$ can have significant antiproliferative activity in their own right [154]. When PPI$_{G3}$ dendrimers are used as synthetic vectors for the systemic delivery of a TNF-α expression plasmid, the overall therapeutic effect is a combination of the activity of the TNF-α plasmid and the dendrimer alone. In a murine xenograft model, treatment with these dendrimers led to a sustained growth delay. Closer examination of the effects of PPI$_{G3}$ showed that the dendrimer alone induced a significant increase in serum levels of soluble TNF receptor 2 (p75), a surrogate maker of TNF-α [209], and quantitative PCR (Q-PCR) confirmed induction of endogenous TNF-α expression in the tumor [154].

13.6 SUMMARY

Dendrimers are unique synthetic molecules with properties that make them particularly suited for drug and gene delivery applications. In particular, it is the intrinsic property of their structures that allows a high density of surface groups, thus enabling exploitation of their multivalency, which is so important for many applications. Furthermore, the various generations of dendrimers occupy a size range that covers the nanoscale (small peptides to large proteins [1 nm G1 … G10 10 nm], and in supramolecular assemblies 100 nm) similar to many biologically important peptides and proteins. Combined with a well-defined structure, flexible chemistry, and broad biocompatibility, these properties make them ideal candidates for the design of drug and gene delivery systems and nanomedicines.

REFERENCES

1. *Explore Chemical History-Polymers Molecular Giants,* 2005, http://www.chemheritage.org/explore/explore.html.
2. Esfand, R. and Tomalia, D.A., Poly(amidoamine) (PAMAM) dendrimers: from biomimicry to drug delivery and biomedical applications, *Drug Discov. Today,* 6(8): 427–436, 2001.
3. Klajnert, B. and Bryszewska, M., Dendrimers: properties and applications, *Acta. Biochim. Pol.,* 48(1): 199–208, 2001.
4. Buhleier, E., Wehner, E., and Vögtle, F., *Synthesis,* 78, 155–158, 1978.
5. Tomalia, D.A. et al., A new class of polymers — starburst-dendritic macromolecules, *Polym. J.,* 17(1): 117–132, 1985.
6. Newkome, G.R. et al., Micelles.1. cascade molecules — a new approach to micelles — a [27]-arborol, *J. Org. Chem.,* 50(11): 2003–2004, 1985.
7. Newkome, G.R. et al., Cascade molecules.2. synthesis and characterization of a benzene[9]3-arborol, *J. Am. Chem. Soc.,* 108(4): 849–850, 1986.
8. Tomalia, D.A. and Frechet, J.M.J., Discovery of dendrimers and dendritic polymers: a brief historical perspective, *J. Polym. Sci. Part A-Polym. Chem.,* 40(16): 2719–2728, 2002.
9. Cloninger, M.J., Biological applications of dendrimers, *Curr. Opin. Chem. Biol.,* 6(6): 742–748, 2002.
10. Tomalia, D.A. and Majoros, I., Dendrimeric supramolecular and supramacromolecular assemblies (reprinted from *Supramolecular Polymers,* Marcel Dekker: New York, pp. 359–434, 2002), *J. Macromolecular Sci.-Polym. Rev.,* C43(3): 411–477, 2003.
11. Boas, U. and Heegaard, P.M., Dendrimers in drug research, *Chem. Soc. Rev.,* 33(1): 43–63, 2004.
12. Grayson, S.M. and Frechet, J.M., A new approach to heterofunctionalized dendrimers: a versatile triallyl chloride core, *Org. Lett.,* 4(19): 3171–3174, 2002.
13. Vinogradov, S.A. and Wilson, D.F., Electrostatic core shielding in dendritic polyglutamic porphyrins, *Chemistry,* 6(13): 2456–2461, 2000.
14. Eichman, J.D. et al., The use of PAMAM dendrimers in the efficient transfer of genetic material into cells, *Pharm. Sci. Technol. Today,* 3(7): 232–245, 2000.
15. Majoral, J.P., Caminade, A.M., and Maraval, V., The specific contribution of phosphorus in dendrimer chemistry, *Chem. Commun. (Camb),* (24): 2929–2942, 2002.
16. Kanaoka, S. et al., Star-shaped polymers by living cationic polymerization. 8. size and shape of star poly(vinyl ether)s determined by dynamic light-scattering and computer-simulation, *J. Polym. Sci. Part B-Polym. Phys.,* 33(4): 527–535, 1995.
17. Uppuluri, S. et al., Rheology of dendrimers. I. Newtonian flow behavior of medium and highly concentrated solutions of polyamidoamine (PAMAM) dendrimers in ethylenediamine (EDA) solvent, *Macromolecules,* 31(14): 4498–4510, 1998.
18. Fischer, R. et al., Adamantanes, nortricyclenes, and dendrimers with extended silicon backbones, *Chemistry,* 10(4): 1021–1030, 2004.
19. Roy, R. and Baek, M.G., Glycodendrimers: novel glycotope isosteres unmasking sugar coding. case study with T-antigen markers from breast cancer MUC1 glycoprotein, *J. Biotechnol.,* 90(3–4): 291–309, 2002.
20. Turnbull, W.B., Kalovidouris, S.A., and Stoddart, J.F., Large oligosaccharide-based glycodendrimers, *Chemistry,* 8(13): 2988–3000, 2002.

21. Turnbull, W.B. and Stoddart, J.F., Design and synthesis of glycodendrimers, *J. Biotechnol.*, 90(3–4): 231–255, 2002.

22. Sadler, K. and Tam, J.P., Peptide dendrimers: applications and synthesis, *J. Biotechnol.*, 90(3–4): 195–229, 2002.

23. Barth, R.F. and Soloway, A.H., Boron neutron capture therapy of primary and metastatic brain tumors, *Mol. Chem. Neuropathol.*, 21(2–3): 139–154, 1994.

24. Gillies, E.R. and Frechet, J.M., Dendrimers and dendritic polymers in drug delivery, *Drug Discov. Today*, 10(1): 35–43, 2005.

25. Bosman, A.W., Janssen, H.M., and Meijer, E.W., About dendrimers: structure, physical properties and applications, *Chem. Rev.*, 99: 1665–1688, 1999.

26. Merino, S. et al., Synthesis and characterization of linear, hyperbranched, and dendrimer-like polymers constituted of the same repeating unit, *Chemistry*, 7(14): 3095–3105, 2001.

27. Boris, D. and Rubinstein, M., A self-consistent mean field model of a starburst dendrimer: Dense core vs. dense shell, *Macromolecules*, 29(22): 7251–7260, 1996.

28. Chai, M. et al., Structure and conformation of DAB dendrimers in solution via multidimensional NMR techniques, *J. Am. Chem. Soc.*, 123(20): 4670–4678, 2001.

29. Topp, A. et al., Probing the location of the terminal groups of dendrimers in dilute solution, *Macromolecules*, 32(21): 7226–7231, 1999.

30. Topp, A. et al., Effect of solvent quality on the molecular dimensions of PAMAM dendrimers, *Macromolecules*, 32(21): 7232–7237, 1999.

31. Rietveld, I.B. et al., Location of the outer shell and influence of pH on carboxylic acid-functionalized poly(propyleneimine) dendrimers, *Macromolecules*, 34(23): 8380–8383, 2001.

32. Jones, J.W. et al., Crowned dendrimers: pH-responsive pseudorotaxane formation, *J. Org. Chem.*, 68(6): 2385–2839, 2003.

33. Frechet, J.M., Functional polymers and dendrimers: reactivity, molecular architecture, and interfacial energy, *Science*, 263(5154): 1710–1715, 1994.

34. Mourey, T.H. et al., Unique behavior of dendritic macromolecules — intrinsic-viscosity of polyether dendrimers, *Macromolecules*, 25(9): 2401–2406, 1992.

35. Alper, J., Rising chemical "stars" could play many roles, *Science*, 251(5001): 1562–1564, 1991.

36. Mammen, M., Choi, S.-K., and Whitesides, G.M., Polyvalent interactions in biological systems: implications for design and use of multivalent ligands and inhibitors, *Angew. Chem. Int. Ed. Engl.*, 37: 2754–2794, 1998.

37. Bielinska, A.U. et al., DNA complexing with polyamidoamine dendrimers: implications for transfection, *Bioconjugate Chem.*, 10(5): 843–850, 1999.

38. Bezouska, K., Design, functional evaluation and biomedical applications of carbohydrate dendrimers (glycodendrimers), *J. Biotechnol.*, 90(3–4): 269–290, 2002.

39. Bhadra, D. et al., A PEGylated dendritic nanoparticulate carrier of fluorouracil, *Int. J. Pharm.*, 257(1–2): 111–124, 2003.

40. Kojima, C. et al., Synthesis of polyamidoamine dendrimers having poly(ethylene glycol) grafts and their ability to encapsulate anticancer drugs, *Bioconjugate Chem.*, 11(6): 910–917, 2000.

41. Gillies, E.R., Jonsson, T.B., and Frechet, J.M., Stimuli-responsive supramolecular assemblies of linear-dendritic copolymers, *J. Am. Chem. Soc.*, 126(38): 11936–11943, 2004.

42. Hawker, C.J., Wooley, K.L., and Frechet, J.M.J., Unimolecular micelles and globular amphiphiles — dendritic macromolecules as novel recyclable solubilization agents, *J. Chem. Soc. Perkin Trans.*, 1, (12): 1287–1297, 1993.

43. Wallimann, P. et al., Steroids in molecular recognition, *Chem. Rev.*, 97(5): 1567–1608, 1997.

44. Smith, D.K. and Diederich, F., Dendritic hydrogen bonding receptors: enantiomerically pure dendroclefts for the selective recognition of monosaccharides, *Chem. Commun.*, (22): 2501–2502, 1998.

45. Twyman, L.J. et al., The synthesis of water soluble dendrimers, and their application as possible drug delivery systems, *Tetrahedron Lett.*, 40(9): 1743–1746, 1999.

46. Watkins, D.M. et al., Dendrimers with hydrophobic cores and the formation of supramolecular dendrimer-surfactant assemblies, *Langmuir*, 13(12): 3136–3141, 1997.

47. SayedSweet, Y. et al., Hydrophobically modified poly(amidoamine) (PAMAM) dendrimers: Their properties at the air-water interface and use as nanoscopic container molecules, *J. Mater. Chem.*, 7(7): 1199–1205, 1997.

48. Jansen, J., Debrabandervandenberg, E.M.M., and Meijer, E.W., Encapsulation of guest molecules into a dendritic box, *Science*, 266(5188): 1226–1229, 1994.

49. Schenning, A. et al., Amphiphilic dendrimers as building blocks in supramolecular assemblies, *J. Am. Chem. Soc.*, 120(32): 8199–8208, 1998.

50. Zimmerman, S.C. et al., Self-assembling dendrimers, *Science*, 271(5252): 1095–1098, 1996.

51. Sakthivel, T., Toth, I., and Florence, A.T., Synthesis and physicochemical properties of lipophilic polyamide dendrimers, *Pharm. Res.*, 15(5): 776–782, 1998.

52. Al-Jamal, K.T., Sakthivel, T., and Florence, A.T., Dendrisomes: vesicular structures derived from a cationic lipidic dendron, *J. Pharm. Sci.*, 94(1): 102–113, 2005.

53. Bielinska, A. et al., Regulation of in vitro gene expression using antisense oligonucleotides or antisense expression plasmids transfected using starburst PAMAM dendrimers, *Nucl. Acids Res.*, 24(11): 2176–2182, 1996.

54. Fischer, D. et al., In vitro cytotoxicity testing of polycations: influence of polymer structure on cell viability and hemolysis, *Biomaterials*, 24(7): 1121–1131, 2003.

55. Ruponen, M., Yla-Herttuala, S., and Urtti, A., Interactions of polymeric and liposomal gene delivery systems with extracellular glycosaminoglycans: physicochemical and transfection studies, *Biochim. Biophys. Acta*, 1415(2): 331–341, 1999.

56. Ottaviani, M.F. et al., Interactions between starburst dendrimers and mixed DMPC/DMPA-Na vesicles studied by the spin label and the spin probe techniques, supported by transmission electron microscopy, *Langmuir*, 18(6): 2347–2357, 2002.

57. Hong, S. et al., Interaction of poly(amidoamine) dendrimers with supported lipid bilayers and cells: hole formation and the relation to transport, *Bioconjugate Chem.*, 15(4): 774–782, 2004.

58. Haensler, J. and Szoka, F.C., Jr., Polyamidoamine cascade polymers mediate efficient transfection of cells in culture, *Bioconjugate Chem.*, 4(5): 372–379, 1993.

59. Zinselmeyer, B.H. et al., The lower-generation polypropylenimine dendrimers are effective gene-transfer agents, *Pharm. Res.*, 19(7): 960–967, 2002.

60. Roberts, J.C., Bhalgat, M.K., and Zera, R.T., Preliminary biological evaluation of polyamidoamine (PAMAM) Starburst dendrimers, *J. Biomed. Mater. Res.*, 30(1): 53–65, 1996.

61. Jevprasesphant, R. et al., The influence of surface modification on the cytotoxicity of PAMAM dendrimers, *Int. J. Pharm.*, 252(1–2): 263–266, 2003.

62. Malik, N. et al., Dendrimers: relationship between structure and biocompatibility in vitro, and preliminary studies on the biodistribution of I-125-labelled polyamidoamine dendrimers in vivo, *J. Controlled Release*, 65(1–2): 133–148, 2000.

63. Uchegbu, I.F. et al., Gene transfer with three amphiphilic glycol chitosans — the degree of polymerisation is the main controller of transfection efficiency, *J. Drug Target*, 12(8): 527–539, 2004.

64. Brownlie, A., Uchegbu, I.F., and Schatzlein, A.G., PEI-based vesicle-polymer hybrid gene delivery system with improved biocompatibility, *Int. J. Pharm.*, 274(1–2): 41–52, 2004.

65. Schatzlein, A.G. et al., Preferential liver gene expression with polypropylenimine dendrimers, *J. Controlled Release*, 101(1–3): 247–258, 2005.

66. Malik, N. et al., Dendrimers: relationship between structure and biocompatibility in vitro, and preliminary studies on the biodistribution of 125I-labelled polyamidoamine dendrimers in vivo, *J. Controlled Release*, 65(1–2): 133–148, 2000.

67. Harris, J.M. and Chess, R.B., Effect of pegylation on pharmaceuticals, *Nat. Rev. Drug Discov.*, 2(3): 214–221, 2003.

68. Molineux, G., Pegylation: engineering improved pharmaceuticals for enhanced therapy, *Cancer Treat. Rev.*, 28(Suppl. A): 13–16, 2002.

69. Chen, H.T. et al., Cytotoxicity, hemolysis, and acute in vivo toxicity of dendrimers based on melamine, candidate vehicles for drug delivery, *J. Am. Chem. Soc.*, 126(32): 10044–10048, 2004.

70. Florence, A.T., Issues in oral nanoparticle drug carrier uptake and targeting, *J. Drug Target*, 12(2): 65–70, 2004.

71. Sakthivel, T., Toth, I., and Florence, A.T., Distribution of a lipidic 2.5 nm diameter dendrimer carrier after oral administration, *Int. J. Pharm.*, 183(1): 51–55, 1999.

72. Florence, A.T., Sakthivel, T., and Toth, I., Oral uptake and translocation of a polylysine dendrimer with a lipid surface, *J. Controlled Release*, 65(1–2): 253–259, 2000.

73. Florence, A.T. and Hussain, N., Transcytosis of nanoparticle and dendrimer delivery systems: evolving vistas, *Adv. Drug Delivery Rev.*, 50(Suppl. 1): S69–89, 2001.

74. Wiwattanapatapee, R. et al., Anionic PAMAM dendrimers rapidly cross adult rat intestine in vitro: a potential oral delivery system? *Pharm. Res.*, 17(8): 991–998, 2000.

75. Wilbur, D.S. et al., Biotin reagents for antibody pretargeting. 3. Synthesis, radioiodination, and evaluation of biotinylated starburst dendrimers, *Bioconjugate Chem.*, 9(6): 813–825, 1998.

76. Rajananthanan, P. et al., Evaluation of novel aggregate structures as adjuvants: composition, toxicity studies and humoral responses, *Vaccine*, 17(7–8): 715–730, 1999.

77. Spetzler, J.C. and Tam, J.P., Self-assembly of cyclic peptides on a dendrimer: multiple cyclic antigen peptides, *Pept. Res.*, 9(6): 290–296, 1996.

78. Matsumura, Y. and Maeda, H., A new concept for macromolecular therapeutics in cancer chemotherapy: mechanism of tumoritropic accumulation of proteins and the antitumor agent smancs, *Cancer Res.*, 46(12 pt. 1): 6387–6392, 1986.

79. Duncan, R., The dawning era of polymer therapeutics, *Nat. Rev. Drug Discov.*, 2(5): 347–360, 2003.

80. Plank, C. et al., Activation of the complement system by synthetic DNA complexes: a potential barrier for intravenous gene delivery, *Hum. Gene Ther.*, 7(12): 1437–1446, 1996.

81. Rosenecker, J. et al., Interaction of bronchoalveolar lavage fluid with polyplexes and lipoplexes: analysing the role of proteins and glycoproteins, *J. Gene Med.*, 5(1): 49–60, 2003.

82. Zeng, F.W. and Zimmerman, S.C., Dendrimers in supramolecular chemistry: from molecular recognition to self-assembly, *Chem. Rev.*, 97(5): 1681–1712, 1997.

83. Hecht, S. and Frechet, J.M., Dendritic encapsulation of function: applying nature's site isolation principle from biomimetics to materials science, *Angew. Chem. Int. Ed. Engl.*, 40(1): 74–91, 2001.

84. Nourse, A., Millar, D.B., and Minton, A.P., Physicochemical characterization of generation 5 polyamidoamine dendrimers, *Biopolymers*, 53(4): 316–328, 2000.

85. Ohshima, A. et al., Ordered structure in ionic dilute solutions: dendrimers with univalent and bivalent counterions, *Phys. Rev. E Stat. Nonlin. Soft. Matter Phys.*, 64(5 pt. 1): 051808, 2001.

86. Tripathi, P.K. et al., Dendrimer grafts for delivery of 5-fluorouracil, *Pharmazie*, 57(4): 261–264, 2002.

87. Purohit, G., Sakthivel, T., and Florence, A.T., Interaction of cationic partial dendrimers with charged and neutral liposomes, *Int. J. Pharm.*, 214(1–2): 71–76, 2001.

88. Khopade, A.J. and Caruso, F., Stepwise self-assembled poly(amidoamine) dendrimer and poly(styrenesulfonate) microcapsules as sustained delivery vehicles, *Biomacromolecules*, 3(6): 1154–1162, 2002.

89. Kono, K., Liu, M., and Frechet, J.M., Design of dendritic macromolecules containing folate or methotrexate residues, *Bioconjugate Chem.*, 10(6): 1115–1121, 1999.

90. Quintana, A. et al., Design and function of a dendrimer-based therapeutic nanodevice targeted to tumor cells through the folate receptor, *Pharm. Res.*, 19(9): 1310–1316, 2002.

91. Patri, A.K. et al., Synthesis and in vitro testing of J591 antibody-dendrimer conjugates for targeted prostate cancer therapy, *Bioconjugate Chem.*, 15(6): 1174–1181, 2004.

92. Malik, N., Evagorou, E.G., and Duncan, R., Dendrimer-platinate: a novel approach to cancer chemotherapy, *Anticancer Drugs*, 10(8): 767–776, 1999.

93. Schätzlein, A.G., Introduction to therapeutic nucleic acids, in *Biomaterials-Based Delivery and Biocompatibility of Proteins and Nucleic Acids*, Mahato, R., Ed., CRC Press, Boca Raton, FL, 2004, pp. 531–568.

94. Nishikawa, M. and Huang, L., Nonviral vectors in the new millennium: delivery barriers in gene transfer, *Hum. Gene Ther.*, 12(8): 861–870, 2001.

95. Anderson, W.F., Human gene therapy, *Nature*, 392(6679 SS): 25–30, 1998.

96. Pearson, S., Jia, H., and Kandachi, K., China approves first gene therapy, *Nat. Biotechnol.*, 22(1): 3–4, 2004.

97. Lehrman, S., Virus treatment questioned after gene therapy death, *Nature*, 517–518, 1999.

98. Kaiser, J., Gene therapy. Panel urges limits on X-SCID trials, *Science*, 307(5715): 1544–1545, 2005.

99. Brown, M.D., Schätzlein, A.G., and Uchegbu, I.F., Gene delivery with synthetic (non viral) carriers, *Int. J. Pharm.*, 229(1–2): 1–21, 2001.

100. Schätzlein, A.G., Non-viral vectors in cancer gene therapy: principles and progress, *Anti-Cancer Drugs*, 12(4): 275–304, 2001.

101. Wagner, E., Kircheis, R., and Walker, G.F., Targeted nucleic acid delivery into tumors: new avenues for cancer therapy, *Biomed. Pharmacother.*, 58(3): 152–161, 2004.
102. Dufes, C., Schätzlein, A.G., and Uchegbu, I.F., Dendritic polymers in gene therapy, *Adv. Drug Delivery Rev.*, 57(15): 2177–2202, 2005.
103. Niven, R. et al., Biodistribution of radiolabeled lipid-DNA complexes and DNA in mice, *J. Pharm. Sci.*, 87(11): 1292–1299, 1998.
104. Mislick, K.A. and Baldeschwieler, J.D., Evidence for the role of proteoglycans in cation-mediated gene transfer, *Proc. Natl. Acad. Sci. USA*, 93(22): 12349–12354, 1996.
105. Schätzlein, A.G., Targeting of synthetic gene delivery systems, *J. Biomed. Biotechnol.*, 2003(2): 149–158, 2003.
106. Bragonzi, A. et al., Comparison between cationic polymers and lipids in mediating systemic gene delivery to the lungs, *Gene Ther.*, 6(12): 1995–2004, 1999.
107. Song, Y.K. and Liu, D.X., Free liposomes enhance the transfection activity of DNA/lipid complexes in vivo by intravenous administration, *Biochim. Biophys. Acta*, 1372(1): 141–150, 1998.
108. Song, Y.K., Liu, F., and Liu, D., Enhanced gene expression in mouse lung by prolonging the retention time of intravenously injected plasmid DNA, *Gene Ther.*, 5(11): 1531–1537, 1998.
109. Coll, J.L. et al., In vivo delivery to tumors of DNA complexed with linear polyethylenimine, *Hum. Gene Ther.*, 10(10): 1659–1666, 1999.
110. Goula, D. et al., Polyethylenimine-based intravenous delivery of transgenes to mouse lung, *Gene Ther.*, 5(9): 1291–1295, 1998.
111. Bielinska, A.U., Kukowska-Latallo, J.F., and Baker, J.R., Jr., The interaction of plasmid DNA with polyamidoamine dendrimers: mechanism of complex formation and analysis of alterations induced in nuclease sensitivity and transcriptional activity of the complexed DNA, *Biochim. Biophys. Acta*, 1353(2): 180–190, 1997.
112. Abdelhady, H.G. et al., Direct real-time molecular scale visualisation of the degradation of condensed DNA complexes exposed to DNase I, *Nucl. Acids Res.*, 31(14): 4001–4005, 2003.
113. Tang, M.X. and Szoka, F.C., The influence of polymer structure on the interactions of cationic polymers with DNA and morphology of the resulting complexes, *Gene Ther.*, 4(8): 823–832, 1997.
114. Chen, W., Turro, N.J., and Tomalia, D.A., Using ethidium bromide to probe the interactions between DNA and dendrimers, *Langmuir*, 16(1): 15–19, 2000.
115. Tang, M.X., Redemann, C.T., and Szoka, F.C., Jr., In vitro gene delivery by degraded polyamidoamine dendrimers, *Bioconjugate Chem.*, 7(6): 703–714, 1996.
116. Kukowska-Latallo, J.F. et al., Efficient transfer of genetic material into mammalian cells using Starburst polyamidoamine dendrimers, *Proc. Natl. Acad Sci. USA*, 93(10): 4897–4902, 1996.
117. Kabanov, V.A. et al., Interpolyelectrolyte complexes formed by DNA and astramol poly(propylene imine) dendrimers, *Macromolecules*, 33(26): 9587–9593, 2000.
118. Ottaviani, M.F. et al., Formation of supramolecular structures between DNA and starburst dendrimers studied by EPR, CD, UV, and melting profiles, *Macromolecules*, 33(21): 7842–7851, 2000.
119. Mitra, A. and Imae, T., Nanogel formation consisting of DNA and poly(amido amine) dendrimer studied by static light scattering and atomic force microscopy, *Biomacromolecules*, 5(1): 69–73, 2004.
120. Schatzlein, A.G. et al., Preferential liver gene expression with polypropylenimine dendrimers, *J. Controlled Release*, 101(1–3): 247–258, 2005.
121. Manunta, M. et al., Gene delivery by dendrimers operates via a cholesterol dependent pathway, *Nucl. Acids Res.*, 32(9): 2730–2739, 2004.
122. Zuhorn, I.S., Kalicharan, R., and Hoekstra, D., Lipoplex-mediated transfection of mammalian cells occurs through the cholesterol-dependent clathrin-mediated pathway of endocytosis, *J. Biol. Chem.*, 277(20): 18021–18028, 2002.
123. Zhang, Z.Y. and Smith, B.D., High-generation polycationic dendrimers are unusually effective at disrupting anionic vesicles: Membrane bending model, *Bioconjugate Chem.*, 11(6): 805–814, 2000.
124. Lai, J.C., Yuan, C., and Thomas, J.L., Single-cell measurements of polyamidoamine dendrimer binding, *Ann. Biomed. Eng.*, 30(3): 409–416, 2002.
125. Sonawane, N.D., Szoka, F.C., Jr., and Verkman, A.S., Chloride accumulation and swelling in endosomes enhances DNA transfer by polyamine-DNA polyplexes, *J. Biol. Chem.*, 278(45): 44826–44831, 2003.
126. Behr, J.P., Gene transfer with synthetic cationic amphiphiles: prospects for gene therapy, *Bioconjugate Chem.*, 5(5): 382–389, 1994.

127. Yoo, H. and Juliano, R.L., Enhanced delivery of antisense oligonucleotides with fluorophore-conjugated PAMAM dendrimers, *Nucl. Acids Res.*, 28(21): 4225–4231, 2000.

128. Godbey, W.T., Wu, K.K., and Mikos, A.G., Tracking the intracellular path of poly(ethylenimine)/DNA complexes for gene delivery, *Proc. Natl. Acad Sci. USA*, 96(9): 5177–5181, 1999.

129. Delong, R. et al., Characterization of complexes of oligonucleotides with polyamidoamine starburst dendrimers and effects on intracellular delivery, *J. Pharm. Sci.*, 86(6): 762–764, 1997.

130. Yoo, H., Sazani, P., and Juliano, R.L., PAMAM dendrimers as delivery agents for antisense oligonucleotides, *Pharm. Res.*, 16(12): 1799–1804, 1999.

131. Helin, V. et al., Uptake and intracellular distribution of oligonucleotides vectorized by a PAMAM dendrimer, *Nucleosides Nucleotides*, 18(6–7): 1721–1722, 1999.

132. Hollins, A.J. et al., Evaluation of generation 2 and 3 poly(propylenimine) dendrimers for the potential cellular delivery of antisense oligonucleotides targeting the epidermal growth factor receptor, *Pharm. Res.*, 21(3): 458–466, 2004.

133. Santhakumaran, L.M., Thomas, T., and Thomas, T.J., Enhanced cellular uptake of a triplex-forming oligonucleotide by nanoparticle formation in the presence of polypropylenimine dendrimers, *Nucl. Acids Res.*, 32(7): 2102–2112, 2004.

134. de Jong, G. et al., Efficient in-vitro transfer of a 60-Mb mammalian artificial chromosome into murine and hamster cells using cationic lipids and dendrimers, *Chromosome Res.*, 9(6): 475–485, 2001.

135. Haensler, J. and Szoka, F.C., Jr., Polyamidoamine cascade polymers mediate efficient transfection of cells in culture, *Bioconjugate Chem.*, 4(5): 372–379, 1993.

136. Gebhart, C.L. and Kabanov, A.V., Evaluation of polyplexes as gene transfer agents, *J. Controlled Release*, 73(2–3): 401–416, 2001.

137. Hudde, T. et al., Activated polyamidoamine dendrimers, a non-viral vector for gene transfer to the corneal endothelium, *Gene Ther.*, 6(5): 939–943, 1999.

138. Marano, R.J. et al., Inhibition of in vitro VEGF expression and choroidal neovascularization by synthetic dendrimer peptide mediated delivery of a sense oligonucleotide, *Exp. Eye Res.*, 79(4): 525–535, 2004.

139. Maruyama-Tabata, H. et al., Effective suicide gene therapy in vivo by EBV-based plasmid vector coupled with polyamidoamine dendrimer, *Gene Ther.*, 7(1): 53–60, 2000.

140. Nakanishi, H. et al., Nonviral genetic transfer of Fas ligand induced significant growth suppression and apoptotic tumor cell death in prostate cancer in vivo, *Gene Ther.*, 10(5): 434–442, 2003.

141. Maksimenko, A.V. et al., Optimisation of dendrimer-mediated gene transfer by anionic oligomers, *J. Gene Med.*, 5(1): 61–71, 2003.

142. Vincent, L. et al., Efficacy of dendrimer-mediated angiostatin and TIMP-2 gene delivery on inhibition of tumor growth and angiogenesis: in vitro and in vivo studies, *Int. J. Cancer*, 105(3): 419–429, 2003.

143. Sato, N. et al., Tumor targeting and imaging of intraperitoneal tumors by use of antisense oligo-DNA complexed with dendrimers and/or avidin in mice, *Clin. Cancer Res.*, 7(11): 3606–3612, 2001.

144. Qin, L. et al., Efficient transfer of genes into murine cardiac grafts by Starburst polyamidoamine dendrimers, *Hum. Gene Ther.*, 9(4): 553–560, 1998.

145. Wang, Y. et al., DNA/dendrimer complexes mediate gene transfer into murine cardiac transplants ex vivo, *Mol. Ther.*, 2(6): 602–608, 2000.

146. Wang, Y. et al., Combination of electroporation and DNA/dendrimer complexes enhances gene transfer into murine cardiac transplants, *Am. J. Transplant.*, 1(4): 334–338, 2001.

147. Turunen, M.P. et al., Efficient adventitial gene delivery to rabbit carotid artery with cationic polymer-plasmid complexes, *Gene Ther.*, 6(1): 6–11, 1999.

148. Rudolph, C. et al., In vivo gene delivery to the lung using polyethylenimine and fractured polyamidoamine dendrimers, *J. Gene Med.*, 2(4): 269–278, 2000.

149. Kukowska-Latallo, J.F. et al., Intravascular and endobronchial DNA delivery to murine lung tissue using a novel, nonviral vector, *Hum. Gene Ther.*, 11(10): 1385–1395, 2000.

150. Kihara, F. et al., In vitro and in vivo gene transfer by an optimized alpha-cyclodextrin conjugate with polyamidoamine dendrimer, *Bioconjugate Chem.*, 14(2): 342–350, 2003.

151. Cassidy, J. and Schätzlein, A.G., Tumor targeted drug and gene delivery: principles and concepts, *Exp. Rev. Mol. Med.*, 6(19): 1–17, 2004.

152. Brown, M.D. et al., Preliminary characterization of novel amino acid based polymeric vesicles as gene and drug delivery agents, *Bioconjugate Chem.*, 11(6): 880–891, 2000.

153. Brown, M.D. et al., In vitro and in vivo gene transfer with poly(amino acid) vesicles, *J. Controlled Release*, 93(2): 193–211, 2003.

154. Dufes, C. et al., Synthetic anti-cancer gene medicine exploits intrinsic anti-tumor activity of cationic vector to cure established tumors, *Cancer Res.*, 65: 8079–8084, 2005.

155. Runge Val, M., *Clinical MRI*, London: Saunders, 2002, 504 p.

156. Merbach, A.E. and Tóth, É., *The Chemistry of Contrast Agents in Medical Magnetic Resonance Imaging*, Chichester: John Wiley & Sons, 2001, 300 p.

157. Winalski, C.S. et al., Magnetic resonance relaxivity of dendrimer-linked nitroxides, *Magn. Reson. Med.*, 48(6): 965–972, 2002.

158. Fischer, M. and Vogtle, F., Dendrimers: From design to application — a progress report, *Angew. Chem. Int. Ed. Engl.*, 38(7): 885–905, 1999.

159. Wiener, E.C. et al., Dendrimer-based metal chelates: a new class of magnetic resonance imaging contrast agents, *Magn. Reson. Med.*, 31(1): 1–8, 1994.

160. Kobayashi, H. and Brechbiel, M.W., Dendrimer-based nanosized MRI contrast agents, *Curr. Pharm. Biotechnol.*, 5(6): 539–549, 2004.

161. Kobayashi, H. et al., Renal tubular damage detected by dynamic micro-MRI with a dendrimer-based magnetic resonance contrast agent, *Kidney Int.*, 61(6): 1980–1985, 2002.

162. Kobayashi, H. et al., Polyamine dendrimer-based MRI contrast agents for functional kidney imaging to diagnose acute renal failure, *J. Magn. Reson. Imaging*, 20(3): 512–518, 2004.

163. Kobayashi, H. et al., Macromolecular MRI contrast agents with small dendrimers: pharmacokinetic differences between sizes and cores, *Bioconjugate Chem.*, 14(2): 388–394, 2003.

164. Kobayashi, H. et al., Comparison of dendrimer-based macromolecular contrast agents for dynamic micro-magnetic resonance lymphangiography, *Magn. Reson. Med.*, 50(4): 758–766, 2003.

165. Kobayashi, H. et al., 3D-micro-MR angiography of mice using macromolecular MR contrast agents with polyamidoamine dendrimer core with reference to their pharmacokinetic properties, *Magn. Reson. Med.*, 45(3): 454–460, 2001.

166. Kobayashi, H. et al., Comparison of the macromolecular MR contrast agents with ethylenediamine-core versus ammonia-core generation-6 polyamidoamine dendrimer, *Bioconjugate Chem.*, 12(1): 100–107, 2001.

167. Sato, N. et al., Pharmacokinetics and enhancement patterns of macromolecular MR contrast agents with various sizes of polyamidoamine dendrimer cores, *Magn. Reson. Med.*, 46(6): 1169–1173, 2001.

168. Kobayashi, H. et al., Positive effects of polyethylene glycol conjugation to generation-4 polyamidoamine dendrimers as macromolecular MR contrast agents, *Magn. Reson. Med.*, 46(4): 781–788, 2001.

169. Kobayashi, H. et al., Novel liver macromolecular MR contrast agent with a polypropylenimine diaminobutyl dendrimer core: comparison to the vascular MR contrast agent with the polyamidoamine dendrimer core, *Magn. Reson. Med.*, 46(4): 795–802, 2001.

170. Konda, S.D. et al., Development of a tumor-targeting MR contrast agent using the high-affinity folate receptor: work in progress, *Invest Radiol.*, 35(1): 50–57, 2000.

171. Konda, S.D. et al., Specific targeting of folate-dendrimer MRI contrast agents to the high affinity folate receptor expressed in ovarian tumor xenografts, *Magma*, 12(2–3): 104–113, 2001.

172. Wiener, E.C. et al., Targeting dendrimer-chelates to tumors and tumor cells expressing the high-affinity folate receptor, *Invest. Radiol.*, 32(12): 748–754, 1997.

173. Patri, A.K., Majoros, I.J., and Baker, J.R., Dendritic polymer macromolecular carriers for drug delivery, *Curr. Opin. Chem. Biol.*, 6(4): 466–471, 2002.

174. Barth, R.F. et al., Molecular targeting of the epidermal growth factor receptor for neutron capture therapy of gliomas, *Cancer Res.*, 62(11): 3159–3166, 2002.

175. Alam, F. et al., Dicesium N-succinimidyl 3-(undecahydro-closo-dodecaboranyldithio)propionate, a novel heterobifunctional boronating agent, *J. Med. Chem.*, 28(4): 522–525, 1985.

176. Barth, R.F. et al., Boronated starburst dendrimer-monoclonal antibody immunoconjugates: evaluation as a potential delivery system for neutron capture therapy, *Bioconjugate Chem.*, 5(1): 58–66, 1994.

177. Sauter, G. et al., Patterns of epidermal growth factor receptor amplification in malignant gliomas, *Am. J. Pathol.*, 148(4): 1047–1053, 1996.

178. Wu, G. et al., Site-specific conjugation of boron-containing dendrimers to anti-EGF receptor monoclonal antibody cetuximab (IMC-C225) and its evaluation as a potential delivery agent for neutron capture therapy, *Bioconjugate Chem.*, 15(1): 185–194, 2004.

179. Huang, S.M., Bock, J.M., and Harari, P.M., Epidermal growth factor receptor blockade with C225 modulates proliferation, apoptosis, and radiosensitivity in squamous cell carcinomas of the head and neck, *Cancer Res.*, 59(8): 1935–1940, 1999.

180. Shukla, S. et al., Synthesis and biological evaluation of folate receptor-targeted boronated PAMAM dendrimers as potential agents for neutron capture therapy, *Bioconjugate Chem.*, 14(1): 158–167, 2003.

181. Mamede, M. et al., Radiolabeling of avidin with very high specific activity for internal radiation therapy of intraperitoneally disseminated tumors, *Clin. Cancer Res.*, 9(10 pt. 1): 3756–3762, 2003.

182. van Bommel, K.J. et al., Water-soluble adamantane-terminated dendrimers possessing a rhenium core, *J. Org. Chem.*, 66(16): 5405–5412, 2001.

183. Thompson, J.P. and Schengrund, C.L., Inhibition of the adherence of cholera toxin and the heat-labile enterotoxin of Escherichia coli to cell-surface GM1 by oligosaccharide-derivatized dendrimers, *Biochem. Pharmacol.*, 56(5): 591–597, 1998.

184. Thompson, J.P. and Schengrund, C.L., Oligosaccharide-derivatized dendrimers: defined multivalent inhibitors of the adherence of the cholera toxin B subunit and the heat labile enterotoxin of E. coli to GM1, *Glycoconjugate J.*, 14(7): 837–845, 1997.

185. Nagahori, N. et al., Inhibition of adhesion of type 1 fimbriated Escherichia coli to highly mannosylated ligands, *Chembiochem*, 3(9): 836–844, 2002.

186. Reuter, J.D. et al., Inhibition of viral adhesion and infection by sialic-acid-conjugated dendritic polymers, *Bioconjugate Chem.*, 10(2): 271–278, 1999.

187. Landers, J.J. et al., Prevention of influenza pneumonitis by sialic acid-conjugated dendritic polymers, *J. Infect. Dis.*, 186(9): 1222–1230, 2002.

188. Witvrouw, M. et al., Polyanionic (i.e., polysulfonate) dendrimers can inhibit the replication of human immunodeficiency virus by interfering with both virus adsorption and later steps (reverse transcriptase/integrase) in the virus replicative cycle, *Mol. Pharmacol.*, 58(5): 1100–1108, 2000.

189. Kensinger, R.D. et al., Novel polysulfated galactose-derivatized dendrimers as binding antagonists of human immunodeficiency virus type 1 infection, *Antimicrob. Agents Chemother.*, 48(5): 1614–1623, 2004.

190. Zhao, H. et al., Polyamidoamine dendrimers inhibit binding of Tat peptide to TAR RNA, *FEBS Lett.*, 563(1–3): 241–245, 2004.

191. Bourne, N. et al., Dendrimers, a new class of candidate topical microbicides with activity against herpes simplex virus infection, *Antimicrob. Agents Chemother.*, 44(9): 2471–2474, 2000.

192. Bernstein, D.I. et al., Evaluations of unformulated and formulated dendrimer-based microbicide candidates in mouse and guinea pig models of genital herpes, *Antimicrob. Agents Chemother.*, 47(12): 3784–3788, 2003.

193. Gong, Y. et al., Evidence of dual sites of action of dendrimers: SPL-2999 inhibits both virus entry and late stages of herpes simplex virus replication, *Antiviral Res.*, 55(2): 319–329, 2002.

194. Razinkov, V. et al., RFI-641 inhibits entry of respiratory syncytial virus via interactions with fusion protein, *Chem. Biol.*, 8(7): 645–659, 2001.

195. Chen, C.Z. et al., Quaternary ammonium functionalized poly(propylene imine) dendrimers as effective antimicrobials: structure-activity studies, *Biomacromolecules*, 1(3): 473–480, 2000.

196. Chen, C.Z. and Cooper, S.L., Interactions between dendrimer biocides and bacterial membranes, *Biomaterials*, 23(16): 3359–3368, 2002.

197. Tam, J.P., Lu, Y.A., and Yang, J.L., Antimicrobial dendrimeric peptides, *Eur. J. Biochem.*, 269(3): 923–932, 2002.

198. Supattapone, S. et al., Elimination of prions by branched polyamines and implications for therapeutics, *Proc. Natl. Acad. Sci. USA*, 96(25): 14529–14534, 1999.

199. Supattapone, S., Nishina, K., and Rees, J.R., Pharmacological approaches to prion research, *Biochem. Pharmacol.*, 63(8): 1383–1388, 2002.

200. Supattapone, S. et al., Branched polyamines cure prion-infected neuroblastoma cells, *J. Virol.*, 75(7): 3453–3461, 2001.

201. Brown, S.B., Brown, E.A., and Walker, I., The present and future role of photodynamic therapy in cancer treatment, *Lancet Oncol.*, 5(8): 497–508, 2004.

202. Battah, S.H. et al., Synthesis and biological studies of 5-aminolevulinic acid-containing dendrimers for photodynamic therapy, *Bioconjugate Chem.*, 12(6): 980–988, 2001.

203. Nishiyama, N. et al., Light-harvesting ionic dendrimer porphyrins as new photosensitizers for photodynamic therapy, *Bioconjugate Chem.*, 14(1): 58–66, 2003.

204. Zhang, G.D. et al., Polyion complex micelles entrapping cationic dendrimer porphyrin: effective photosensitizer for photodynamic therapy of cancer, *J. Controlled Release*, 93(2): 141–150, 2003.
205. Kasai, S. et al., Design and synthesis of antiangiogenic/heparin-binding arginine dendrimer mimicking the surface of endostatin, *Bioorg. Med. Chem. Lett.*, 12(6): 951–954, 2002.
206. Shaunak, S. et al., Polyvalent dendrimer glucosamine conjugates prevent scar tissue formation, *Nat. Biotechnol.*, 22(8): 977–984, 2004.
207. Baird, E.J. et al., Highly effective poly(ethylene glycol) architectures for specific inhibition of immune receptor activation, *Biochemistry*, 42(44): 12739–12748, 2003.
208. Vannucci, L. et al., Effects of N-acetyl-glucosamine-coated glycodendrimers as biological modulators in the B16F10 melanoma model in vivo, *Int. J. Oncol.*, 23(2): 285–296, 2003.
209. Curnis, F., Sacchi, A., and Corti, A., Improving chemotherapeutic drug penetration in tumors by vascular targeting and barrier alteration, *J. Clin. Invest.*, 110(4): 475–482, 2002.
210. Tomalia, D.A. et al., Dendritic macromolecules — synthesis of starburst dendrimers, *Macromolecules*, 19(9): 2466–2468, 1986.
211. Hawker, C.J. and Frechet, J.M.J., Preparation of polymers with controlled molecular architecture — a new convergent approach to dendritic macromolecules, *J. Am. Chem. Soc.*, 112(21): 7638–7647, 1990.
212. Worner, C. and Mulhaupt, R., Polynitrile-functional and polyamine-functional poly(trimethylene imine) dendrimers, *Angew. Chem. Int. Ed. Engl.*, 32(9): 1306–1308, 1993.
213. Debrabandervandenberg, E.M.M. and Meijer, E.W., Poly(propylene imine) dendrimers — large-scale synthesis by hetereogeneously catalyzed hydrogenations, *Angew. Chem. Int. Ed. Engl.*, 32(9): 1308–1311, 1993.
214. Debrabandervandenberg, E.M.M. et al., Large-scale production of polypropylenimine dendrimers, *Macromolecular Symposia*, 77: 51–62, 1994.
215. Milhem, O.M. et al., Polyamidoamine starburst dendrimers as solubility enhancers, *Int. J. Pharm.*, 197(1–2): 239–241, 2000.
216. Chauhan, A.S. et al., Dendrimer-mediated transdermal delivery: enhanced bioavailability of indomethacin, *J. Controlled Release*, 90(3): 335–343, 2003.
217. Chauhan, A.S. et al., Solubility enhancement of indomethacin with poly(amidoamine) dendrimers and targeting to inflammatory regions of arthritic rats, *J. Drug Target*, 12(9–10): 575–583, 2004.
218. Ooya, T., Lee, J., and Park, K., Effects of ethylene glycol-based graft, star-shaped, and dendritic polymers on solubilization and controlled release of paclitaxel, *J. Controlled Release*, 93(2): 121–127, 2003.
219. Ooya, T., Lee, J., and Park, K., Hydrotropic dendrimers of generations 4 and 5: synthesis, characterization, and hydrotropic solubilization of paclitaxel, *Bioconjugate Chem.*, 15(6): 1221–1229, 2004.
220. Morgan, M.T. et al., Dendritic molecular capsules for hydrophobic compounds, *J. Am. Chem. Soc.*, 125(50): 15485–15489, 2003.
221. Kolhe, P. et al., Drug complexation, in vitro release and cellular entry of dendrimers and hyperbranched polymers, *Int. J. Pharm.*, 259(1–2): 143–160, 2003.
222. Devarakonda, B., Hill, R.A., and de Villiers, M.M., The effect of PAMAM dendrimer generation size and surface functional group on the aqueous solubility of nifedipine, *Int. J. Pharm.*, 284(1–2): 133–140, 2004.
223. Namazi, H. and Adeli, M., Dendrimers of citric acid and poly (ethylene glycol) as the new drug-delivery agents, *Biomaterials*, 26(10): 1175–1183, 2005.
224. Vandamme, T.F. and Brobeck, L., Poly(amidoamine) dendrimers as ophthalmic vehicles for ocular delivery of pilocarpine nitrate and tropicamide, *J. Controlled Release*, 102(1): 23–38, 2005.
225. Liu, M., Kono, K., and Frechet, J.M., Water-soluble dendritic unimolecular micelles: their potential as drug delivery agents, *J. Controlled Release*, 65(1–2): 121–131, 2000.
226. Wang, F. et al., Synthesis and evaluation of a star amphiphilic block copolymer from poly(epsilon-caprolactone) and poly(ethylene glycol) as a potential drug delivery carrier, *Bioconjugate Chem.*, 16(2): 397–405, 2005.
227. Yang, H., Morris, J.J., and Lopina, S.T., Polyethylene glycol-polyamidoamine dendritic micelle as solubility enhancer and the effect of the length of polyethylene glycol arms on the solubility of pyrene in water, *J. Colloid Interface Sci.*, 273(1): 148–154, 2004.
228. Khopade, A.J. et al., Effect of dendrimer on entrapment and release of bioactive from liposomes, *Int. J. Pharm.*, 232(1–2): 157–162, 2002.

229. Zhuo, R.X., Du, B., and Lu, Z.R., In vitro release of 5-fluorouracil with cyclic core dendritic polymer, *J. Controlled Release*, 57(3): 249–257, 1999.
230. Padilla De Jesus, O.L. et al., Polyester dendritic systems for drug delivery applications: in vitro and in vivo evaluation, *Bioconjugate Chem.*, 13(3): 453–461, 2002.
231. Ihre, H.R. et al., Polyester dendritic systems for drug delivery applications: design, synthesis, and characterization, *Bioconjugate Chem.*, 13(3): 443–452, 2002.
232. Wiwattanapatapee, R., Lomlim, L., and Saramunee, K., Dendrimers conjugates for colonic delivery of 5-aminosalicylic acid, *J. Controlled Release*, 88(1): 1–9, 2003.
233. D'Emanuele, A. et al., The use of a dendrimer-propranolol prodrug to bypass efflux transporters and enhance oral bioavailability, *J. Controlled Release*, 95(3): 447–453, 2004.
234. Khandare, J. et al., Synthesis, cellular transport, and activity of polyamidoamine dendrimer-methyl-prednisolone conjugates, *Bioconjugate Chem.*, 16(2): 330–337, 2005.

Glossary

Absorption band: The wavelength of electromagnetic radiation absorbed by a molecule or atom.

Active targeting: Targeting of drug conjugates and other drug delivery systems to cells based on the ability of homing devices or ligands to specifically bind to a complementary structure present at the target site.

Amphiphiles: Molecules with distinct hydrophobic and hydrophilic domains that usually self assemble, above a critical concentration, in aqueous media.

Angiogenesis: Complex process by which the growth of new blood vessels is induced and regulated.

Atomic force microscopy (AFM): A form of microscopy which relies on the measurement of local properties, such as height for example, of a sample by using a sharp tip of a cantilever to scan along the surface of the material. When in close proximity the attractive forces between the tip and sample surface can be measured as a deflection of the cantilever; feedback from the force measurement may be used to build up a surface profile of the sample.

Bilayer membrane: A membrane formed from the self assembly of amphiphilic molecules in which the molecules are arranged in two layers with the hydrophobic portion of the molecule constituting the interior of the membrane and the hydrophilic portion of the molecule constituting both sides of the exterior of the membrane.

Bioavailability: The amount of a drug that is available in the systemic circulation; depends on the specific route of administration and the physicochemical properties of the drug.

Biocompatibility: Describing the ability of materials to be tolerated by or be non-toxic to a biological system.

Biodegradable linkers: Covalent chemical linker groups binding drug molecules to other non-drug groups, with the ability to release drug molecules in specific biological environments; typical examples are prodrugs with linkers which are cleaved in the presence of a specific enzyme.

Block copolymers: Polymers that are organised in blocks so that one series of monomer repeat units is followed immediately by a second series of alternative monomer repeat units.

Blood brain barrier: Specialised layer of cells at the interface between the systemic blood circulation and the interstitium of the brain; this barrier tightly controls the passage of substances into the brain.

Bone engineering: Tissue engineering of materials to produce a material with the functional properties of bone.

Cancer xenograft models: Experimental model tumours comprising human cancer cells grown typically in immune deficient mice; cells are frequently grown as subcutaneous tumours in the flank of the animal.

Cationic polymers: Polymers which are protonated at physiological pH (pH = 7.4); such polymers frequently contain amine functional groups.

Cell differentiation: The process by which cells change morphology to specialise according to cell type and lineage and fulfil the typical functions within the context of a specific tissue; frequently linked to a reduction in proliferation potential of a cell.

Cell proliferation: Increase in the number of cells through repeated cycles of cell division.

Cellular efflux pump: Group of cellular membrane transporters which efficiently lower the intracellular concentrations of substrates such as drugs, thus potentially leading to drug resistance.

Chelating agents: Organic compounds which form ionic complexes with metal ions.

Chemical shift: A term used in nuclear magnetic resonance spectroscopy to denote the frequency of the resonance signal of an atom; the position of the resonance signal in the spectrum is heavily dependant on the electron density and magnetic field around the atom in question and is given relative to the solvent signal or an internal standard such as tetra methyl silane as parts per million of the applied magnetic field.

Clonal expansion: Cell proliferation deriving from a single cell.

Coacervation: The formation of a microcapsule around a colloid or droplet in which the coacervate encapsulates the droplet; the coacervate is a macromolecule-rich phase which has separated from a macromolecule-poor phase on desolvation of the macromolecule in solution.

Colloids: Particles in the nanometre size range (10^{-9} m; nm).

Complement activation: The activation of the complement system occurs through a biochemical cascade along the classical, the alternative, or the lectin mediated pathway; complement activation leads to increased activity of various elements of the immune system including opsonisation and phagocytosis.

Copolymer: A polymer prepared from more than one monomer unit.

Critical micelle concentration (CMC): The concentration at which amphiphiles start to self-assemble into closed structures (micelles) in the nanometre range; within micelles the hydrophobic parts of the amphiphilic molecules constitute the interior of the structure whereas the hydrophilic parts of the molecules constitute the exterior of the structure.

Cross-linking density: The density of covalent or physical linkages between polymer chains that are physically or covalently linked to each other.

Denaturation: Typically describes a change in the three dimensional conformation of a molecule brought about by physicochemical changes that may modify the molecule's solubility and/or adversely affect its function.

Differential Scanning Calorimetry (DSC): A thermal analytical technique based on measurement of the heat flow in a test sample compared to the heat flow in a control sample; useful for determining the temperature of polymer thermal transitions and whether such processes are endothermic (require heat) or exothermic (release heat).

Discomes: Large closed bilayer membrane bound self assemblies with an aqueous core and up to 100 μm in size, which arise on the addition of soluble surfactants to non-ionic surfactant vesicles.

Dissolution: The process of a substance ("solute") dissolving in a solvent.

Drug targeting: Pharmaceutical approaches to improve the specificity of a medical treatment by increasing the amount of drug at the desired site of action, i.e. the diseased tissue, and/or reduction of its concentration in healthy tissues.

Dynamic Mechanical Analysis (DMA): An analytical technique for determination of the elastic modulus of a sample.

Elastic modulus (G′): A measure of the hardness, stiffness or resistance to deformation of a material; the ratio of the stress (applied force per unit area) to strain (deformation or increase in length).

Emulsion: A dispersion of one liquid inside another liquid; when both liquids are ordinarily immiscible.

Endocytosis: Process of uptake of material from either the fluid surrounding the cell (fluid phase endocytosis), after adsorption to the cell membrane, or binding to membrane receptors (receptor medicated endocytosis), uptake occurs by formation of membrane invaginations that become intracellular vesicles, so called endosomes; intracellular processing of these vesicles depends on their exact nature but unless the endocytosed material can leave the endosome it may ultimately be degraded in the lysosomes.

Endosomal buffering: Ability of some polymeric materials to buffer the pH change that would otherwise result from the continuous influx of protons during endosome acidification.

Endosomal escape: Ability of some drug- or gene delivery systems to facilitate destruction of the endosome thus avoiding lysosomal degradation of the cargo.

Endosome: Intracellular transport vacuole or intracellular transport vesicle.

Enhanced permeability and retention (EPR) effect: Describes the tendency of tumours to act like a sieve by allowing localised extravasation of macromolecules and particulates into the tumour where they may then become trapped within the tumour interstitium; can be exploited to allow passive targeting to tumours.

Environment-sensitive hydrogel: A hydrogel that by virtue of its chemistry is able to alter the release rate of drugs contained in the hydrogel matrix in response to environmental changes.

Extravasation: The ability of macromolecules and nanomedicines to leave the blood vessels; the blood vessel lining (endothelium) in most organs prevents this; in the tumour 'leaky' tumour blood vessels facilitate extravasation; this forms the basis for the Enhanced permeability and retention (EPR) effect.

Fab' fragment: An antibody fragment derived from the 'arms' of the Y-shaped antibody that defines its binding specificity.

First order drug release: Drug release that is proportional to the level of drug contained within the drug releasing matrix.

Fluid-phase endocytosis: See Endocytosis.

Freeze drying: See Lyophilisation

Gadolinium: Rare earth metal that provides enhanced contrast as a paramagnetic contrast agent in magnetic resonance imaging but because of its toxicity requires chelating when used in the body.

Gamma scintigraphy: An analytical technique based on monitoring a gamma emitting radioisotope.

Gel permeation chromatography (GPC): A separation technique that relies on the difference in molecular size of an analyte for its separation; used to separate polymers of differing molecular weight.

Gene: Double stranded DNA sequence coding for the expression of a specific protein.

Glass transition temperature: The temperature below which the polymer molecules have a reduced mobility and the mechanical properties of the polymer change from being rubbery to being brittle.

Growth factors: Endogenous substances that function to control cell proliferation, differentiation and survival.

Hydrodynamic diameter: The diameter of a hydrated particle suspended in an aqueous liquid.

Hydrogels: A gel prepared by the cross-linking of hydrophilic polymer chains; the gel is able to absorb water, encapsulate drug and release drug in a controlled manner.

Hydrophilic: Having an affinity with water by virtue of being able to form polar bonds with water molecules.

Hydrophobic: Materials that are immiscible with water

Immunoconjugates: Covalent conjugates of a drug or a drug-polymer conjugate with an antibody that is susceptible to immunotargeting.

Immunoliposomes: Liposomes that contain antibodies, typically tethered to lipid anchors in the vesicle membrane, and that are susceptible to immunotargeting.

Immunotargeting: Active targeting that utilises antibodies or antibody fragments as the targeting ligand.

Infrared spectroscopy: An analytical tool used to determine chemical structure, which utilises the fact that specific chemical groups absorb electromagnetic radiation in different regions of the infrared spectrum.

Intrinsic viscosity: A measure of the capability of a polymer to enhance the viscosity of a solvent when in solution; intrinsic viscosity [η] is obtained by determining the specific viscosity (η_{sp}) at zero concentration via the intercept of a plot of specific viscosity divided by concentration (η_{sp}/c) vs. concentration; $\eta_{sp} = \eta_{rel}-1$, where η_{rel} = the viscosity of the solution relative to the viscosity of the solvent.

Ion-exchange: The exchange of analyte ions for ions available within an ion exchange resin; useful for the removal of unwanted ions from a polymer sample.

Kupffer cells: Specialised liver cells with phagocytotic activity that frequently take up and filter significant amounts of particulate materials from the blood stream; part of the mononuclear phagocyte system (MPS).

Light scattering: The scattering of an incident beam by a sample in solution; used for the analysis of polymer molecular weight.

Lower critical solution temperature (LCST): The temperature at which a polymer begins to precipitate from solution.

Lyophilisation: The process of drying at low temperatures and under a vacuum

Lysosomes: Intracellular vacuoles or vesicles containing degradative enzymes.

Macromolecule: A large molecule comprising covalently linked repeating monomer units of similar or identical chemical structure.

Magic bullet: Concept first proposed by Paul Ehrlich for antimicrobials; describes the ability of a drug to only target the disease causing cells and avoid healthy cells.

Magnetic Resonance Imaging (MRI): Non-invasive imaging procedure that gives high resolution three dimensional images, in particular of soft tissues; the signal detected is based on the spin of hydrogen nuclei. In a strong homogenous magnetic field the spin angle of these protons is parallel or anti-parallel to the direction of the magnetic field; the spin axis of these protons can be deflected by radiofrequency pulses. The relaxation process, i.e. the return of the spin angle to the starting position once the pulse is switched off, can be detected and the location of the particular hydrogen nuclei in space determined.

Mark-Houwink equation: The equation that relates the intrinsic viscosity of a polymer to its relative molar mass ($[\eta] = KM^{\alpha}$) where $[\eta]$ = intrinsic viscosity, M = viscosity averaged molecular weight and both K and α are constants for a particular polymer-solvent system.

Metastable: A molecular or supramolecular state that has a shorter lifetime than the most stable state but a longer lifetime than the most unstable state

Micelle: A self assembled closed system of a few nanometres in size, composed of amphiphilic molecules in which the interior of the micelle consists of the hydrophobic moieties of the amphiphile and the exterior of the micelle consists of the hydrophilic moieties of the amphiphiles.

Micelle core: The interior of the micelle that consists of the hydrophobic moieties of the micelle forming amphiphiles.

Micelle corona: The exterior section of a micelle that consists of the hydrophilic moieties of the micelle forming amphiphiles.

Microparticle: A particle in the micrometre (μm) size range that is usually formed by the controlled precipitation of polymers.

Microsphere: A spherical particle in the micrometre (μm) size range that is usually formed by controlled precipitation of polymers.

Monogenetic disease: Disease caused by the failure of a single gene to produce the correct amount or correct type of functional protein; such a disease is typically hereditary in nature.

Mononuclear phagocyte system (MPS): Specialised collection of cells with high phagocytotic activity in different parts of the body (also known as reticuloendothelial system, RES) and includes various macrophages and monocytes; an example are the Kupffer cells in the liver.

Mucoadhesive hydrogel: A hydrogel with the ability to adhere to mucous membranes.

Mucoadhesive: A material with the ability to adhere to mucous membranes.

Multidrug resistance: A resistance to cancer chemotherapeutics induced by cancer treatment; treatment with certain cancer chemotherapeutics leads to the overproduction of certain cellular efflux pumps and the broad substrate specificity of such cellular efflux pumps means that the treatment of cancer cells with one drug frequently leads to resistance of these cells to a number of other drugs.

Multigenetic disease: A disease caused by the failure of a complex network of multiple genes; cancer is an example of an acquired multigenetic disease.

Nano: Describing structures in the nanometre size range (nm = 10^{-9}m).

Nanocapsules: Particles within the nanometre size range that consist of a solid shell enclosing a liquid, semisolid or alternative solid interior.

Nanomedicines: Nanometre-sized therapeutics comprising delivery systems based on macromolecular and other colloidal drug carriers.

Nanoparticles: Particles in the nanometre size range.

Nanospheres: Spherical particles in the nanometre size range.

Nuclear Magnetic Resonance (NMR) Spectroscopy: An analytical tool used for chemical structure determination, based on the ability of atomic nuclei to adopt one of two orientations in the presence of an applied magnetic field; such nuclei are able to absorb a radio frequency signal and thus be promoted from a low energy orientation to a high energy orientation; the resonance frequency (on relaxation from the high energy orientation to the low energy orientation) depends on both the applied magnetic field and the nature of the nucleus; the resonance frequency and may be used to identify the atom.

Oil-in-water emulsions: The dispersions of oil droplets in water.

Oligonucleotides: Short single-stranded nucleic acids that can form complex tertiary structures and/or interact specifically with other nucleic acids; may be exploited for diagnostic or therapeutic purposes.

Opsonization: Process by which the binding of endogenous factors (opsonins) tags particulates for efficient phagocytosis.

Passive targeting: Accumulation of medicines in specific areas of the body.

P-glycoprotein: The product of the gene mdr1 that functions as a cellular efflux pump.

Phagocytosis: The ability of cells to engulf and take up other particles; such particles may be bacteria, other single celled organisms or synthetic particles.

Photodynamic therapy (PDT): The use of a 'prodrug' activated by light, typically of high intensity e.g. from a laser source, to produce cytotoxic substances such as free radicals that may destroy the targeted tissues such as skin tumours.

pH-sensitive hydrogel: A hydrogel that by virtue of its chemistry is able to react to a change in environmental pH and alter the release rate of encapsulated drug in response to pH changes.

Pluronics: Block copolymers based on poly(ethylene oxide) and poly(propylene oxide).

Polymer: A large molecule comprising covalently linked repeating monomer units of similar or identical chemical structure.

Polymer-directed enzyme prodrug therapy (PDEPT): A two-step tumour targeting strategy using a combination of a polymeric prodrug and polymer-enzyme conjugate to generate cytotoxic drug selectively at the tumour site.

Polymer monomer: A chemical unit that is covalently bound in a repeating and similar manner to form a larger molecule known as a polymer.

Polymeric bilayer vesicles: Vesicles formed from the self assembly of amphiphilic polymers.

Polymeric micelles: Micelles formed from the self assembly of amphiphilic polymers.

Polymeric vesicles: Vesicles formed from the self assembly of amphiphilic polymers.

Polymersomes: Vesicles formed from the self assembly of amphiphilic polymers.

Protein transduction domains: Peptide or protein sequences that facilitate passage of the protein through the cell membrane directly into the cytoplasm.

Proton sponge: Hypothetical mechanism by which the buffering of endosomal protons by cationic polymers such as poly(ethylenimine), which are used in gene delivery leads to osmotic swelling of the endosome and ultimately disruption of its membrane with concomitant release ('escape') of the endosome contents into the cytoplasm.

Raman spectroscopy: An analytical technique based on the measurement of Raman scattering by a molecule; Raman or inelastic light scattering occurs when the molecule encounters electromagnetic radiation of a particular wavelength and the molecule can lose or gain energy to the electromagnetic radiation; Raman spectroscopy is used for the structural analysis of molecules

Receptor mediated endocytosis: see Endocytosis

Reticuloendothelial system (RES): see Mononuclear phagocyte system (MPS)

RNAi: Double stranded ribonucleic acid (RNA) molecules with the ability to down-regulate expression of complementary gene sequences after intracellular processing.

Scanning Electron Microscopy (SEM): An electron microscopy imaging technique in which electron beams are scanned across a conductive sample; sample is made conductive by coating with gold for example.

Scanning Probe Microscopy (SPM): An imaging technique in which a probe is scanned across the surface of a sample and the image is built up by the probe registering changes in the samples height profile for example; atomic force microscopy (AFM) is a scanning probe technique.

Self assembly: The physical aggregation of single molecules into larger structures that are sometimes referred to as supramolecular structures.

Short interfering RNA (siRNA): Short double stranded ribonucleic acid (RNA) molecules that can down regulate gene expression based on RNA interference (RNAi)

Side effects: Unintended and harmful pharmacological effects of a drug that can limit its useful dose or wider medical use.

Size exclusion chromatograph (SEC): A chromatographic separation technique that separates molecules according to their size; see also gel permeation chromatography (GPC).

Small angle x-ray scattering (SAXS): An analytical technique useful for studying the structure of colloids and which is based on the analysis of X-ray scattering by a sample at low scattering angles (1 - 10°); the scattering pattern obtained is based on the electron density heterogeneities within a sample.

Sol-gel phase transition: The transition from a polymer solution to a polymer gel that is marked by an increase in viscosity of the system.

Spray-drying: A powder processing technique involving the drying of a powder slurry after it has been forced through an orifice; the spray-dried powder normally presents as spherical particles.

Stealth liposomes: Liposomes with a hydrophilic polymer covering the surface; the hydrophilic polymer by steric repulsion effectively creates an exclusion layer that limits the ability of other molecules to interact with the vesicle surface; this covering reduces opsonisation and macrophage uptake that in turn dramatically increases plasma half life of these 'long circulating' liposomes.

Steric repulsion: A repulsion experienced by neighbouring colloids due to the presence of a space filling hydrophilic polymer on the surface of the colloid.

Supercritical carbon dioxide: Supercritical carbon dioxide exists above a critical temperature (31.1°C) and pressure (72.9 atmospheres), known as the critical point, and has both gaseous and liquid properties; useful for the solubilisation of materials during processing.

Supramolecular structures: Structures composed of physically bonded molecules.

Tat peptide: A small 9 amino acid basic peptide derived from the HIV virus that acts as a protein transduction domain.

Thermo gravimetric analysis (TGA): An analytical procedure in which the change in weight of a sample is monitored as the sample is heated in a controlled environment; useful for determining polymer degradation temperatures and the polymer water content.

Tissue engineering: Application of engineering technology to the development of homogenous and heterogeneous multicellular assemblies that is aimed at recreating the physiological functions of tissues.

Transmission Electron Microscopy (TEM): An electron microscopy imaging technique in which electron beams are transmitted through a sample; an image is built up by the scattering of electrons by the sample.

Tumours: Accumulation of genetic changes in cells leads to cell transformation with deregulation of cell proliferation, suppression of apoptosis and unchecked clonal expansion of somatic cells into a solid tumour mass that can displace and/or invade normal tissue.

Van der Waals interactions: An attractive force between two non-polar molecules or atoms due to the progressive creation of temporary dipoles.

Vesicle: A self assembled system composed of amphiphilic molecules in a closed bilayer membrane structure that contains an aqueous core.

Viscometry: The analysis of the flow properties of liquids and semi-solids.

Water-in-oil emulsion: The dispersion of water droplets in oil.

Water-in-oil-in-water emulsion: The dispersion of water droplets within oil droplets that are subsequently dispersed in water.

Wide angle x-ray scattering (WAXS): An analytical technique useful for studying the structure of polymers, which is based on the analysis of X-ray scattering at wide scattering angles ($7-60°$).

Zero order drug release: Drug release that is constant irrespective of the level of drug contained within the releasing matrix.

Index

Printed and bound by CPI Group (UK) Ltd, Croydon, CR0 4YY

23/10/2024

01778250-0007